Mastering
Medisoft

D0166162

Mastering Medisoft

BONNIE J. FLOM

CONTRIBUTOR: LORRAINE M. PAPAZIAN-BOYCE, MS, CPC

Pearson

Boston   Columbus   Indianapolis   New York   San Francisco   Upper Saddle River
Amsterdam   Cape Town   Dubai   London   Madrid   Milan   Munich   Paris Montreal   Toronto
Delhi   Mexico City   Sao Paulo   Sydney   Hong Kong   Seoul Singapore   Taipei   Tokyo

Library of Congress Cataloging-in-Publication Data

Flom, Bonnie J.
  Mastering Medisoft / Bonnie J. Flom.
    p. ; cm.
  ISBN-13: 978-0-13-513022-3
  ISBN-10: 0-13-513022-0
  1. MediSoft. 2. Medical informatics. 3. Medical offices—Automation. I. Title.
  [DNLM: 1. MediSoft. 2. Office Automation—Problems and Exercises. 3. Practice Management—Problems and Exercises.
4. Office Management—Problems and Exercises. 5. Software—Problems and Exercises. W 18.2 F629m 2010]
  R858.F575 2010
  610.285—dc22

                                                                                2009009574

Publisher: Julie Levin Alexander
Publisher's Assistant: Regina Bruno
Editor-in-Chief: Mark Cohen
Executive Editor: Joan Gill
Associate Editor: Bronwen Glowacki
Editorial Assistant: Mary Ellen Ruitenberg
Development Editor: Alexis Ferraro
Director of Marketing: Karen Allman
Senior Marketing Manager: Harper Coles
Marketing Specialist: Michael Sirinides
Marketing Assistant: Judy Noh
Managing Production Editor: Patrick Walsh
Production Liaison: Julie Li

Production Editor: Stacy Proteau
Senior Media Editor: Amy Peltier
Media Project Manager: Lorena Cerisano
Manufacturing Manager: Ilene Sanford
Manufacturing Buyer: Pat Brown
Creative Director: Jayne Conte
Senior Art Director: Maria Guglielmo
Art Director: Christopher Weigand
Cover Designer: Karen Quigley
Cover Image: istock photo
Composition: Laserwords
Printing and Binding: Edwards Brothers
Cover Printer: Phoenix Color Corporation

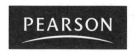

www.pearsonhighered.com

10 9 8 7 6 5 4 3 2 1
ISBN-10:   0-13-513022-0
ISBN-13: 978-0-13-513022-3

This book is dedicated to my parents, Bill and Marijane Pearce, who have always given me love, joy, and guidance throughout my life. It is also dedicated to my former spouse, Tim Nentl, who first supported my vision for a billing agency and has the patience and love of a saint. To my children, Bill and Jordan Nentl, of whom I am very proud and delighted to witness their daily growth and maturity, you give me joy to anticipate the gifts you will share with the world.

Finally, this book is dedicated to my husband, David Flom, who gave me back to me in too many ways to define. He has given me the ability to slow down and appreciate each and every day and to rest in the safety of his love.

Contents

Chapter 4

Chapter 7   **Data Backup and Data Maintenance**   **163**

Chapter 8   **Billing Charges, Security Setup, and Other Little-Known Features**   **183**

Chapter 9

Reporting and Accounts Receivable Management   205

Chapter 12

Office Work Flow Using Medisoft   283

Mastering Medisoft was created specifically to help students learn the skill of medical billing through the use of Medisoft. In addition, *Mastering Medisoft* is also a useful text for clinics and billing services to train their employees. Medisoft has a large number of users, and therefore will be one of the software programs most frequently encountered by the student. This text is designed to allow the reader to first master the "must-know" tasks such as patient, charge, and payment entry, and then move on to the less frequently used, but "good to know" features such as setting up a new practice.

This text is structured to present the tasks the student will use most frequently at the beginning of the book—daily tasks such as entering patient information, entering charges and payments, and proofing the day. Next, the tasks that the student would do less frequently are presented, such as File Maintenance, processing billing charges, and Designing Custom Reports. Finally, those Medisoft functions that are good to know, but that the student may rarely use in a medical office, such as create a new set of data and set up a clinic to transmit electronically are presented.

Over the years, many medical offices have stated that they encounter the same issue when hiring new medical office specialists: They often have difficulty finding individuals who know how to work with Medisoft and "do billing." It takes much effort and training just to get employees to learn the basics of the program and to be able to function in their job. Because Medisoft is one of the most frequently encountered software programs in medical practices, it is imperative that the student have a solid understanding of the functions of this powerful program.

The goal of this text is to create sought-after, dependable students with a working knowledge of Medisoft whom healthcare providers want to hire. This text provides the foundation students need to feel confident that they can enter the work environment able to perform the essential tasks of their job with little or no additional training.

PEDAGOGICAL FEATURES IN THIS TEXTBOOK

The following special features appear throughout this textbook:

- **Learning Objectives:** Specific learning objectives appear at the beginning of each chapter, stating what will be achieved upon successful completion of the chapter.

- **Key Terminology and Abbreviations:** Terms and their definitions appear at the beginning of each chapter as well as in the narrative and the comprehensive glossary. Abbreviations that are used in the text are listed at the beginning of each chapter.

- **Billing Insights:** These boxes appear throughout the chapters. They provide additional information on key topics relevant to medical billing.

- **Medisoft Quick Tips:** These boxes provide additional tips/shortcuts that pertain specifically to the use of Medisoft software.

- **Test Your Knowledge:** In-chapter questions that require students to pause and apply the concepts presented appear in most chapters.

- **Practice Exercises:** These exercises appear within the body of the chapters, and provide step-by-step instruction for the student.

- **Figures:** Numerous Medisoft screen captures and relevant forms appear throughout the book to support the textual material presented and to reinforce key concepts.

- **Chapter Review Questions:** End-of-chapter questions are provided in multiple-choice, true/false, and short-answer format to help to reinforce learning. The review questions measure the student's understanding of the material presented in the chapter. These tools are available for use by the student or by the instructor as an outcome assessment.

- **Resources:** This listing provides organization contact information, websites, and additional resources related to the chapter content and available for student research.

- **Mock Clinic:** A mock clinic simulation appears in Appendix A of the text. This simulation is designed to allow students to create a new data set for a fictional clinic, Sunny Life Clinic. The exercises in this appendix test the knowledge students have gained by reading the text and applying the practice exercises contained within each chapter. The exercises simulate the process of setting up Medisoft in a new clinic and performing tasks from entering the practice information, to performing the Medisoft daily basics, to developing follow-up and backup procedures. Unlike the practice exercises within each chapter, the exercises in this appendix provide minimal guidance; therefore, the reader must rely on his or her knowledge of Medisoft and critical thinking skills to create the new data set. This appendix can serve as a comprehensive review of material learned, or instructors may choose to use it for examination purposes.

TYPES OF MEDISOFT SOFTWARE

It is important for the instructor and student to understand at the outset of learning Medisoft and medical billing that there are several variations of the program that may be installed in the learning centers. In addition, students may encounter many variations of Medisoft while working in the field. The look and feel of the program is consistent; however, the text will point out where there may be differences based upon the type of Medisoft used.

Mastering Medisoft will review Medisoft and the many utilities contained within, including the scheduling utility, Office Hours. There are three types of Medisoft: Basic, Advanced, and Network Professional, and there are two versions of Office Hours, the free version included within Medisoft and an add-on version that can be purchased separately, which is known as Office Hours Professional.

The Medisoft Basic program is designed for a cash practice and works on a single workstation. The Advanced program is designed for an insurance practice and also works on a single workstation. The Network Professional program is designed for offices that have more than one employee working on the program at the same time. It has the most features of all the programs and will serve both a cash and/or insurance practice.

The free version of Office Hours allows the practice to schedule one patient, one day at a time. Office Hours Professional allows practices to view multiple doctors and days at the same time. If a clinic has more than one provider, it is advisable to use Office Hours Professional.

Each college will vary in installation, configuration, and utilization of the Medisoft program, so each student's experience may vary. Be aware that the print screens and instructions contained within this manual are created from Medisoft Advanced and Office Hours Professional. In addition, it is noteworthy to state that the text was created using Version 14 of Medisoft. Features new to Version 14 can be found on the Help menu.

Contained within this text is an installation CD. If you choose to do so, you may install the Medisoft student version directly onto your laptop, thereby simulating an exact experience that is portrayed in the text. The installation instructions are included on the CD. Note that the installation CD contains a tutorial database with mock patients and charges, as well as procedure and diagnosis codes. Because official procedure and diagnosis codes change annually, some codes in the tutorial database may no longer be current. As this book is about how to use Medisoft, it was important to show the photos of Medisoft screens exactly the way they are shown in the tutorial. For that reason, the codes were not updated in the book. This does not affect the functionality of the tutorial.

Students will use the Medical Group Tutorial data to complete many of the practice exercises contained within the text. In addition, they will use the source documents provided in Appendices B and C to complete the exercises. When necessary, specific direction for utilization of the source documents is provided in the exercises.

If any reader has comments, questions, or suggestions, I would be delighted to respond to you via email at bonnie.ph@billingbuddies.com.

Sincerely,
Bonnie J. Flom

Bonnie J. Flom's passion for medical billing and Medisoft began in February 1984 while working in the accounts receivables department at St. Joseph's Medical Center. While there, she served on the Blue Shield EDI committee, United Way Committee, and Benedictine Mission Committee. In 1994, Bonnie decided to break out on her own and started Rapid Return Medical Billing. Medisoft was used in the billing agency, and in 1995, Bonnie became a Medisoft dealer. Her billing agency grew quickly and employed up to seventeen people at one time. Then in 2000, Rapid Return Medical Billing served Blue Cross Blue Shield of Minnesota in testing their Optical Character Reader (OCR), which automatically converted paper claims to National Standard Format (NSF) files. In 2001, Bonnie began serving on the Medicare Advisory committee for the State of Minnesota (PCOM). In 2001, Rapid Return Medical Billing won the Medisoft contest for setting up the first 100 clinics to transmit electronically. In 2002, Bonnie joined the HBMA (Healthcare Billing and Management Association). In 2006, Bonnie began focusing solely on Medisoft by starting a separate company called Softouch Software and a billing company known as Billing Buddies. Bonnie is also the creator and host of the Google group called Medisoft and Medical Billing.

Acknowledgments

First of all, my deepest gratefulness and love go to Carry Schuety. This book would not be in print without her. She was the first person who ignited my passion for medical billing 25 years ago while working at a small hospital in northern Minnesota, and she has been a mentor and dear friend throughout the years.

I would like to acknowledge Joan Gill of Pearson Education and Alexis Breen Ferraro of Triple SSS Press Media Development—Joan and Pearson Education for placing their trust and faith in me to create this first book, and Alexis for her guidance, patience, and great suggestions. Finally, thanks to Joey Borane formerly of Medisoft and now of Successfully Using Medisoft. Joey gave me the fervor to learn, love, and appreciate technology and not get left behind.

The author and publisher would like to thank the following reviewers for their valuable feedback:

Roxanne Abbott, MBA, Certified Instructor of Business Technology Education
Department Chair
Sarasota County Technical Institute, FL

Dolly Horton
Medical Assisting Coordinator
Mayland Community College, NC

Shirley Jelmo, BS, CMA, RMA
MA Program Director
Pima Medical Institute, CO

Angel Moore, RHIA
Medical Office Administration Instructor
Craven Community College, NC

Julie Lindstrom Myhre, CMT
Instructor
Century College, MN

Letitia Patterson, MPA, CPC, CCS-P
Olive Harvey College, IL

Kimberly Pettigrew, CMBS
Lead Allied Health Instructor
Southwestern College, OH

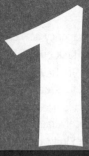

Chapter One

Medisoft Daily Tasks, Patient Charts, and Appointments

Learning Objectives

After completing this chapter, you should be able to:

- ◆ Define and spell the key terms in this chapter.
- ◆ Describe daily Medisoft tasks, including scheduling appointments, entering charges and payments, and follow-up.
- ◆ Explain other tasks a medical office specialist may perform.
- ◆ Understand the forms of help offered by and within Medisoft.
- ◆ Explain the three icons created on the desktop by installing Medisoft.
- ◆ Describe the differences between Office Hours and Office Hours Professional.
- ◆ Demonstrate how to enter patient charts and appointments.
- ◆ Demonstrate how to schedule breaks.
- ◆ Move, edit, and delete appointments.
- ◆ Identify the fields on the CMS-1500 form affected by the patient information in Medisoft.
- ◆ Demonstrate how to print the patient schedule and superbills.

Key Terms

accounts receivable (AR)   money owed to the clinic for services provided.

appointment   time assigned in the schedule for patients to be seen at the clinic.

backup   a second copy of the original data in case the first copy is destroyed.

backup mediums   any form of data storage device such as RW-CDs, zip disks, flash drives, and external hard drives.

beneficiary   patient covered under a health insurance plan.

break   time assigned in the schedule where patients will not be seen.

Centers for Medicare and Medicaid Services (CMS)   a government agency formerly known as HCFA. CMS is part of the U.S. Department of Health and Human Services and is responsible for administering Medicare and Medicaid.

CMS-1500 form   the standard claim form used by physicians and other healthcare professionals to bill for services rendered.

CPT* code   Current Procedural Terminology code; a five-digit code used to describe what procedures were performed.

daily Medisoft tasks   the six typical Medisoft tasks performed daily at offices.

*CPT is a registered trademark of the American Medical Association.

diagnosis   the disease, condition, illness, or accident that is the reason for services provided.

diagnosis codes   ICD-9-CM codes that identify a patient's injury and/or illness or reason for routine or preventive services.

eligibility   verifying insurance coverage for a patient.

Health Care Financing Administration (HCFA)   a government agency now called CMS.

hotkeys   keys that are set up as shortcuts to accomplish a desired task quickly.

ICD-9-CM   abbreviation for International Classification of Diseases, 9th Revision, Clinical Modification. A coding system used to identify signs, symptoms, injuries, diseases, and conditions.

Medisoft   practice management software commonly used by medical offices that allows practices to track patient information, appointments, and accounts receivable.

modifier   a two-digit number placed after the five-digit CPT* code to indicate that the description of the service or procedure has been altered.

Office Hours   software within Medisoft used to track patient appointments.

Patient Day Sheet   Medisoft report used to proof daily transactions, showing all transactions posted on patient accounts for the selected time frame.

patient information   personal information provided by the patient to the medical office in order for the office to treat the patient and obtain reimbursement for services.

practice management system (PMS)   software that allows a clinic to manage its daily tasks via a computer.

right-click keys   shortcuts that can be used inside of Medisoft by clicking the right button on the mouse (see hotkeys).

scheduling   the process of entering breaks and appointments into the schedule.

superbill   a form used by clinics to track the patient's visit, procedures performed, and the diagnoses assigned to the visit.

Transaction Entry   utility inside of Medisoft that allows the user to enter charges, payments, adjustments, comments, and track balances.

Work Administrator   utility in Medisoft used to assign, track, and manage clinic work.

Abbreviations

CMS   Centers for Medicare and Medicaid Services
CPT*   Current Procedural Terminology
HCFA   Health Care Financing Administration
PMS   practice management system
SCHIP   State Children's Health Insurance Program

■ ■ ■ ■

INTRODUCTION

Medical offices and clinics are financially dependent upon their medical billing assistants and therefore are in desperate need of well-trained employees. **Medisoft** is a **practice management system (PMS)** commonly used by medical offices that allows practices to track **patient information, appointments,** and **accounts receivable.** A PMS allows a clinic to manage its daily tasks via a computer. Patient information is the personal information provided by the patient to the medical office in order for the office to treat that patient and obtain reimbursement for services. Appointments are the time assigned in the schedule for patients

*CPT is a registered trademark of the American Medical Association.

to be seen at the clinic, and accounts receivable is outstanding money owed to the clinic for services provided. *Mastering Medisoft* is a guide for anyone working in a medical office to effectively handle the patient information, scheduling, and accounts receivable. In this chapter, you will become acquainted with the daily Medisoft tasks as well as learn patient and appointment entry.

OVERVIEW OF THE DAILY MEDISOFT TASKS AND OFFICE PROCEDURES

A clinic has several options to manage daily tasks within the office. First, it could do it the "old-fashioned" way by using paper and pen and/or possibly a typewriter. With the computer age, the majority of clinics have become enlightened and realize that the old-fashioned way is the most costly and inefficient choice. The more efficient option is for the office to become computerized and process its tasks via a computer and software program. Computerization saves both time and money. There are dozens of PMS programs to choose from; in this book, Medisoft is the PMS studied.

Medisoft was created in 1982, making it a forerunner to other practice management systems. Medisoft allows medical offices with one provider or with groups of fifty or more the ability to track patient information, appointments, and account receivables. The typical medical specialist will work in an office with one to three doctors and will be expected to handle many tasks. It is important to understand the **daily Medisoft tasks** in order to effectively use the program. Let's briefly review the six daily Medisoft tasks (Figure 1-1).

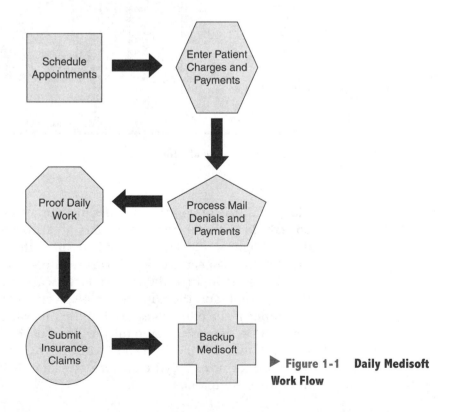

▶ **Figure 1-1   Daily Medisoft Work Flow**

Scheduling Appointments and Developing Superbills

Scheduling appointments and **breaks** is essential to running an organized clinic. Every time a patient is seen at a clinic, whether a new patient or an existing patient, the clinic needs to track his or her appointments. The clinic must also track when patients will not be seen; these time slots are called breaks. Within Medisoft, there is another program known as **Office Hours** that handles these functions. As discussed in the Preface, Medisoft offers two types of Office Hours. One is the free version that is installed with every Medisoft installation, and the other is Office Hours Professional that is purchased separately. It is recommended that Office Hours Professional be installed from the demo CD. For simplicity, the terms Office Hours Professional and Office Hours will be used interchangeably (Figure 1-2).

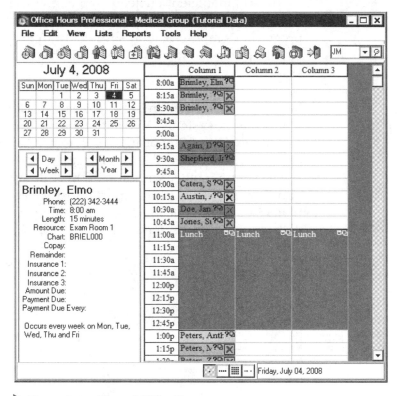

▶ **Figure 1-2** **View of Office Hours**

Along with the appointment schedule, clinics develop charge slips or **superbills** to track the patient visits and provide a worksheet for the doctor (Figure 1-3). The superbill contains the patient's name and chart number, date of service, and boxes to check for the services provided and payments made. In addition, the doctor can list the patient diagnosis on the superbill, and the patient can be given a copy to submit to his or her insurance if the clinic does not bill the insurance directly. However, sometimes insurance companies will not accept the superbill and will return it to the clinic for a **CMS-1500 form.** The CMS-1500 form is the standard form used by healthcare providers to submit claims to insurance companies.

1023	Happy Valley Medical Clinic 5222 E. Baseline Rd. Gilbert, AZ 85234 (800)333-4747	

AGADW000	Again, Dwight	9/4/2008	9:15:00 AM

EXAM	FEE	PROCEDURES	FEE	LABORATORY		FEE
New Patient		Anoscopy	46600	Aerobic Culture	87070	
Problem Focused	99201	Arthrocentesis/Aspiration/Injection		Amylase	82150	
Expanded Problem, Focused	99202	Small Joint	*20600	B12	82607	
Detailed	99203	Interm Joint	*20605	CBC & Diff	85025	
Comprehensive	99204	Major Joint	*20610	CHEM 20	80019	
Comprehensive/High Complex	99204	Audiometry	92552	Chlamydia Screen	86317	
Initial Visit/Procedure	99025	Cast Application		Cholesterol	82465	
Well Exam Infant (up to 12 mos.)	99318	Location Long Short		Digoxin	80162	
Well Exam 1 – 4 yrs.	99382	Catherization	*53670	Electrolytes	80005	
Well Exam 5 – 11 yrs.	99383	Circumcision	54150	Ferritin	82728	
Well Exam 12 – 17 yrs.	99384	Colposcopy	*57452	Folate	82746	
Well Exam 18 – 39 yrs.	99385	Colposcopy w /Biopsy	*57454	GC Screen	87070	
Well Exam 40 – 64 yrs.	99386	Cryosurgery Premalignant Lesion		Glucose	82947	
		Location(s):		Glucose 1 HR	82950	
Established Patient		Cryosurgery Warts		Glycosylated HGB (A1C)	83036	
Minimum	99211	Location(s):		HCT	85014	
Problem Focused	99212	Curettement Lesion w /Biopsy	CTF	HDL	83718	
Expanded Problem Focused	99213	Curettement Lesion w o/ Biopsy		Hep BSAG	86278	
Detailed	99214	Single	*11050	Hepatitis Profile	80059	
Comprehensive/High Complex	99215	2 – 4	*11051	HGB & HCT	85014	
Well Exam Infant (up to 12 mos.)	99391	> 4	*11052	HIV	86311	
Well Exam 1 – 4 yrs.	99392	Diaphram Fitting	*57170	Iron & TBC 83540	83550	
Well Exam 5 – 11 yrs.	99393	Ear Irrigation	69210	Kidney Profile	80007	
Well Exam 12 – 17 yrs.	99394	ECG	93000	Lead	83655	
Well Exam 18 – 39 yrs.	99395	Endometrial Biopsy	*58100	Liver Profile	82977	
Well Exam 40 – 64 yrs.	99396	Exc. Lesion w /Biopsy	CTF	Mono Test	86308	
		w /o Biopsy		Pap Smear	88155	
Obstetrics		Location Size		Pregnancy Test	84703	
Total OB Care	59400	Exc. Skin Tags (1 – 15)	*11200	Prenatal Profile	80055	
Obstetrical Visit	99212	Each Additional 10	*11201	Pro Time	85610	
Injections		Fracture Treatment		PSA	84153	
Administration Sub. / IM	90782	Loc		RPR	86592	
Drug		w /Reduc	w /o Reduc	Sed. Rate	85651	
Dosage		Fracture Treatment F/U	99024	Stool Culture	87045	
Allergy	95155	I & D Abscess Single/Simple	*10060	Stool O & P	87177	
Cocci Skin Test	86490	Multiple or Comp	*10061	Strep Screen	86403	
DPT	90701	I & D Pilonidal Cyst Simple	*10080	Theophylline	80198	
Haemophilus	90737	Pilonidal Cyst Complex	10081	Thyroid Profile	80091	
Influenza	90724	IV Therapy – To One Hour	90780	TSH	84443	
MMR	90707	Each Additional Hour	*90781	Urinalysis	81000	
OPV	90712	Laceration Repair		Urine Culture	87088	
Pneumovax	90732	Location Size Sim/Comp		Drawing Fee	36415	
TB Skin Test	86585	Laryngoscopy	31505	Specimen Collection	99000	
TD	90718	Oximetry	94760			
Unlisted Immun	90749	Punch Biopsy	CTF			
		Rhythm Strip	93040			
		Treadmill	93015			
		Trigger Point or Tendon Sheath Inj.	*20550			
		Tympanometry	92567			

Diagnosis / ICD – 9

I acknowledge receipt of medical services and authorize the release of any medical information necessary to process this claim for healthcare payment only.

I ☐ do ☐ do not authorize payment to the provider

Patient Signature

Tax ID Number:

Total Estimated Charges:
Payment Amount:

▶ Figure 1-3 **Sample Superbill**

PRACTICE EXERCISE 1-1   Scheduling Patients

In the first exercise, we are going to schedule a series of patients into Office Hours. Remember that it is recommended to install Office Hours Professional from the demo disk included with the manual.

In this exercise, use the current date for the appointment and the Medical Group Tutorial Data as you proceed. Pay close attention to each patient's name, attending provider, and appointment time. If there are already preexisting appointments in the time slots, delete them.

Patient Name	Attending Provider	Time
Dwight Again	Mallard, J.D.	10:00 am
Jane S. Doe	Mallard, J.D.	11:00 am
Zimmerman, Anthony	Mallard, J.D.	12:00 am
Clinger, Wallace	Morris, Melvin	9:00 am
Peters, Anthony	Morris, Melvin	2:00 pm
Simpson, Tanus J.	Lee, Robert	9:00 am
Wagnew, Jeremy	Lee, Robert	10:00 am
Shepard, Jarem	Lee, Robert	12:00 pm
Jasper, Stephanie L.	Lee, Robert	3:00 pm
Koseman, Chadwick	Hinckle, Wallace	11:00 am
Nielsen, Lindsey	Hinckle, Wallace	1:00 pm

1   Open Office Hours Professional. (If Medisoft and Office Hours Professional are not yet installed, please refer to the Preface.)

2   Change the view to see the schedule of all the doctors. This can be done by clicking on View from the menu bar, Multi View from the drop-down menu, and Complete from the side menu. **Note:** There are four buttons at the lower right corner of Office Hours Professional next to the date. One of them offers the same option. Experiment with them now to find the one that offers this option (Figure 1-4).

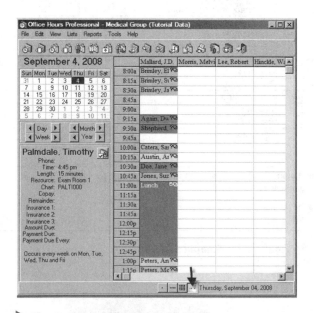

▶ Figure 1-4   **Office Hours Multi View**

3 Next, right-click on the appropriate field for each appointment time under the provider's name and select New Appointment (Figure 1-5).

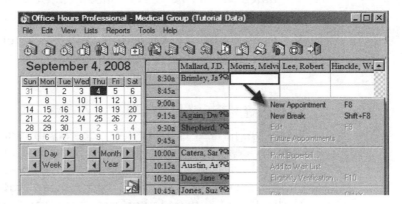

► Figure 1-5 **Adding a New Appointment**

4 Enter the patient's chart number by keying the first three letters of the patient's last name. Or, by clicking the magnifying glass, a drop-down list will display the patients to choose from.

5 After the patient is chosen, verify that the provider names and appointment time are valid and then click save. Allow the default amount of time to remain.

6 Repeat this process until all appointments have been entered for all providers.

PRACTICE EXERCISE 1-2   Print a Schedule for Each Doctor

In this exercise, we are going to print a schedule for each doctor. In a clinical setting, healthcare providers often receive a copy of their schedule at the beginning of each day. This schedule will also serve as a way to check your work from Practice Exercise 1-1.

1 Select Reports from the menu bar of Office Hours and Appointment List from the drop-down menu, then press Start. This will create a pop-up screen (Figure 1-6).

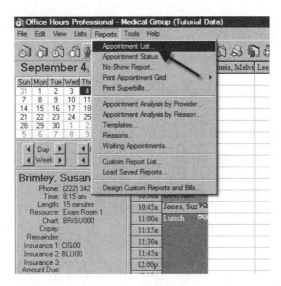

► Figure 1-6 **Printing an Appointment List**

2 The pop-up screen that appears will default to the current date. If Practice Exercises 1-1 and 1-2 are completed on the same day, the dates will not need to be modified. However, if they are done on separate days, enter the appointment date and click ok.

3 Preview the appointment lists to check your work. **Note:** There should be a separate list for each provider.

Entering Patient Charges and Payments

While the patient is being seen, doctors and staff members will record the services provided and payments made on the superbill. After the patient has been seen, the medical office specialist will enter the services and payments into Medisoft. **Transaction Entry** is the utility inside of Medisoft that is used to perform these functions (Figure 1-7).

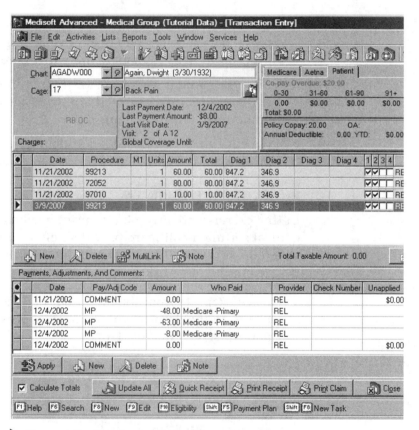

▶ Figure 1-7   **Transaction Entry Screen**

Processing Mail Denials and Payments

Clinics receive mail each day. Inside the mail there are patient and insurance payments and correspondence from patients and insurance companies, including denial letters. Medisoft has a function called Enter Deposit/Payments that quickly processes these items. This function displays the name Deposit List at the top of the screen. It allows the user to post payments and denials, bill secondary and tertiary claims, and send patient statements all from one entry screen. Tracking unpaid accounts, or follow-up, is a critical function in accounts receivable management, and this feature streamlines the process. **Note:** In the Basic version of Medisoft, this Deposit List is not available. In this instance, the office uses Transaction Entry to process mail payments and denials. As discussed in the Preface, the Basic program was outlined as a program used for cash practices. Hence, the Deposit List features are not necessary (Figure 1-8).

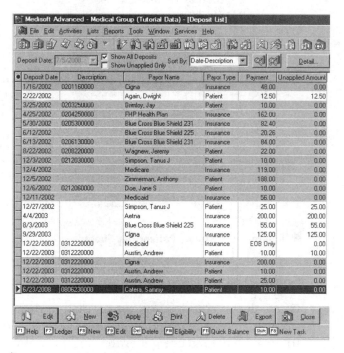

▶ **Figure 1-8   Deposit List**

Proofing Daily Work

Every well-run organization has a check-and-balance system in place to make sure charges and payments are properly entered. Medisoft has a report called the **Patient Day Sheet** used to balance the daily activities in Medisoft. The Patient Day Sheet allows the office to match the charges against the appointment list and the receipts against the Deposit List. This proves the funds have been posted correctly and that every patient has been charged and accounted for (Figure 1-9).

Happy Valley Medical Clinic
Patient Day Sheet
July 05, 2008
ALL

Entry	Date	Document	POS	Description	Provider	Code	Modifiers	Amount
AGADW000 Again, Dwight								
46	9/3/2002	0209030000	11	X-Ray, Hand, Min 3 Views	REL	73130		45.00
47	9/3/2002	0209030000	11	Office Visit Est. Patient EEL	REL	99213		60.00
22	11/21/2002	0211210000	11	Office Visit Est. Patient EEL	REL	99213		60.00
23	11/21/2002	0211210000	11	X-Ray, Spinal, Complete	REL	72052		80.00
24	11/21/2002	0211210000	11	Hot/Cold Pack Therapy	REL	97010		10.00
26	12/4/2002	0211210000		#23664	REL	MP		-48.00
27	12/4/2002	0211210000		#23664	REL	MP		-63.00
28	12/4/2002	0211210000		#23664	REL	MP		-8.00
91	3/9/2007	0703090000	11	Office Visit Est. Patient EEL	REL	99213		60.00

Patient's Charges	Patient's Receipts	Insurance Receipts	Adjustments	Patient Balance
$315.00	$0.00	-$119.00	$0.00	$196.00

Entry	Date	Document	POS	Description	Provider	Code	Modifiers	Amount
AUSAN000 Austin, Andrew								
85	12/22/2003	0312220000	11	Cash Payment--Thank You!	JM	CASH		-10.00
86	12/22/2003	0312220000	11	Personal Check Payment	JM	CHECK		-25.00

Patient's Charges	Patient's Receipts	Insurance Receipts	Adjustments	Patient Balance
$0.00	-$35.00	$0.00	$0.00	-$35.00

Entry	Date	Document	POS	Description	Provider	Code	Modifiers	Amount
BORJO000 Bordon, John								
87	2/9/2006	0602090000	11	Office Visit Est. Patient DDM	JM	99214		65.00

▶ **Figure 1-9   Sample Patient Day Sheet**

Submitting Insurance Claims

Once all the charges and payments are entered and proofed, the insurance claims must be submitted to the insurance companies. Insurance claims are generated for patients who have primary, secondary, and tertiary coverage. Medisoft has a feature called Claims Management that processes the insurance claims either by printing them on a form called the CMS-1500 form or by transmitting the claims electronically to the payers (Figure 1-10).

> **Billing Insight**   The CMS-1500 Claim Form
>
> The CMS-1500 form is used by all medical offices to submit claims to insurance companies. The current version of the CMS-1500 form, created to accommodate the National Provider Identifier, was approved in August of 2005. Clinics could begin using it October 1, 2006; it is now required for all claims. **CMS** is an acronym for Centers for Medicare and Medicaid Services, which is the U.S. federal agency which administers Medicare, Medicaid, and the State Children's Health Insurance Program (**SCHIP**). Previously, this agency was known as the Health Care Financing Administration (**HCFA**). Hence, the old form is known as the HCFA-1500 form; you may hear this terminology in the field.

1500

HEALTH INSURANCE CLAIM FORM

APPROVED BY NATIONAL UNIFORM CLAIM COMMITTEE 08/05

| | PICA | | | | | | | PICA | |

1. MEDICARE ☐ (Medicare #) MEDICAID ☐ (Medicaid #) TRICARE CHAMPUS ☐ (Sponsor's SSN) CHAMPVA ☐ (Member ID#) GROUP HEALTH PLAN ☐ (SSN or ID) FECA BLK LUNG ☐ (SSN) OTHER ☐ (ID)

1a. INSURED'S I.D. NUMBER (For Program in Item 1)

2. PATIENT'S NAME (Last Name, First Name, Middle Initial)

3. PATIENT'S BIRTH DATE MM | DD | YY SEX M ☐ F ☐

4. INSURED'S NAME (Last Name, First Name, Middle Initial)

5. PATIENT'S ADDRESS (No., Street)

6. PATIENT RELATIONSHIP TO INSURED Self ☐ Spouse ☐ Child ☐ Other ☐

7. INSURED'S ADDRESS (No., Street)

CITY   STATE

8. PATIENT STATUS Single ☐ Married ☐ Other ☐

CITY   STATE

ZIP CODE   TELEPHONE (Include Area Code) ( )

Employed ☐ Full-Time Student ☐ Part-Time Student ☐

ZIP CODE   TELEPHONE (Include Area Code) ( )

9. OTHER INSURED'S NAME (Last Name, First Name, Middle Initial)

10. IS PATIENT'S CONDITION RELATED TO:

11. INSURED'S POLICY GROUP OR FECA NUMBER

a. OTHER INSURED'S POLICY OR GROUP NUMBER

a. EMPLOYMENT? (Current or Previous) YES ☐ NO ☐

a. INSURED'S DATE OF BIRTH MM | DD | YY SEX M ☐ F ☐

b. OTHER INSURED'S DATE OF BIRTH MM | DD | YY SEX M ☐ F ☐

b. AUTO ACCIDENT? PLACE (State) YES ☐ NO ☐

b. EMPLOYER'S NAME OR SCHOOL NAME

c. EMPLOYER'S NAME OR SCHOOL NAME

c. OTHER ACCIDENT? YES ☐ NO ☐

c. INSURANCE PLAN NAME OR PROGRAM NAME

d. INSURANCE PLAN NAME OR PROGRAM NAME

10d. RESERVED FOR LOCAL USE

d. IS THERE ANOTHER HEALTH BENEFIT PLAN? YES ☐ NO ☐ *If yes*, return to and complete item 9 a-d.

READ BACK OF FORM BEFORE COMPLETING & SIGNING THIS FORM.
12. PATIENT'S OR AUTHORIZED PERSON'S SIGNATURE I authorize the release of any medical or other information necessary to process this claim. I also request payment of government benefits either to myself or to the party who accepts assignment below.

SIGNED _____ DATE _____

13. INSURED'S OR AUTHORIZED PERSON'S SIGNATURE I authorize payment of medical benefits to the undersigned physician or supplier for services described below.

SIGNED _____

14. DATE OF CURRENT: ILLNESS (First symptom) OR INJURY (Accident) OR PREGNANCY(LMP) MM | DD | YY

15. IF PATIENT HAS HAD SAME OR SIMILAR ILLNESS. GIVE FIRST DATE MM | DD | YY

16. DATES PATIENT UNABLE TO WORK IN CURRENT OCCUPATION FROM MM | DD | YY TO MM | DD | YY

17. NAME OF REFERRING PROVIDER OR OTHER SOURCE

17a.

17b. NPI

18. HOSPITALIZATION DATES RELATED TO CURRENT SERVICES FROM MM | DD | YY TO MM | DD | YY

19. RESERVED FOR LOCAL USE

20. OUTSIDE LAB? YES ☐ NO ☐ $ CHARGES

21. DIAGNOSIS OR NATURE OF ILLNESS OR INJURY (Relate Items 1, 2, 3 or 4 to Item 24E by Line)

1. ⌊___.___⌋   3. ⌊___.___⌋
2. ⌊___.___⌋   4. ⌊___.___⌋

22. MEDICAID RESUBMISSION CODE _____ ORIGINAL REF. NO. _____

23. PRIOR AUTHORIZATION NUMBER

24. A. DATE(S) OF SERVICE From MM DD YY To MM DD YY **B.** PLACE OF SERVICE **C.** EMG **D.** PROCEDURES, SERVICES, OR SUPPLIES (Explain Unusual Circumstances) CPT/HCPCS | MODIFIER **E.** DIAGNOSIS POINTER **F.** $ CHARGES **G.** DAYS OR UNITS **H.** EPSDT Family Plan **I.** ID. QUAL. **J.** RENDERING PROVIDER ID. #

1 .... NPI
2 .... NPI
3 .... NPI
4 .... NPI
5 .... NPI
6 .... NPI

25. FEDERAL TAX I.D. NUMBER SSN ☐ EIN ☐

26. PATIENT'S ACCOUNT NO.

27. ACCEPT ASSIGNMENT? (For govt. claims, see back) YES ☐ NO ☐

28. TOTAL CHARGE $

29. AMOUNT PAID $

30. BALANCE DUE $

31. SIGNATURE OF PHYSICIAN OR SUPPLIER INCLUDING DEGREES OR CREDENTIALS (I certify that the statements on the reverse apply to this bill and are made a part thereof.)

SIGNED _____ DATE _____

32. SERVICE FACILITY LOCATION INFORMATION

a. NPI   b.

33. BILLING PROVIDER INFO & PH # ( )

a. NPI   b.

NUCC Instruction Manual available at: www.nucc.org   **PLEASE PRINT OR TYPE**   APPROVED OMB-0938-0999 FORM CMS-1500 (08-05)

Sidebar labels: CARRIER | PATIENT AND INSURED INFORMATION | PHYSICIAN OR SUPPLIER INFORMATION

▶ **Figure 1-10   CMS-1500 Form**

Backing Up Medisoft

Finally, no day would be complete unless a **backup** was done of Medisoft. A backup is a second copy of your data in case the first copy is damaged or destroyed. It is best to back up on an external device that can be brought to an offsite location and to develop a backup cycle of rotating your backup disks. Procedures should be established to ensure that transportation and storage of backup media are HIPAA compliant. Typical **backup mediums** are burnable CDs, zip disks, flash drives, and external hard drives. Medisoft has its own backup utility and makes a copy of all Medisoft and Office Hours data for the practice. Occasionally, clinics may have more than one set of data—i.e., each doctor has a separate tax identification number and therefore a separate dataset within Medisoft. If this is the case, each dataset must be backed up separately (Figure 1-11).

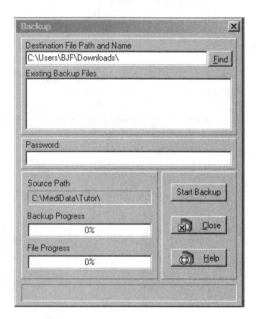

▶ Figure 1-11   **Medisoft Backup**

PRACTICE EXERCISE 1-3   Backing Up Medisoft

It is often said to only back up your data as often as you don't want to reenter it; therefore, backups should be done frequently. Data is very valuable, and we all depend upon it more and more each day. Medisoft has a great utility within the program that assists the user in creating backups. In this exercise, we are going to create a backup of the Medical Group Tutorial Data on the local drive (C drive) of the computer.

1   Open Medisoft and select File on the menu bar and Backup data on the drop-down menu. This will bring a pop-up box titled Backup.

2   Next, select the Find button on the right side of the screen. This in turn will give another pop-up box that allows the user to select where to create the backup. All of the resources available on the computer will be listed. For this exercise, select the "C:" drive and ok, then press Start Backup. The backup will be created. **TIP:** Some computers, particularly those with the Vista operating system, do not allow backups to be created on the C drive. If that issue is

encountered, choose another location, such as Documents. The error message that will be given if the location you chose is not available is "Please insert disk 2 of the set."

3 After the backup has completed, notice that the backup name will default to mwXX-XX-XXXX.mbk. The Xs stand for today's date. This can come in handy if the backup needs to be restored. Each office should have numerous backups, and if there aren't any data issues, the most recent one would be the appropriate one to restore (Figure 1-12).

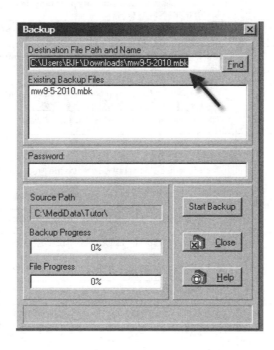

▶ Figure 1-12 **Medisoft Backup with File Name**

Medisoft Toolbar

Below the Menu bar is the toolbar, which contains buttons to open files for data entry segments of the program.

Button	Definition
	The Transaction Entry icon opens the Transaction Entry window where most of the transactions for the practice are maintained.
	The Claim Management icon opens the Claim Management window where claims are prepared, edited, and sent for payment.
	The Statement Management icon opens the Statement Management window where statements are prepared, edited, and sent for payment.
	The Collection List icon opens the Collection List window where you manage collection items.
	The Add Collection List Item icon opens the Add Collection List Items , which you can use to create collection items.
	The Appointment Book icon opens the Office Hours Patient Appointment Scheduler where appointments for the practice are scheduled.
	The Eligibility icon opens the Eligibility Verification Results window where you can check patient insurance eligibility.
	The Patient Quick Entry icon opens the Patient Quick Entry window. This feature provides another method for creating patient and case records. For more information on this feature, see the topic Patient Quick Entry Overview .
	The Patient List icon opens the Patient List window and access to patient case information.
	The Insurance Carrier List icon opens the Insurance Carrier List window and access to carrier information.
	The Procedure Codes List icon opens the Procedure/Payment/Adjustment List window.
	The Diagnosis Codes List icon opens the Diagnosis List window.
	The Provider List icon opens the Provider List window.
	The Referring Provider List icon opens the Referring Provider List window.
	The Address List icon opens the Address List window.
	The Patient Recall Entry icon opens the Patient Recall: (new) window.
	Clicking the Custom Report List icon displays the Open Report window and lets you print any of the documents listed, such as Statements, Walkout Receipts, Patient Lists, CMS- or HCFA-1500, Superbills, etc. See Custom Report List .
	The Quick Ledger icon opens the Quick Ledger . You can access the ledger by clicking this icon or pressing F7 at almost any time the program is open. If you have already selected a chart number, the Quick Ledger defaults to that chart number.
	The Quick Balance icon opens the Quick Balance window, which displays a selected guarantor's remainder balance.
	The Enter Deposits and Apply Payments icon opens the Deposit List window where you can create and print deposit lists and apply payments to patient transactions.
	The Show/Hide Hints icon is a toggle on/off icon. A Hint is a context-sensitive help feature that displays a short description of that portion of the program or window on which the pointer is resting. A written description of the function is also displayed in the Status bar at the bottom of the window.
	The Help icon opens the Help files.
	The Advanced Reporting icon opens the Advanced Reporting program where you can create and/or modify custom reports.
	The Launch Work Administrator icon opens the Work Administrator program where you can create tasks for users and/user groups.
	The Edit Patient Notes in Final Draft icon opens the Final Draft program. It is a word processing program that is integrated with your patient accounting program and can be used for creating letters, notices, notes, etc., using data already stored in the patient accounting database.
	Clicking Exit takes you out of the program entirely. If you have the Remind to Backup on Program Exit option activated in Program Options , you are reminded to back up your files before the program is shut down.

▶ **Figure 1-13   Medisoft Toolbar**

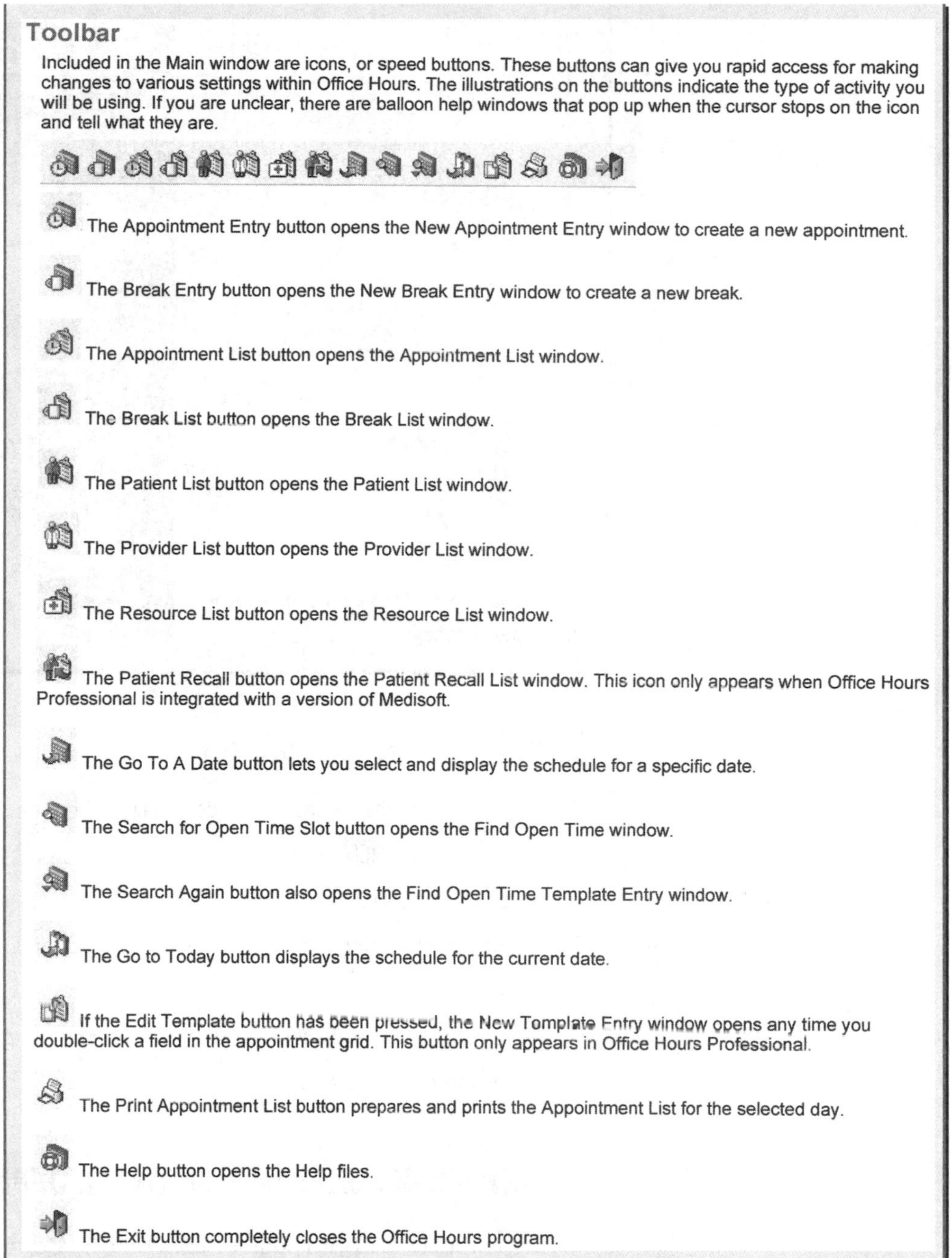

Toolbar

Included in the Main window are icons, or speed buttons. These buttons can give you rapid access for making changes to various settings within Office Hours. The illustrations on the buttons indicate the type of activity you will be using. If you are unclear, there are balloon help windows that pop up when the cursor stops on the icon and tell what they are.

The Appointment Entry button opens the New Appointment Entry window to create a new appointment.

The Break Entry button opens the New Break Entry window to create a new break.

The Appointment List button opens the Appointment List window.

The Break List button opens the Break List window.

The Patient List button opens the Patient List window.

The Provider List button opens the Provider List window.

The Resource List button opens the Resource List window.

The Patient Recall button opens the Patient Recall List window. This icon only appears when Office Hours Professional is integrated with a version of Medisoft.

The Go To A Date button lets you select and display the schedule for a specific date.

The Search for Open Time Slot button opens the Find Open Time window.

The Search Again button also opens the Find Open Time Template Entry window.

The Go to Today button displays the schedule for the current date.

If the Edit Template button has been pressed, the New Template Entry window opens any time you double-click a field in the appointment grid. This button only appears in Office Hours Professional.

The Print Appointment List button prepares and prints the Appointment List for the selected day.

The Help button opens the Help files.

The Exit button completely closes the Office Hours program.

▶ **Figure 1-14   Office Hours Toolbar**

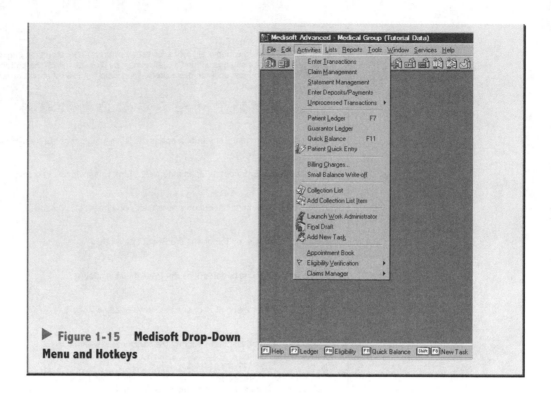

▶ **Figure 1-15 Medisoft Drop-Down Menu and Hotkeys**

▶ Test Your Knowledge 1-1

1. List and define the six basic tasks done daily in Medisoft.

2. Define CMS and HCFA.

3. What are breaks used for?

4. Name the form used to track patient visits and provide a worksheet for each doctor.

5. Define follow-up.

6. What is the name of the form used to bill insurance companies?

7. Name three shortcut keys in Medisoft.

OTHER TASKS WITHIN A MEDICAL OFFICE

While the title and purpose of this text is *Mastering Medisoft,* it is important to note that other functions are performed by the medical office specialist that are outside of the scope of using Medisoft. The following is a brief discussion of some of these additional tasks.

Verify Eligibility of Insurance Coverage

When a new or existing patient calls to schedule an appointment, offices will sometimes have a procedure in place to collect the patient's insurance information and call to determine **eligibility** and financial responsibility. There are a variety of ways to determine insurance eligibility. First, the medical office specialist can call the insurance company, or if the insurance company has the availability, eligibility can be verified online or through an electronic transaction. There are pros and cons for an office that offers this service to patients and doctors. First, patients may miss appointments, causing the time-consuming task of determining eligibility to seem wasted. In addition, the insurance company always offers a disclaimer that benefits given are a quote and not a guarantee. Therefore, the data cannot be absolutely relied upon for determining coverage of services. Another perceived drawback is the doctor and/or patient may make utilization of care decisions based upon inaccurate information. Nonetheless, many offices choose to verify eligibility because the advantages of knowing potential coverage limitations outweigh the concerns.

Review Proper Coding and Billing Procedures

In order to properly complete the CMS-1500 form, various codes are required, such as **CPT* codes, diagnosis codes,** and **modifiers.** (In later chapters, we will review the CMS-1500 form in greater detail and the coding systems applied on it.) What is crucial to understand is that the coding must be valid and correct, and certain insurance companies require additional modifiers and information in order to process the claims. It is the medical office specialist's duty to stay abreast of any changes in the billing industry and to review the claim information to ensure proper payment.

Review of Contract Payments

Some insurance companies require contracts with medical offices in order for the office to treat their **beneficiaries.** Beneficiaries are the people entitled to coverage under a health insurance plan. The most common companies to require contracting are Medicare, Medicaid, and Blue Cross Blue Shield. Other insurance companies may offer incentives to becoming contracted providers such as patient referrals. It is important to know that anytime there is a contract, the payment rates are outlined. And, like most things involving money, there may be discrepancies between what is paid and what should be paid. It is the medical office specialist's responsibility to ensure that the clinic is properly paid according to the contract. Typically, a specialist will have a grid of contracted rates available at the time payments are posted and review them for accuracy.

MEDISOFT PATIENT CHARTS AND APPOINTMENT ENTRY

Now that we have reviewed the daily Medisoft tasks, the rest of this chapter covers in detail how to create a patient chart and appointment. **Note:** There are two parts to entering a patient into Medisoft: the Chart and the Case. In this section we will cover only the Chart. This is the most typical office flow since all insurance data is not gathered or verified the moment an appointment is scheduled.

---

*CPT is a registered trademark of the American Medical Association.

We will now add patient charts and appointments to Medisoft. First, we want to make sure that we are using the Medisoft tutorial database.

Now that Medisoft has been installed, please note that there will be three icons on your desktop: the Medisoft icon is red in color, Office Hours has a clock on it, and the **Work Administrator** will have a pencil on it (Figure 1-16).

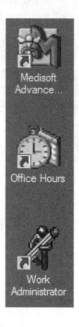

▶ Figure 1-16   **Medisoft, Office Hours, and Work Administrator Icons**

We will enter the charges and payments and track the accounts receivable in the Medisoft portion of the program. Office Hours is where the clinic's schedule is kept, and Work Administrator is an excellent tool for managing work within the office. Patient charts and cases are flexible and may be entered into either Medisoft or Office Hours.

PRACTICE EXERCISE 1-4   Entering Appointments and Patient Charts

In this exercise, we are going to add appointments for both existing and new patients. This will simulate the typical job of a scheduler in a healthcare clinic. For this exercise, you will need to reference the source documents in Appendix B.

1   Open Office Hours by left-double-clicking on the icon on the desktop, or, if you already have Medisoft open, you will see there is an Office Hours icon on the toolbar. You can also click on this.

2   For our exercises, we are going to work with Dr. J.D. Mallard. He has several patients already on the schedule, and we are going to add several new patients. To view Dr. Mallard's schedule, click on the initials on the top right of the screen. Office Hours will give you a drop-down box of all the providers available, JM being Dr. Mallard (Figure 1-17).

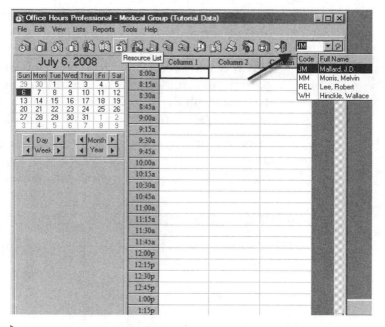

▶ Figure 1-17   **Office Hours Provider Selection**

3   Next, we want to select the day we are scheduling for. You can do this by clicking on the date on the calendar on the upper left side. For this example, select September 4, 2008 (Figure 1-18).

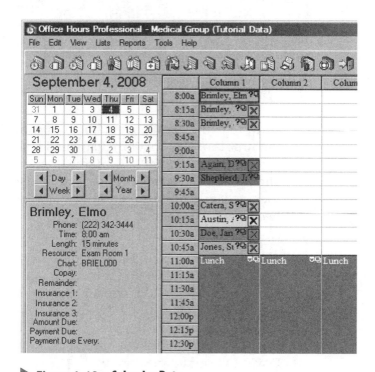

▶ Figure 1-18   **Calendar Date**

4 We want to add two existing patients to the schedule: Wallace Clinger at 9:00 am and Stephanie Jasper at 3:00 pm. In addition, we want to add three new patients to the schedule: William Johnson at 8:45 am, David Lyle at 10:30 am, and Jane Jordan at 1:15 pm. The new patient information can be found in Appendix B: Source Documents, 1-3. Make all five appointments 15 minutes in length. Remember, accuracy is a must. Always double-check your work.

5 Adding a new appointment for an existing patient is quite simple: Just point to the spot to add the new appointment (i.e., 9:00 am), right-click, and select new appointment (Figure 1-19).

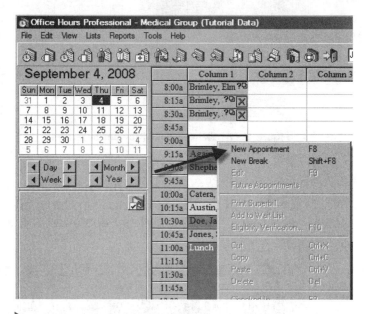

▶ Figure 1-19   **Adding a New Appointment**

6 Next, to add the patient's name to the appointment, just start typing the first three letters of the patient's last name, and Office Hours will drop-down to the patient's name (Figure 1-20). If there is more than one patient with the same last name, use the arrow keys to move to the one you wish to select. Now add appointments for the remaining two existing patients.

7 Next, to add the three new patients to the schedule, there is a two-part process for each. First, right-click or hit F8 on 8:45 am for William Johnson. When the new appointment box appears, right-click (or hit F8) to add a new patient. A Patient/Guarantor New box will appear. Complete the Name, Address and Other Information tabs for William Johnson (Figures 1-21 and 1-22). Also, add and complete the appointment and patient information for our other two patients, David Lyle and Jane Jordan.

Note: A new patient and new appointment may also be added by going to the List menu at the top of Office Hours and selecting the appropriate item.

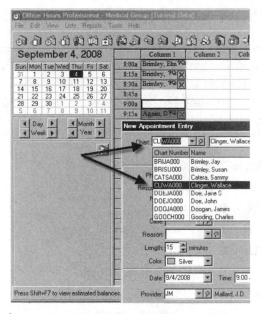

▶ **Figure 1-20** **Selecting an Existing Patient**

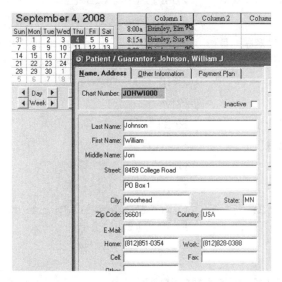

▶ **Figure 1-21** **Add a New Patient; Patient/Guarantor Tab**

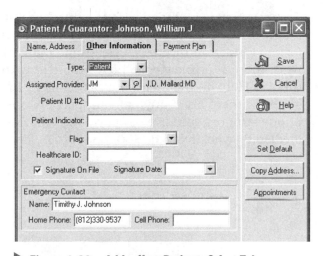

▶ **Figure 1-22** **Add a New Patient; Other Tab**

MEDISOFT SHORTCUTS AND HOTKEYS

Medisoft has integrated many of Microsoft's operating system shortcuts into the program. One handy shortcut is the **right-click** feature. On any blank that you need to fill, just single-right-click in the field. The program will display the options available to you. In addition, next to the option, the hotkey will be displayed for that function. The following are some hotkeys that are available to you in Office Hours:

CTRL + X	Cut
CTRL + V	Paste
CTRL + C	Copy
CTRL + T	Go to today
CTRL + G	Go to date
CTRL + F	Find open time
CTRL + N	Find next open time
CTRL + D	Show/Hide Calendar
CTRL + I	Zoom appointment grid in
CTRL + O	Zoom appointment grid out
CTRL + S	Save view. This command is only applicable when using Office Hours Professional.
F1	Help
F3	Save
F5	Refresh
F6	Search
F8	New
F9	Edit
F12	Office Messenger- Integrated with Medisoft Network Professional Only

MEDISOFT SUPPORT

Free support is included with the purchase of most software programs, and Medisoft is no exception. With Medisoft, free support takes three forms. First, you receive an electronic manual on the installation CD; next, there is a Knowledge Base online at www.medisoft.com; and finally, there is Help on the menu bar of Medisoft. In addition to the free support, there are many paid support options, including a training DVD, phone support, and live support. You can find these options on Medisoft's website or at (800) 333-4747.

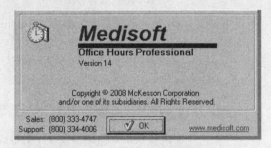

▶ **Figure 1-23**   **Determining the Version of Office Hours**

▶ ## Test Your Knowledge 1-2

1. List the steps for adding an existing patient to the schedule.

2. Describe the steps for adding a new patient to the schedule.

3. List the shortcut keys most applicable to adding an appointment.

4. Name three forms of free support that comes with Medisoft.

Help Within Medisoft

Each appointment field contains required information and optional information. Required information includes the name of the doctor, the date and time, and patient's chart. There are numerous fields for optional information such as reason, status and notes. Medisoft has an incredible resource within it. Wherever you are in the program, if you hit function key F1, Help will pop up for the area you are viewing (Figure 1-24).

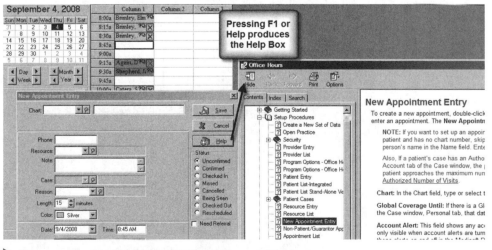

▶ **Figure 1-24**   **Medisoft Help Within the Program**

PRACTICE EXERCISE 1-5 **Accessing Help Within Medisoft**

As previously discussed, Medisoft offers a great help feature within the program. Help is customized by the area in which you are working at the time it is deployed. This same feature can be found in many software programs; remembering this tip can be very valuable on the job site.

1 For this exercise, hit F1 in the New Appointment Entry Window. Notice this brings specific help to the user for adding a new appointment. Read through the detail now.

2 Next, hit F1 in the Patient/Guarantor New window. Read through the definitions for each field. Some of these fields will be included in the Chapter Review section.

LINKING THE PATIENT INFORMATION TO THE CMS-1500 FORM

A critical function of Medisoft is billing insurance companies. So, it is imperative that we understand where the information for the CMS-1500 form is pulled from in Medisoft. So far, we have entered a few of these critical fields when we entered the new patient information. It is essential for this information to be double-checked and accurate in order for the clinic to be properly reimbursed for its services. Review the CMS-1500 form found in Figure 1-25 and the following grid to identify the patient chart fields affecting the billing form.

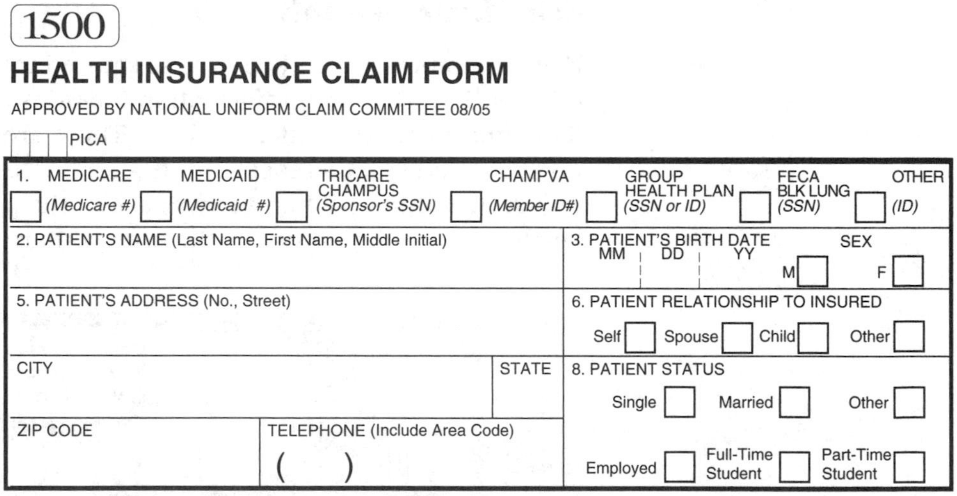
1500

HEALTH INSURANCE CLAIM FORM

APPROVED BY NATIONAL UNIFORM CLAIM COMMITTEE 08/05

PICA

1. MEDICARE (Medicare #) MEDICAID (Medicaid #) TRICARE CHAMPUS (Sponsor's SSN) CHAMPVA (Member ID#) GROUP HEALTH PLAN (SSN or ID) FECA BLK LUNG (SSN) OTHER (ID)

2. PATIENT'S NAME (Last Name, First Name, Middle Initial)

3. PATIENT'S BIRTH DATE MM DD YY SEX M F

5. PATIENT'S ADDRESS (No., Street)

6. PATIENT RELATIONSHIP TO INSURED Self Spouse Child Other

CITY STATE

8. PATIENT STATUS Single Married Other

ZIP CODE TELEPHONE (Include Area Code) ( )

Employed Full-Time Student Part-Time Student

▶ **Figure 1-25** **CMS-1500 Form—Boxes 2 through 5**

CMS-1500 Form Box	Field in Medisoft - Patient Chart
Box 2	Patient's Last Name, First Name, and Middle Initial
Box 3	Birthdate and Sex
Box 5	Street, City, State, Zip, and Home Telephone Number

SCHEDULING BREAKS

Along with scheduling appointments, the doctor will also need his or her specialist to schedule breaks. Breaks are periods of times that patients will not be seen. It may be for lunch, a meeting, or any variety of reasons. In Practice Exercise 1-6, breaks will be entered into the schedule.

PRACTICE EXERCISE 1-6   Entering Breaks

1   Adding a break is very similar to adding appointments. Just point to the time on the schedule where you want to add the new break and right-click the mouse. The drop-down menu will display the options available: Select New Break and add the name for the break. Again, click on the Help button to the right (or click F1 - Help) to see the definitions for each field (Figure 1-26).

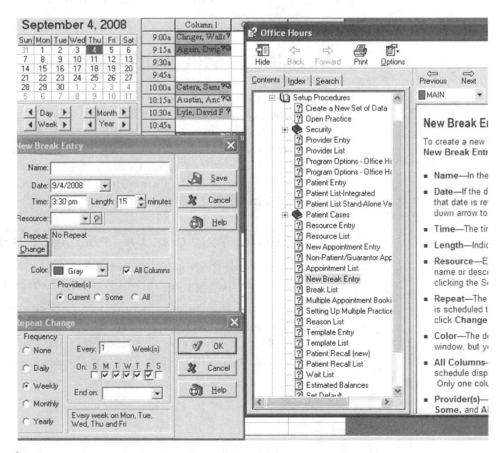

▶ Figure 1-26   Break Entry and Repeat Appointments

2 With both appointments and breaks, the user has the option to repeat the entry. This option is used more frequently with breaks since the doctor will tend to repeat the same lunchtime or break time each day. Review the notes under Help for Repeat Appointment/Break.

3 Add a 30-minute break beginning at 3:30 pm on September 4, 2008, and repeat it indefinitely Monday through Friday.

MOVING, EDITING, AND DELETING

As with any situation, there is the chance that changes will need to be made to the schedule. In this exercise, appointments will be modified by moving, editing, or deleting them. Any appointment or break can be moved, edited, or deleted by right-clicking on the appointment and selecting the appropriate option from the drop-down menu. To move an appointment or break, you can also drag the appropriate appointment from one time slot to another.

PRACTICE EXERCISE 1-7   Moving, Editing, and Deleting

1 For this exercise, let's move the appointment for Dwight Again from 9:15 am to 9:30 am. **Note:** Once we move the appointment, the program will ask us if we want all appointments to be changed or only the current appointment. This is because this patient has a "Repeat" appointment setup. Choose the option to only change the current appointment.

PRINTING SCHEDULES AND SUPERBILLS

At the end of each day, medical office specialists print a schedule and superbills for each of the following day's appointments. The staff uses this information to prepare the patients' charts and gives it to the doctor to record the visits. As discussed earlier, superbills allow the provider to check the services given to the patient and the diagnosis codes attributed to the services. With Office Hours, there are some great reports that will assist in these tasks.

PRACTICE EXERCISE 1-8   Printing the Schedule

1 To print the appointment list for our exercise, go to Reports on the main menu and Appointment Lists on the drop-down menu (Figure 1-27).

2 Under the Data Selection box, choose the information for our current example. Choose the date of service of 09/04/08 and the provider JM. This will give you the report that most clinics will utilize to pull the charts in preparation for the next day.

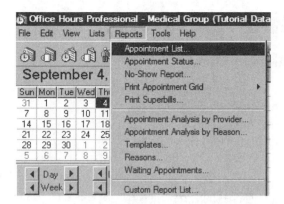

▶ **Figure 1-27**   **Printing the Schedule**

PRACTICE EXERCISE 1-9   **Printing the Superbills**

1   To print the superbills for our exercise, go to Reports on the main menu and Print Superbills, and then select the Superbill (numbered) from the Open Report box (Figure 1-28).

2   Again, enter the date of service 09/04/08 and the provider JM. This will give you a superbill for each patient on the schedule. This is the form the doctor uses during the patient visit to record the patient services and diagnoses.

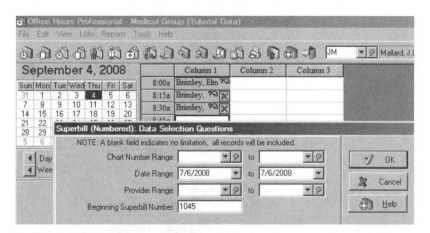

▶ **Figure 1-28**   **Printing Superbills**

Medisoft Quick Tip   Design Custom Reports

Any report that is found under the Custom Report List, such as the Superbill (numbered), can be customized under the Design Custom Reports and Bills feature. With superbills this is especially helpful because each type of practice offers different types of services and will need to customize its superbill in order to have it work for its practice type.

CHAPTER REVIEW

Multiple Choice

1. What is the name of the free version of Office Hours?
   a. Office Hours Professional
   b. Office Hours
   c. Office Work Administrator
   d. Medisoft Office Hours

2. What is the name of the current claim form?
   a. CMS-1500 Form
   b. HCFA-1500 Form
   c. Superbill
   d. Claim form

3. What is the superbill used for?
   a. Billing insurance companies
   b. A worksheet for the doctor and office staff
   c. A form used by the patient to bill insurance companies.
   d. Both b and c

4. What does the F1 key give you in Medisoft?
   a. A new appointment
   b. Help
   c. A new break
   d. All of the above

5. Which report do you run at the end of the day to proof your charges and payments?
   a. Patient day sheet
   b. Appointment list
   c. Superbill report
   d. Proofing report

6. Which information do you enter in the patient's chart that goes on the CMS-1500 form?
   a. Patient's insurance information
   b. Patient's name, address, and date of birth
   c. Patient's diagnoses
   d. Patient's policy number

7. How do you add a new appointment?
   a. Right-click on the time slot and select new appointment
   b. Select the time slot and hit the F8 key
   c. Go to List and Appointment on the top of the screen
   d. All of the above

8. How often should you back up Medisoft?
   a. Weekly
   b. Daily
   c. Monthly
   d. Hourly

9. What is the purpose of Medisoft in the clinic?
   a. To track patient information, schedules, and accounts receivable
   b. To track patient information, medical records, and superbills
   c. To track appointment lists, enter patients, and produce superbills
   d. Both a and c

10. What can the Work Administrator do in Medisoft?
    a. Track the work for the doctor
    b. Track the work for the office
    c. Track work entered by the staff
    d. All of the above

11. Which are tasks that are done daily?
    a. Schedule appointments, enter finance charges, bill insurance companies
    b. Proof daily work, process payments and denials, back up Medisoft
    c. Back up Medisoft, schedule appointments, print medical records
    d. All of the above

12. Which of these reports will be run from Office Hours?
    a. Superbills
    b. Appointment lists
    c. Patient day sheet
    d. Both a and b

True/False

Identify each of the following statements as true or false.

1. Medisoft is used to track patient medical records.

2. The CMS-1500 form is the current form being used to bill insurance companies.

3. To view the options available inside of Medisoft, you left-click on the blank field.

4. The superbill is the form used by doctors that shows all the patients on the same page.

5. If you get stuck in Medisoft and need help, you should hit the function key F2.

6. Medisoft backups should be made once a week.

7. After creating claims, it is important to proof the charges and payments.

8. If repeat appointment is modified, Office Hours will ask if all the appointments or only the current appointment should be modified.

9. Medisoft Basic has a Deposit List.

10. Office Hours Professional must be purchased separately.

Short Answer

1. Imagine yourself working at local clinic. Describe your day, including the six daily Medisoft tasks.

2. List the names and types of reimbursement that may be received by a clinic.

3. Explain the difference between an appointment and a break.

4. List the default naming convention for a Medisoft backup.

5. List three things to consider when managing Medisoft backups.

Resources

Medisoft Knowledgebase: **www.medisoft.com**

(Click on Support and Knowledge Base) This site is updated on a daily basis and includes material on the program as well as changes in the healthcare industry. Listed are the latest updates and patches, Latest Articles, Hot Topics, and Top 10 Frequently Asked Questions, as well as a search area to type in topics and questions.

Centers for Medicare and Medicaid Services (CMS): **www.cms.gov**

This is an excellent resource for billing regulations. The main page gives you CMS Programs & Information, CMS Highlights, Top 10 Links, and much more, as well as a search bar.

The National Uniform Claim Committee (NUCC): **www.nucc.org**

This organization is responsible for developing the CMS-1500 form. It is chaired by the American Medical Association (AMA) and by the Centers for Medicare and Medicaid Services (CMS). It is an excellent resource for the CMS-1500 claim form manual and directions.

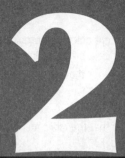

Chapter Two

Patient Information

Learning Objectives

After completing this chapter, you should be able to:

♦ Define and spell the key terms in this chapter.

♦ Explain the purpose of the Case and demonstrate how to create Case information in Medisoft.

♦ Describe each of the tabs within a Case.

♦ Show how to create custom Patient and custom Case information.

♦ Describe the different types of Medisoft.

♦ Describe the three forms of help in Medisoft.

♦ Understand signatures and assignments and explain their importance in billing.

Key Terms

adjudicate   the process an insurance company uses to process a claim and determine the applicable benefits.

Assignment of Benefits   a form signed by the insured whereby he or she directs the insurance company to send payment directly to the provider.

Case   a grouping of transactions associated to the patient's chart information that is linked to a common billing scenario such as diagnosis, insurance, facility, or provider.

Case Description   a field inside the Case that defines the different information for the Case, such as insurance coverage, diagnosis, provider, or facility.

Cash Case   a patient Case whereby there is no insurance coverage for the services and only the patient will be billed.

Centers for Disease Control and Prevention (CDC)   the government agency that promotes health and quality of life by preventing and controlling disease, injury, and disability.

courtesy billing   billing that occurs when clinics request that patients pay for their services on the day of service, and the clinics give the patients a claim form to submit to their insurance. The insurance will then process this and reimburse the patient as specified in the patient's policy.

Custom Case data   Case information that is added to the screen and customized by the Medisoft user.

Custom Patient data   patient information that is added to the screen and customized by the Medisoft user.

guarantor   person who is financially responsible for the account and will receive the statement.

ICD-9-CM   abbreviation for International Classification of Diseases, 9th Revision, Clinical Modification. A coding system used to identify signs, symptoms, injuries, diseases, and conditions.

insured   person who owns the insurance policy, also known as subscriber.

Knowledge Base   Medisoft's online collection of articles to provide help to users.

Multimedia tab   the Medisoft Network Professional feature that allows the user to save media in patient cases, such as pictures, X-rays, and medical records.

National Center for Health Statistics (NCHS)   the government office that provides U.S. public health statistics, including information on diseases, pregnancies, births, aging, and mortality.

National Provider Identifier (NPI)   the lifetime provider number that uniquely identifies a healthcare provider in standard transactions, such as healthcare claims.

patient   the person receiving healthcare services.

signature on file (SOF)   indicates to the insurance company that the clinic has a copy of the required signature on file for CMS-1500 claim form boxes 12 and 13.

Abbreviations

CDC   Centers for Disease Control and Prevention

NCHS   National Center for Health Statistics

NPI   National Provider Identifier

■ ■ ■ ■

INTRODUCTION

Case information complements the Chart information reviewed in Chapter 1. Case information holds data that can change frequently, such as insurance information, diagnosis, and referring doctor, to name a few. The Case information in Medisoft completes the entry of the patient information. The majority of the billing information that completes the CMS-1500 form can be found in the Case. Medisoft uses the Case to define specific billing scenarios such as different insurance coverage, diagnosis, providers, or facilities. In addition, Medisoft allows the user to create additional information that can be added to the Chart or to the Case. This information is customizable by the user and is called **Custom Patient Data** and **Custom Case Data.** Custom Patient Data is available in Advanced Medisoft, while both Custom Patient Data and Custom Case Data are available in Network Professional Medisoft. The goal of this chapter is to learn how to set up the Case information, learn all of the fields of the CMS-1500 form, and create Custom Case Data and Custom Patient Data inside of Medisoft.

OVERVIEW OF THE CASE INFORMATION

Each time a patient is seen at a clinic, the visit may have unique circumstances. The patient may have a different reason for going to the clinic—for example, strep throat or a broken arm. The patient may have different insurance coverage for different visits—for example, health insurance or auto insurance. The patient may even be seen by different doctors or providers or at different locations (facilities) at the clinic. Each one of the scenarios could warrant creating a new Case. The CMS-1500 form requires the utmost attention to detail in order for the claim to be processed properly by the insurance. The claim form has 33 boxes on it, and most of the information comes from the Medisoft Case information. Figure 2-1 shows the link between the information in Medisoft and the CMS-1500 form.

CMS-1500 Form Locations in Medisoft

CMS Box	Claim Form Box	Data Source	Location in Medisoft
Top of form	Insurance Name and Address	Insurance	Case, Insurance Carrier Name and Address
1	Insurance Type	Insurance	Case, Insurance Carrier, Options, Type
1a	Insured's I.D. Number	Case	Case, Policy 1, 2, or 3, Policy Number
2	Patient's Name	Patient	Patient/Guarantor Name
3	Patient Birthday, Sex	Patient	Patient/Guarantor Date of Birth and Sex
4	Insured's Name	Case	Case, Policy Holder 1, 2, or 3, Name
5	Patient's Address	Patient	Patient/Guarantor Address
6	Patient Relationship to Insured	Case	Case, Policy 1, 2, or 3, Relationship to Insured
7	Insured's Address	Patient	Case, Policy 1, 2, or 3, Insured Address
8	Patient Status	Case	Case, Personal, Marital, Student and Emp. Status
9	Other Insured's Name	Case	Case, Policy 2 or 3, Insured
9a	Other Policy/Group Number	Case	Case, Policy 2 or 3, Group Number
9b	Other Insured's Date of Birth	Patient	Patient/Guarantor Date of Birth and Sex
9c	Employer's Name or School	Patient	Patient/Guarantor, Other Information, Employer
9d	Insurance Plan Name	Insurance	Insurance Carrier, Options, Plan Name
10a	Condition Related to Employment	Case	Case, Condition, Employment Related
10b	Related to: Auto Accident	Case	Case, Condition, Accident Related to Auto
10c	Related to: Other Accident	Case	Case, Condition Accident Related to Yes
10d	Local Use A	Case	Case, Miscellaneous, Local Use A
11	Insured's Policy Group Number	Case	Case, Policy 1, Group Number
11a	Date of Birth	Patient	Case, Insured, Date of Birth
11b	Employer/School	Patient	Case, Insured, Other Information, Employer
11c	Insurance Plan Name/Program Name	Insurance	Insurance Carrier, Options, Plan Name
11d	Is there another benefit plan	Case	Case, Policy 2 or 3
12	Patient or Authorized Signature	Patient	Patient/Guarantor, Other Information Signature on File
13	Insured's Signature	Patient	Patient/Guarantor, Other Information Signature on File
14	Date of Current Illness, Injury or LMP	Case	Case, Condition, Injury/Illness/LMP Date
15	If Patient had Same or Similar Illness	Case	Case, Condition, Date of Similar Symptoms
16	Dates Patient Unable to Work	Case	Case, Condition, Dates Unable to Work
17	Name of Referring Provider	Case	Case, Account, Referring Provider
17a	ID Qualifier and ID	Case	Case, Account, Referring Provider PIN and Qualifier
17b	Referring Provider NPI	Case	Case, Account, Referring Provider National Identifier
18	Hospital Dates Related to Current	Case	Case, Condition, Dates of Hospitalization
19	Local Use B	Case	Case, Miscellaneous, Local Use B
20	Outside Lab?	Case	Case, Miscellaneous, Outside Lab Work
21	Diagnosis Codes	Case	Case, Diagnosis, Default 1, 2, 3, 4
22	Medicaid Resubmission	Case	Case, Medicaid and Tricare, Resubmission Number
23	Prior Authorization	Case	Case, Miscellaneous, Prior Authorization Number
24A	Dates of Service	Transaction	Transaction Entry, Date From, Date To
24B	Place of Service	Transaction	Transaction Entry, Place of Service
24C	EMG	Case	Case, Condition, Emergency Check Box
24D	Procedure Codes/Modifiers	Transaction	Transaction Entry, Procedure, M1, M2, M3, M4
24E	Diagnosis Codes	Transaction	Transaction Entry, Diag 1, Diag 2, Diag 3, Diag 4
24F	$ Charges	Transaction	Transaction Entry, Amount
24G	Days or Units	Transaction	Transaction Entry, Units
24H	EPSDT Family Plan	Case	Case, Medicaid and Tricare, ESPDT
24I	ID Qualifier	Transaction	Transaction, Provider, Pins, ID Qualifier
24J	Rendering Provider ID #	Transaction	Transaction, Provider, Pins and National Identifier
25	Federal Tax ID	Practice	Provider, Default Pins, SSN/Federal Tax ID
26	Patient's Account No.	Patient	Patient/Guarantor Chart Number
27	Accept Assignment?	Case	Case, Policy 1, 2, or 3, Assignment of Benefits
28	Total Charge	Transaction	Calculated Field
29	Amount Paid	Transaction	Transaction Entry, Payment
30	Balance Due	Transaction	Calculated Field
31	Physician's Signature	Insurance	Insurance Carrier, Options, Physicians Signature on File
32	Facility Address	Case	Case, Account, Facility
32a	Facility NPI	Case	Case, Account, Facility, National ID
32b	Facility ID Qualifier and Pin	Case	Case, Account, Facility, Pins, Pin and Qualifier
33	Billing Provider Info and Pin	Provider	Case, Provider, Address and Phone
33a	Billing Provider NPI	Provider	Case, Provider, Default Pins, National Identifier
33b	Billing Provider ID Qualifier and Pin	Provider	Case, Provider, Pins, Group ID and Qualifier

▶ Figure 2-1   Medisoft and CMS-1500 Linkage

Billing Insight   Providers Versus Doctors

Medical services may be provided by individuals from a variety of disciplines; at least half of those individuals are not medical doctors. Medisoft is used by all sorts of medical providers that need to be reimbursed for their services such as ambulance companies, medical supply companies, chiropractors, and mental health professionals. Remember that the terms *doctor* and *provider* are used interchangeably throughout this book; therefore, any entity that could be using Medisoft to bill on the CMS-1500 form is being referred to.

CREATING A CASE

Once a patient has arrived at the clinic, completed the registration form, and has been seen by the doctor or provider of services, the Case can be created (Figure 2-2). To create the Case, simply right-click in the Case box and select New Case or hit one of the hot keys (F8 for New Case, F9 for Edit Case, or F4 for Copy Case). This will bring up a box that has up to thirteen tabs in it. Let's review those tabs now (Figure 2-3).

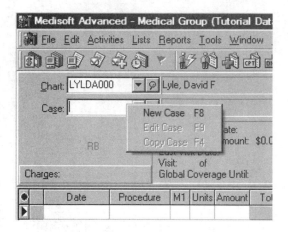

▶ Figure 2-2 Case Created

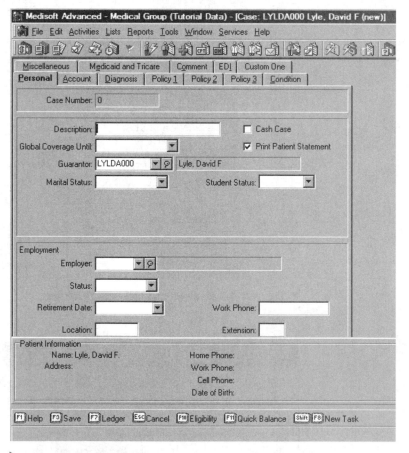

▶ Figure 2-3 Case Tabs

Personal Tab: Includes the **Case Description, Cash Case** checkbox, Guarantor Information, Marital and Student Status, and Employment Information.

Account Tab: Includes the Assigned, Referring, and Supervising Provider; Referral Source; Attorney; and Facility. Also, includes the Case Billing Code and Treatment Authorization and Series Information.

Diagnosis: Stores up to four default diagnoses, the pop-up information for Medisoft and Office Hours and EDI information.

Medisoft Quick Tip Diagnosis Entry

The diagnosis information that is put in the case prints in Box 21, fields 1-4. All of the patient's presenting diagnoses can be placed here. However, on the charge line in Transaction Entry, we will link the appropriate diagnosis(es) to the specific charge. The linkage will be shown in box 24E lines, 1-6.

Policy 1: Stores the information for the patient's primary insurance coverage.

Policy 2: Stores the information for the patient's secondary insurance coverage.

Policy 3: Stores the information for the patient's tertiary insurance coverage.

Condition: Contains information related to the patient's visit; date of injury or illness, dates unable to work, hospitalization dates, etc.

Miscellaneous: Outside Lab Work and Charges, Local Use A and B, Prior Authorization Number, and Primary Care Provider

Medicaid and Tricare: Stores information related specifically to Medicaid and Tricare insurance companies.

EDI: Stores Electronic Data Interchange (EDI) information related to sending claims electronically for specific specialties; lab, X-ray, vision, and home health, to name a few.

Multimedia: The **multimedia tab** is available only in the Network-Professional version of Medisoft. It stores a variety of files from image—X-rays, lab results—to sound and video. Clinics often store X-rays or pictures of their patients in this area.

Billing Insight The Three Parties to Every Visit

With each office visit, there are three possible parties that may need to be tracked within Medisoft. First, there is the **patient** who is receiving services. Next, there is the **insured** or subscriber (these terms are used interchangeably by the healthcare industry) who has insurance coverage for the visit, and finally there is the **guarantor**, who agrees to be responsible for the bill. In some cases, patients may have more than one insured and there could potentially be more than three parties. This can be seen with blended families or when both spouses are working and have family insurance coverage. The following is a "cheat sheet" for looking at the possible parties involved in each office visit:

Patient Person receiving the service.
Insured (Subscriber) Person having insurance coverage for the service.
Guarantor Person guaranteeing payment of service (receives statement).

Comment: This is an area that gives the user free text to document information specific to the case.

Custom Case Data: This tab is created by the Medisoft user and may contain dozens of fields the user has deemed necessary to track by case.

PRACTICE EXERCISE 2-1 Creating a New Case

In this exercise, a Case will be added for one of the new patients, David F. Lyle. Please refer to Source Document 2 in Appendix B and have Dave F. Lyle ready to enter.

1   To begin, go into Transaction Entry in Medisoft. To do this, go to Activities and Enter Transactions (Figure 2-4).

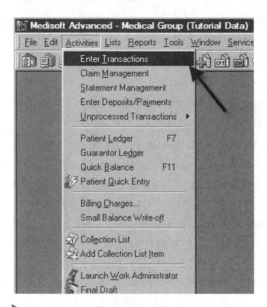

▶ **Figure 2-4   Transaction Entry**

2   After the Transaction Entry screen pops up, you can start entering the patient's last name in the Chart box. Enter David F. Lyle first by entering the first three letters of his last name, LYL (Figure 2-5).

3   Once that Chart comes up, you can right-click next to Case and select New Case.

4   Inside the Case, we have several tabs. Please refer to Source Document 2, which is the patient information form for David F. Lyle (found in Appendix B) and note the information that is available to enter on the first tab, Personal. On the Personal tab, there is a description tab to assign the name of the Case, a checkbox for Cash Case, and other personal information. To start with, since the patient came in with a broken arm, we will call the case "Broken

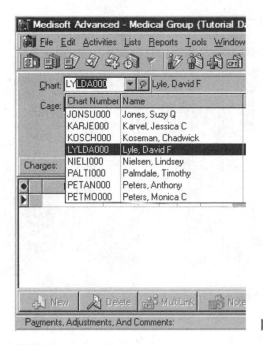

▶ Figure 2-5 **Patient Lookup**

Arm – Dr. Mallard." The Description field inside the Case is critical. It defines the unique billing scenario associated with this Case. This may be different insurance coverage, diagnosis, provider, or facility. This is a good tool for you to track transactions and associate them to the correct Case. For example, if David F. Lyle comes in next week with strep throat, you would not want to add transactions to his case with the diagnosis Broken Arm. The lab test for strep throat would be denied with a diagnosis broken arm because it does not meet the criteria of medical necessity.

5   Next, the patient does not have insurance, so check the box Cash Case. This is a really important box because it does several things inside Medisoft. First, it assigns the payment as due from the patient and prints remainder statements. Next, it tells Medisoft that there is no insurance coverage; therefore, Medisoft will not remind you during each and every transaction that insurance information is missing.

6   Add the marital and student status if known. **Note:** Many registration forms at clinics do not ask every question that is found in Medisoft. The general guideline is to enter as much information as possible.

7   Add the Employer information (Figure 2-6). Start typing the name of the employer in the Provider box or hit F6 to search for the employer. If you do not have the employer information, you can right-click for your options. As you can see, F8 adds a new employer.

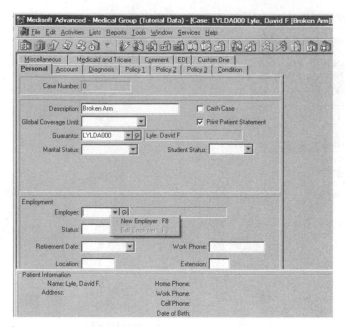

► Figure 2-6   **Employer Information**

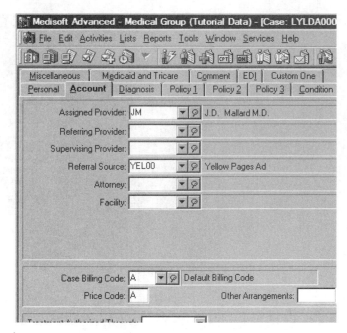

► Figure 2-7   **Account Tab**

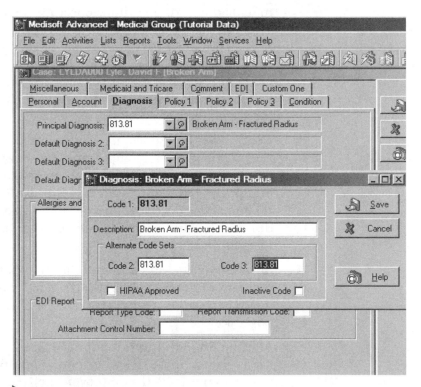

► Figure 2-8   **Diagnosis Tab**

8 Next, complete the Account tab. On David F. Lyle's intake, we can see that he was referred by the Yellow Pages. Add that information as well as Dr. Mallard's being the assigned provider (Figure 2-7).

9 Next, complete the Diagnosis tab. The diagnosis will be given to you by the provider making the diagnosis or by a coding specialist as directed by the provider. The diagnosis for broken arm is 813.81. You can type that in or hit F6 to search for the diagnosis. In this example, the diagnosis does not exist in our dataset. Therefore, we will need to right-click and add a New Diagnosis or hit F8 to add (Figure 2-8).

10 Finally, the other tabs within the case are related more to completing the claim form. Policy 1, 2, or 3 boxes do not apply to David F. Lyle, because he is a Cash Case, and the Condition tab shows the injury and illness information. The Miscellaneous, EDI, Medicaid, and Tricare tab have more billing information fields. This leaves only the Comment, Multimedia, and Custom tabs as possible tabs we have to complete. As a general rule, enter everything that you can into the case. With Cash Cases, it is important to get information that may be used later in collection if the patient does not pay. In some instances, if the patient does have insurance coverage and you do not have enough information, you will need to call the patient or insurance company to get the information.

Billing Insight ICD-9-CM Codes

The diagnoses that are used in box 21, fields 1–4 on the CMS-1500 form come from the International Classification of Diseases, 9th Revision, Clinical Modification. Hence, they are called the **ICD-9-CM** codes. The ICD-9-CM codes may have three to five digits. They are maintained by the **U.S. National Center for Health Statistics (NCHS)** and the **Centers for Disease Control and Prevention (CDC)**. Diagnosis codes must be coded to the proper digit and accurate coding is absolutely required for proper documentation and claim reimbursement. Generally, the provider of service or a certified coding specialist will assign the proper code(s) to the patient's chart and claim.

▶ **Test Your Knowledge 2-1**

In Medisoft, there are several hotkeys that perform the same functions over and over, only in different locations. Enter the hotkey below that performs the function listed.

F4   **F6**   **F8**   **F9**

_____ Adds New Data
_____ Edits Data
_____ Searches Data
_____ Copies Data

There are three types of the Medisoft program: Basic, Advanced, and Network Professional. While working in a healthcare provider's office, you may encounter any one of these programs. Network Professional has the most features and reports and allows the user to share the database on multiple computers. Advanced works on only one computer, but has almost all the features and reports as Network Professional. Basic has the fewest features and reports and is designed for a cash practice. Keep in mind as you read through this text and go into the business world that you may encounter different programs. In order to know which program is installed on your computer, open Medisoft and go to Help and About Medisoft. Here is the translation of the program types:

Medisoft Patient Accounting = Basic
Medisoft Advanced Patient Accounting = Advanced
Medisoft Network Professional = Network Professional

In addition, under the Help menu, in the Medisoft manual, and in the Knowledge Base, different features will be listed as only available in certain types of the program.

In addition to the different types of Medisoft, there are also different versions of Medisoft. Each version of Medisoft contains different features. The higher the version number, the more features contained in the program. See Figure 2-9 for a sampling of the feature evolution of Medisoft.

medisoft™
Version 14 Feature Matrix

Accounting/Billing	Medisoft Version						
	v7	v8	v9	v10	v11	v12	V14
Customized Aging Buckets	X	X	X	X	X	X	X
Withhold Code Type for Procedure Codes	X	X	X	X	X	X	X
Automatic Rebill for Claims	X	X	X	X	X	X	X
Serialized Superbills	X	X	X	X	X	X	X
Multi-link Treatment Plans	X	X	X	X	X	X	X
Deactivate Codes		X	X	X	X	X	X
Color-coding Transactions and Quick Ledger		X	X	X	X	X	X
Dunning Messages for Statements		X	X	X	X	X	X
Statement Management			X	X	X	X	X
Cycle Billing				X	X	X	X
Rules-based Collection Assignments				X	X	X	X
Actionable Collection Work List				X	X	X	X
Task or Date-driven Collection Workflow				X	X	X	X
On-demand Collection Letters				X	X	X	X
Insurance Groupings for Reporting and Analysis				X	X	X	X
Automatic Recalculation of Patient Remainder Balance					X	X	X
Automatic Small Balance Write-off					X	X	X
Remittance Tracking for Secondary Claims					X	X	X
Integrated Electronic Eligibility Checking					X	X	X
Missed Copay Tracking						X	X
Unprocessed Transactions (Holding Tank)						X	X
Aging View in Transaction Entry						X	X
CCI/LMRP Claim Edits*						X	X
Claim Level Response Reporting*						X	X
Timely Filing Letters*						X	X
Custom Claim Edits*						X	X
UB-04 Paper and Print Image							X
Custom Dates on ERA Posting							X
Global Days							X
Billing for 8 Diagnosis Codes							X
*Available with Claims Manager Subscription							

Usability	Medisoft Version						
	v7	v8	v9	v10	v11	v12	V14
Set Default Data Fields	X	X	X	X	X	X	X
Customizable Tool Bar	X	X	X	X	X	X	X
Option to Display Subtotals	X	X	X	X	X	X	X
Customized Data Screens	X	X	X	X	X	X	X
Warn on Duplicate Patient	X	X	X	X	X	X	X
Auto Tax Entry	X	X	X	X	X	X	X
Streamlined Transaction Entry		X	X	X	X	X	X
Field Data Checking		X	X	X	X	X	X
Patient Flagging			X	X	X	X	X

▶ **Figure 2-9   Medisoft Feature Evolution**

PRACTICE EXERCISE 2-2   Determining the Version of Medisoft on Your Computer

Because of the importance of knowing the version of Medisoft in use, in this exercise you will determine the version on your system.

1   Within Medisoft, click on Help.

2   After the drop-down menu appears, select About Medisoft.

3   Compare the name of the version to Figure 2-9 and note the version number.

PRACTICE EXERCISE 2-3   Creating a Case for Jane N. Jordan

In this exercise, a Case will be created for Jane N. Jordan. Refer to Source Document 3 in Appendix B for the information needed to complete this exercise.

1   Now let's enter a case for Jane N. Jordan. She is coming in for fatigue, and her health insurance will be billed. She will be seeing Dr. Mallard. Since her health insurance will be billed for any other health-related/non-accident visits, we are going to name this case using her health insurance and assigned doctor. Enter the pertinent personal information from the Source Document into Medisoft now (Figures 2-10 and 2-11). **Note:** Insurance will be processing the

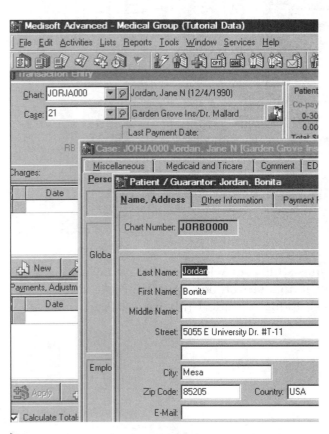

▶ Figure 2-10   **Personal Information – Entering the Guarantor**

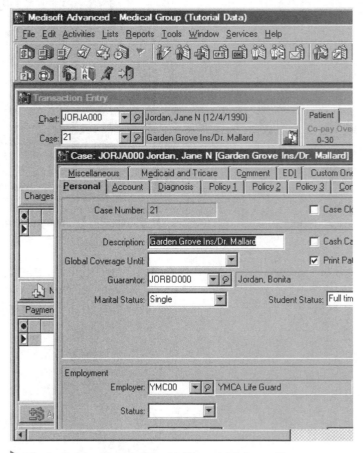

▶ Figure 2-11   **Completing the Personal Information**

charges for these services, so Cash Case will not be checked. However, the person responsible for her account is her mother, Bonita Jordan. Make sure to add the guarantor to this tab. In addition, see the option to Copy Address. This is a time-saving feature whereby you can pick the address of another family member to copy from. Choose to copy from Jane Jordan's address.

2   Next, go to the Account tab and select Dr. Mallard as the Assigned Provider (Figure 2-12).

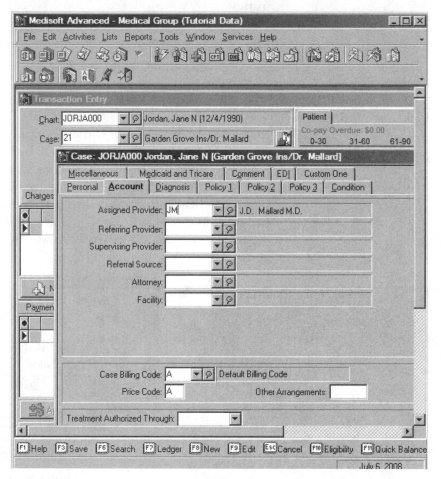

▶ Figure 2-12   Account Tab

3   Now click on the Diagnosis tab and select the diagnosis 780.7 Fatigue. **Note:** F6 brings up a search box, and diagnosis can be searched either by Description or Code 1 (Figure 2-13).

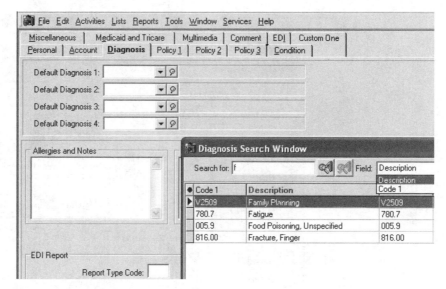

▶ Figure 2-13 Diagnosis Tab

4   Inside the Diagnosis tab, there is a box called Allergies and Notes. In this box, you can add notes that will pop up in two places. They will pop up in Transaction Entry and in Appointment Entry in Office Hours. In this spot, add a note that "the patient needs a copy of the medical records for her school" (Figures 2-14 and 2-15).

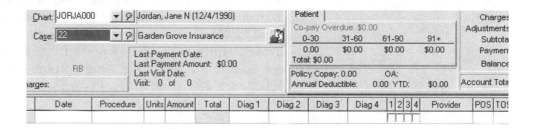

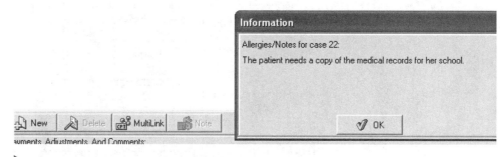

▶ Figure 2-14 Allergies and Notes in Medisoft

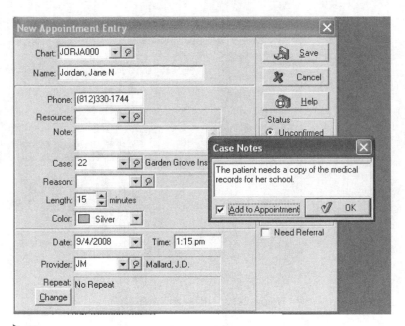

▶ Figure 2-15   Allergies and Notes in Office Hours

5   Next, select Policy 1 and enter the policy information. In each box, right-click the mouse to see the options available for the field. You can either create New information or Edit information. Also, hitting F6 or clicking on the magnifying glass will give you the ability to search for existing information. You should always search for the information prior to adding new information to prevent duplicate records. So, first we want to add the insurance information "Garden Grove Insurance" to Jane's account. Click F6 to make sure it does not exist in our database. After you have confirmed that it does not exist, click F8 to add a new insurance (Figure 2-16).

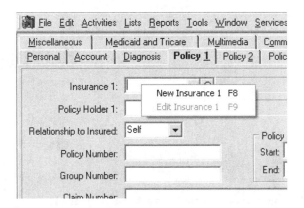

▶ Figure 2-16   New Insurance

6 After the Insurance Carrier (New) box pops up, note there are five tabs at the top of the screen. Complete the insurance information in the Address tab, leaving the Code box empty. Medisoft will automatically assign a code to the new insurance (Figure 2-17).

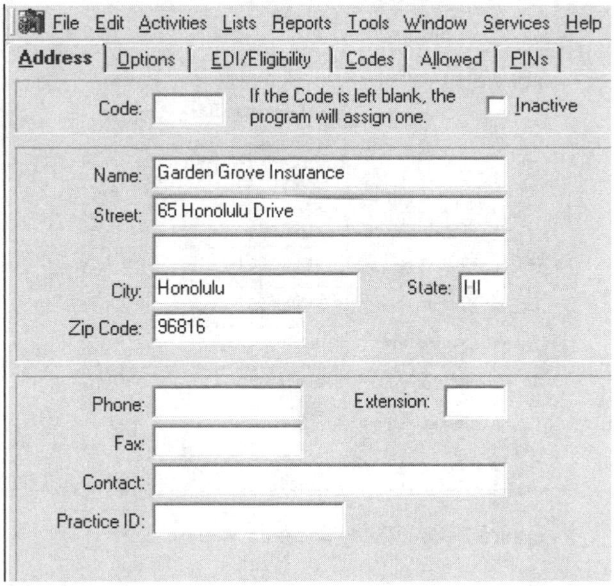

▶ **Figure 2-17 Complete Insurance**

The second tab in the insurance screen is the Options tab. This tab is very important because it relates to the fields on the insurance form that tell the insurance company what signatures are on file and whether they are to pay the clinic or the patient for the billed services. The term **Signatures on File (SOF)** refers to whether the patient and insured signed the appropriate forms applicable to boxes 12 and 13 on the claim form. The clinic may have some or all of the signatures. By entering SOF in any one of the boxes, the clinic saves time by not having the person(s) sign the form again. In addition, if requested, the clinic can provide the insurance company with a copy of the actual signature. It is important to be certain the physical signature has been obtained and is, in fact, "on file" when SOF is indicated. Within Medisoft, there are two places the user can trigger the signatures for boxes 12 and 13. The first is accessed through Chart, Other Information, then Signature on File. The second is accessed through Insurance, Options, Patient, then Signature on File. Utmost attention must be paid to those areas in order for the clinic to be reimbursed properly. Both locations must have signature on file indicated in order for it to print properly in the boxes. The other tab, EDI/Eligibility, Codes, Allowed, and Pins will be discussed in later chapters.

After adding the insurance, click Save. **Note:** Delay Secondary Billing is a time-saving feature that can be found in the Advanced and Network Professional versions of Medisoft. It allows the users to run secondary insurance bills on a daily basis but only the bills where the primary has paid will print (Figure 2-18).

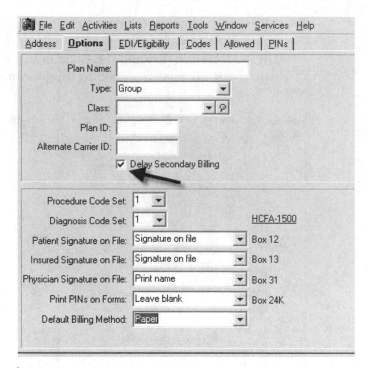

▶ Figure 2-18 **Delay Secondary**

7 Next, enter Jane's policy number and group number. Pay attention to who the policy holder of the insurance is and the relationship to the insured. **Note:** The person who has the insurance is often referred to as the Subscriber, Policy Holder, or Insured. These terms can be used interchangeably.

We know her co-payment per visit is $10.00. Enter that on this screen as well. The $10.00 co-payment will display on the transaction entry screen and make it easy for the clinic to collect money at the time of service from the patient. Remember, if the clinic wants to be paid by the insurance company, check the **Assignment of Benefits/Accept Assignment box.** The term assignment of benefits means that the insured assigned the medical benefits from her insurance to be paid directly to the healthcare provider (Figures 2-19 and 2-20).

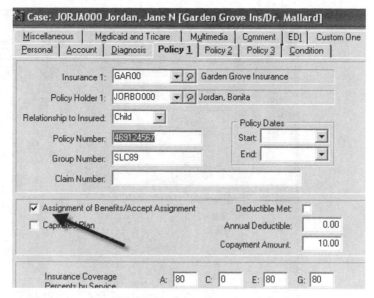

Figure 2-19   Entering Policy 1

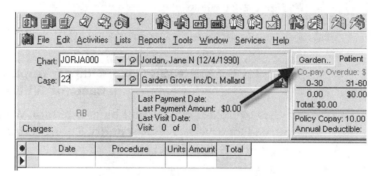

Figure 2-20   Viewing Policy 1 from Transaction Entry

8   That completes the required information that we need to add to Jane
     N. Jordan's account. However, there are other tabs that are available
     for entry. Click the Help button within the case and review the avail-
     able tabs. You will be tested on your knowledge later in the chapter
     (Figure 2-21).

Billing Insight   National Provider Identification (NPI)

Some of the features that are built into Medisoft, such as the Type in the Options tab and the Pins tab
that can be seen in insurance entry have become obsolete since May 23, 2007. On May 23, 2007, the
National Provider Identifier (NPI) became required. The NPI is a lifetime number assigned to
each provider that is accepted by all insurance companies. Prior to this, each insurance company could
assign each provider a unique number. Hence, each provider could literally have dozens of provider
numbers. This became a management nightmare. The provider and insurance companies had up to
one year (May 23, 2008) to become compliant.

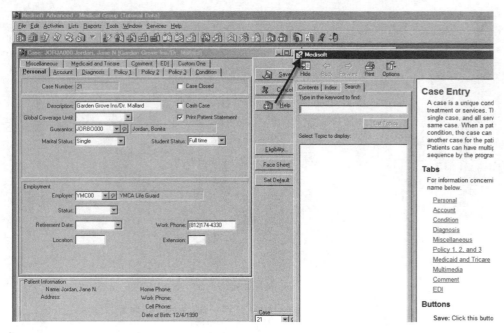

▶ **Figure 2-21 Help.**

**PRACTICE EXERCISE 2-4   Chapter Application: Creating a New
Case for William Jon Johnson**

In this exercise, a Case will be created for William Jon Johnson. Refer to
Source Document 1 in Appendix B for the information needed to
complete this exercise.

1   Now, we are going to test your abilities. Using the information presented in this chapter and your experience completing the practice
exercises presented earlier in this chapter, enter the case for William
Jon Johnson. His doctor is Dr. Robert Lee, and he is being seen for a
toe injury. See Figures 2-22 to 2-25 for the tabs referenced to complete this exercise.

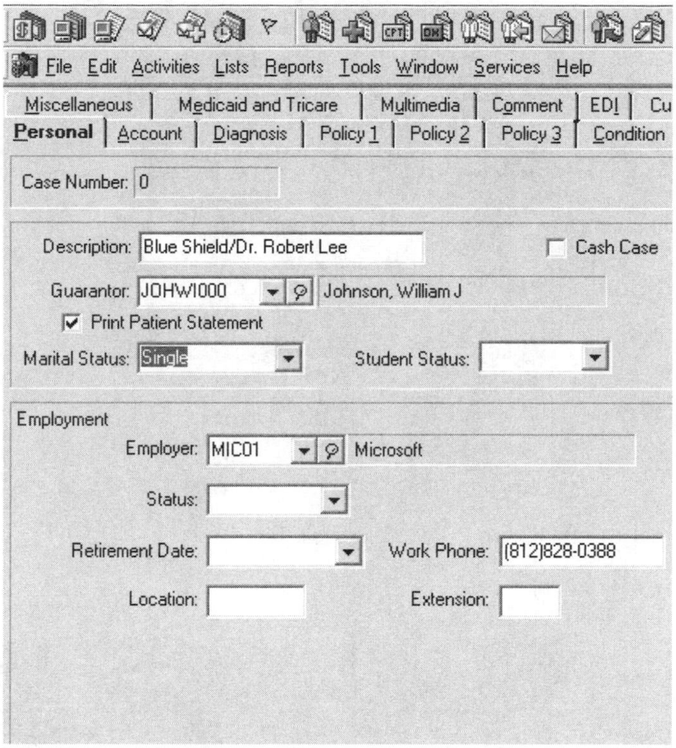

▶ **Figure 2-22 Personal Tab**

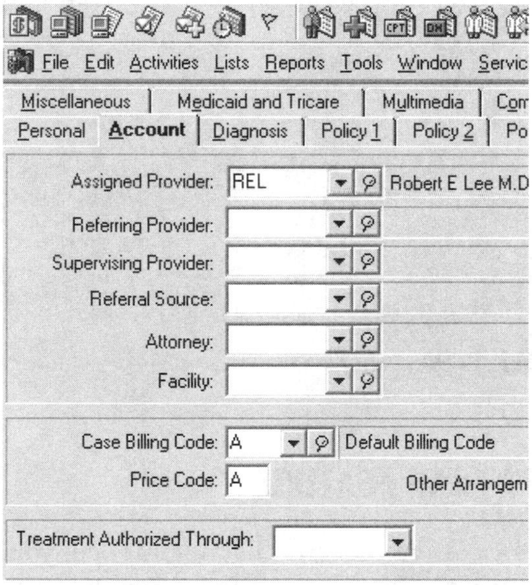

▶ **Figure 2-23 Account Tab**

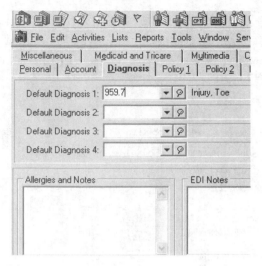

▶ **Figure 2-24   Diagnosis Tab**

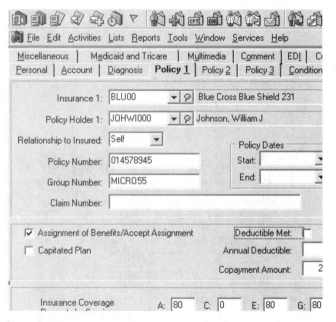

▶ **Figure 2-25   Policy 1 Tab**

COPY CASE FEATURE

Once a patient is set up in the practice, you will want to create a new Case any time you have a new provider, insurance, diagnosis, facility, and prior authorization. This can easily be done using the Copy Case feature. Just right-click and copy the Case or hit the F4 key. Then, you only need to change the information that has changed and not reenter all the information (Figure 2-26).

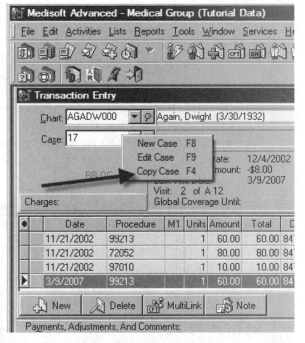

▶ Figure 2-26   **Copy Case**

PRACTICE EXERCISE 2-5   Copying a Case

In this exercise, William Jon Johnson will present a new insurance card, so we want to copy and edit his Case. You will refer to Source Document 1 in Appendix B for the information needed on William Jon Johnson; however, you must change the insurance information from Blue Shield to Medicare, change the Policy number to 473124578A, and change the group number to NONE.

1   Open the Chart for William Jon Johnson.

2   Right click on the Case information and select Copy Case. Note the drop-down menu. F4 will also allow a Case to be copied.

3   Click on the Policy 1 tab and make the desired changes.

CREATING CUSTOM PATIENT AND CASE DATA

In Medisoft Advanced, the user has the ability to create another screen in the Chart area called Custom Patient Data. Medisoft Network Professional allows the user to create both Custom Patient Data and Custom Case Data. When setting up the data fields for these two areas, the user should keep in mind how the information will be used. If it is information that is consistent to the patient and does not change, it should be created in the Custom Chart tab. Examples of this are tracking race or religion for reporting purposes (e.g., many nonprofit organizations are required to report who utilizes their services). If the information being tracked can vary depending upon the patient's situation, it should be created in the Custom Case tab. Examples of this are payment arrangements and insurance authorization information.

PRACTICE EXERCISE 2-6   Creating Custom Patient Data

In this exercise, we will review the Custom Patient Data screen and add a field named Religion to the Custom Patient Data.

1   Let's begin by selecting Tools on the menu bar and Design Custom Patient Data. **Note:** This same exercise could be used to demonstrate how to add Custom Case Data (Figure 2-27). For the purposes of this demonstration, select Design Custom Patient Data, which can be viewed under the Chart field of the Transaction Entry screen.

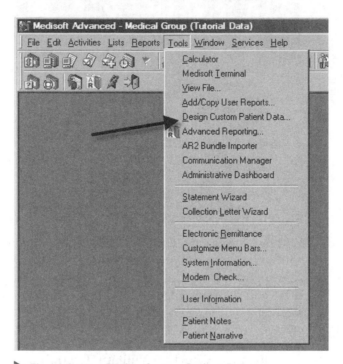

▶ Figure 2-27   **Design Custom Patient Data**

2   Once this screen has been opened, you will see the data that Medisoft created for the tutorial data. To explore modifying or adding a field, go to Help and Contents and detailed instructions will be displayed (Figure 2-28).

3   Next, select several custom fields on the right and watch as the property editor changes the definitions on the left for each of the fields. This will familiarize you with the structure of the data.

4   Per the instructions in the Help screen, add a Custom Data Field named Religion to the View/Custom Datafield List.

5   Once the field is created, insert it into the screen again following the directions in Help.

6   Next, insert a Text field labeling the new field as Religion.

7   Save your work and review it under Chart in Transaction Entry.

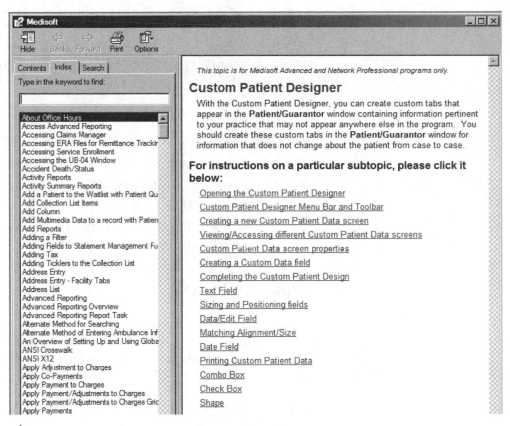

▶ Figure 2-28 **Help Custom Patient Designer**

THREE FORMS OF HELP IN MEDISOFT

Most software programs, including Medisoft, come with three forms of free help. These are valuable tools and will enhance your daily use of the program.

Medisoft Manual

The manual is electronic and comes with the installation CD. It can either be viewed directly from the CD or copied to your desktop or hard drive. The advantage of having an electronic manual is that it enables you to easily search for topics.

Help Within Medisoft

There are two ways to access Help within Medisoft. First, it can be located on the menu bar and you can select the topic you want to view. Or, you can hit F1 wherever you are in the program, and Medisoft will bring you help for that area.

Knowledge Base

The online Medisoft **Knowledge Base** can be found by going to the website www.medisoft.com and selecting Support on the top menu bar and then Knowledge Base. Next, you can enter the topic you are looking for in the Search bar, or you can search for information by article number.

In this exercise, you will retrieve article number 129790 from the Medisoft Knowledge Base to learn how to set up a patient properly in Medisoft.

1   Access the Internet and go to www.medisoft.com.

2   Select Support on the left side of the screen.

3   Select Knowledge Base from the drop-down options.

4   In the Search bar, type in 129790. The article for how to set up a patient properly will appear.

5   Review the article to gain a thorough understanding of entering a patient into Medisoft.

SIGNATURES AND ASSIGNMENTS

Since signatures and assignments are so critical to proper billing, we will review this topic again in this section. There are four places on the CMS-1500 form that address signatures and assignments: boxes 12, 13, 27, and 31.

Box 12 states the patient or authorized person's signature is on file to release any medical information or other information necessary to process or **adjudicate** the claim. Adjudication is the process by which the insurance company determines and/or pays any applicable benefits due on a claim. Box 12 will be affected by two places in Medisoft. First, pay attention to the signature on file under the Chart information, Other Information and also under List, Insurance Carrier, and the Option tab. If the clinic is billing the insurance, a signature should always be on file to release confidential information.

Box 13 states the insured or authorized person's signature is on file for payment of medical services to the undersigned physician or supplier for services described below. Box 13 will be affected by two places in Medisoft. The first area is the Signature On File check box under the Chart information. Since this box must always be checked to bill insurance and the clinic may not always want to receive payment, the Option tab under List and Insurance Carrier needs to be adjusted based on whether the clinic wants to be paid. If the clinic does not want to be paid, make sure that Insured's Signature on File says to "Leave Blank"; if the clinic does want to be paid, make sure it says "Signature on File" (Figure 2-29).

Box 27 states that the provider agrees to accept assignment under the terms of the Medicare program. This information comes from the Case and Policy 1, 2, or 3 tabs and the Assignment of Benefits/Accept Assignment. Even though by definition this refers to Medicare and government programs, in practice clinics check "Yes" to accept assignment if they want to receive the payment and "No" if they want the patient to receive the payment for the services provided.

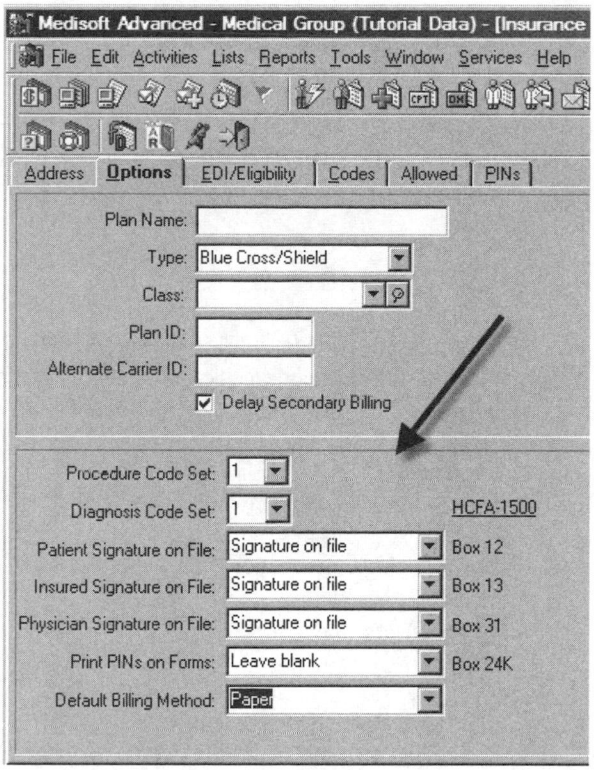

▶ **Figure 2-29   Signatures on File**

Billing Insight   Courtesy Billing

Since billing has become more difficult and time consuming, there is a new trend arising among clinics to do **courtesy billing**. This means that the clinic wants the patient to pay for his or her services on the day of service, and the clinic will give the patient a claim form to submit to his or her insurance. The insurance will then process this to the patient. To do this type of billing, Box 12 must be marked "Signature on File," Box 13 must be blank, and Box 27 must be marked "No."

Finally, Box 31 states the provider certifies the services shown on the CMS form were medically indicated and necessary for the health of the patient and were personally furnished by the provider or incident to professional supervision. Again, like boxes 12 and 13, two areas in Medisoft can affect the completion of box 31. The first area is under Provider information found under the List menu. The signature on file needs to be checked in the Address tab. This will print the provider's name and credentials in box 31, as SOF is not allowed in this field. **Note:** There is a Date field. If completed, this date will print in box 31. If not, the date the claim was created will print in box 31.

CHAPTER REVIEW

Multiple Choice

1. How many numbered boxes are there on the new CMS-1500 form?
   a. 33
   b. 26
   c. 45
   d. 69

2. Which box on the claim form tells the insurance that the patient or authorized person signed a statement to release any medical or other information necessary to process the claim?
   a. Box 13
   b. Box 12
   c. Box 27
   d. All of the above

3. Which field in the Case creates pop-up messages in Medisoft and Office Hours?
   a. Allergies and Notes
   b. Popup Notes
   c. Remarks and Comments
   d. Notes Now

4. Which tab in the Case contains the pop-up messages?
   a. Diagnosis
   b. Condition
   c. Pop-up
   d. Miscellaneous

5. What are the free forms of help that come with Medisoft?
   a. Online Knowledge Base, Help within the program
   b. Manual that comes with Medisoft
   c. Electronic Manual, Help within the program, Knowledge Base Online
   d. Medisoft Technical Support at 1-800-333-4747

6. Who creates the Custom Patient and Custom Case tabs?
   a. User
   b. Medisoft
   c. Patient
   d. Doctor

7. Who receives the statement?
   a. Insured
   b. Patient
   c. Guarantor
   d. Parent

8. Which hotkey creates a new case?
   a. F4
   b. F8
   c. F9
   d. F1

9. Which hotkey copies a case?
   a. F9
   b. F4
   c. F8
   d. F1

10. Which hotkey edits a case?
    a. F8
    b. F4
    c. F9
    d. F1

11. According to the Knowledge Base article 129790, which tab do you use to report the injury date?
    a. Miscellaneous Tab
    b. Account Tab
    c. Condition Tab
    d. Personal Tab

12. When do you select the option Cash Case?
    a. When there is no insurance coverage
    b. When you want the patient to pay cash
    c. When you want the patient to pay prior to his or her visit
    d. b and c

13. What does ICD-9-CM stand for?
    a. International Classification of Diagnosis, 9th Copy
    b. International Classification of Diagnosis, 9th Revision, Clinical Modification
    c. International Classification of Diseases, 9th Revision, Clinical Modification
    d. Internal Case of Diseases, 9th Term

14. What does NPI stand for?
    a. National Provider Identifier
    b. National Physician Identifier
    c. National Provider Identification
    d. Nationwide Provider ID

15. Where in Medisoft does it say which version of the program you have?
    a. Under Help and Program Type
    b. Under Help and About Medisoft
    c. Under File and Program Type
    d. Under File and About Medisoft

True/False

Identify each of the following statements as true or false.

1. Each patient should have at least one Case in Medisoft.

2. The patient's date of birth is in the personal information of the Case tab.

3. If the insured signs an assignment of benefits form for the clinic, that means the clinic will be paid the insurance benefits.

4. The majority of the billing information can be found in the Case.

5. If the patient's social security number changes, you need to create a new Case.

6. There can be up to six digits in an ICD-9-CM code.

7. When you enter the co-payment per visit amount in the Case, it shows the amount the patient owes on the main transaction entry screen.

8. To copy a Case, hit the F5 key.

9. Medisoft gives each user a paper manual.

10. Courtesy billing means the clinic submits a bill to the patient's insurance, but expects the patient to pay the clinic and the insurance to pay the patient.

Short Answer

1. How would you complete the Chart and Case information to accomplish courtesy billing?

2. Provide a brief explanation of the three types of Medisoft and their differences. How can you determine which version you are working with and where to find the features exclusive to certain types?

3. Prepare a list of at least five types of healthcare providers that could utilize Medisoft.

Resources

Each medical specialty area has an association or board that assists its members. These are excellent sources for billing and healthcare regulations that are pertinent to the specific specialty. The boards and associations often have state and national chapters. To find the applicable group, just go to **www.google.com** or your favorite search engine and type a search for an association or a board: e.g., Chiropractic Association or Board of Chiropractic.

Medicare, Medicaid, and Blue Shield often have state specific regulations for healthcare professionals. There are valuable resources and training tools available on their websites. To find your state's websites, go to **www.google.com** or your favorite search engine and search for your local government carriers: e.g., Medicare, Medicaid, or Blue Shield.

The American Medical Association is an excellent resource for training and coding materials. Information can be found at its website at **www.ama-assn.org**.

3

Transaction Entry

Learning Objectives

After completing this chapter, you should be able to:

◆ Define and spell the key terms in this chapter.

◆ Understand and define the components of Transaction Entry.

◆ Define and demonstrate the entry of Charges, Payments, Adjustments, and Comments.

◆ Modify grid columns.

◆ Understand CPT* codes, modifiers, diagnosis linkage, POS (place of service), and MultiLink codes.

◆ Create a checks-and-balance report to proof transactions.

Key Terms

adjustment   a transaction, other than a charge or payment, that is entered into a Case either adding to or subtracting from the outstanding balance.

billing charge   interest or finance charge added to a patient's account.

charge   a transaction added to a Case for services rendered, adding to the patient's balance.

comment   a transaction added to the Case giving the user further clarification about the account.

Current Procedural Terminology (CPT)*   a five-digit coding system designed by the American Medical Association (AMA) to report the service or supply received by the patient.

diagnosis   the disease, condition, illness, or accident that is the reason for services provided.

diagnosis codes   ICD-9-CM codes that identify a patient's injury and/or illness or reason for routine or preventive services.

EDI comments   notes that provide additional information to the insurance company as to the services provided.

Electronic Data Interchange (EDI)   the process of exchanging data electronically between healthcare covered entities: the clinic, the clearinghouse, and the insurance company.

EOB comments   notes that contain additional information provided by the insurance company on the EOB, such as coverage terminated, no full-time student letter received, or insurance premium not paid/coverage terminated.

Explanation of Benefits (EOB)   a statement given to the clinic by the insurance company to explain how the patient's claim was adjudicated.

grid column   fields within each Medisoft table that store data.

*CPT is a registered trademark of the American Medical Association.

hardship and bad debt write-offs   adjustments made to the accounts of patients who cannot pay or those who refuse to pay for which the clinic deems it acceptable to cancel the debt.

Healthcare Common Procedure Coding System (HCPCS)   a five-digit coding system beginning with an alpha character created by CMS; a standard code set for reporting professional services, procedures, and supplies.

insurance contractual adjustments   write-offs made to the patient's account under the agreement of the contract between the healthcare provider and the insurance company.

internal notes   comments entered into Medisoft that help the user to handle the patient and the account more effectively.

modifier   a two-digit number placed after the five-digit CPT* code to indicate that the description of the service or procedure has been altered.

MultiLink Codes   a feature within Medisoft that allows the user to create multiple transactions at the same time.

Patient Day Sheet   Medisoft report used to proof daily transactions, showing all transactions posted on patient account for the selected time frame.

payment   money received from insurance, or patients, lowering the patient's balance.

statement notes   comments entered into Medisoft that will print on the patient statements.

Transaction Entry   utility inside Medisoft that allows the user to enter charges, payments, adjustments, comments, and track balances.

Abbreviations

AMA   American Medical Association

CMS   Centers for Medicare and Medicaid Services

CPT*   Current Procedural Technology

EDI   Electronic Data Interchange

EOB   Explanation of Benefits

HCPCS   Healthcare Common Procedure Coding System

ICD-9-CM   International Classification of Diseases, 9th Revision, Clinical Modification

POS   Place of service

TOS   Type of service

■ ■ ■ ■

INTRODUCTION

One of the primary objectives for using Medisoft is to produce a reliable cash flow. Medisoft gives the user all of the tools necessary to easily and efficiently enter and track **charges**, **payments**, **adjustments** and **comments**, the backbone of the clinic's reimbursement. Charges are fees charged to patients for services rendered. Payments are compensation received by the clinic for its service either from the patient or an insurance company. Adjustments are the amount the provider needs to write off according to the contract with the insurance company or an amount added or subtracted from a patient's account such as billing charges, write-offs or refunds. Comments are notes created by the user and held within Transaction Entry that allow the office to document pertinent information. This chapter demonstrates the workings of the **Transaction Entry**

*CPT is a registered trademark of the American Medical Association.

function, which is the tool inside of Medisoft that allows the user to view patient accounts and balances and enter charges, payments, adjustments, and comments. This chapter provides tools for staying abreast of changes in Medisoft and the healthcare industry, in order to give the user confidence that he or she is accurately entering charges and payments.

OVERVIEW OF TRANSACTION ENTRY

Transaction entry is all about accuracy. First, the user must choose the correct patient and case, and then utmost attention to detail must be paid to add the patient's correct charge including **modifier**, **diagnosis**, provider, and units. If a payment or adjustment is being entered, accuracy to the type and amount must be attended to. In addition, the comments and notes added to Medisoft are instrumental in problem-solving future dilemmas. Let's take a closer look at the definition of each transaction type:

Charges: Transactions in which the person is assessed fees for services or products received. Besides the provider fees, clinics many times will offer supplies such as crutches or vitamins. Some charges may be submitted to insurance and some will not depending upon insurance coverage.

Payments: Transactions in which either the patient or insurance pays for services or products received.

Adjustments: An amount that is either added to or subtracted from the patient's account. Typical adjustments are insurance contractual adjustments, hardship or bad debt writeoffs, and billing or finance charges.

Comments: Notes that are added to the case with information pertinent to the account such as payment arrangements or follow-up calls.

The Components of a Charge

Each type of transaction entry has its own components. With all of the transaction types, you first need to make sure you have the correct patient's Chart and Case. With a charge entry, you must pay attention to the details of the charge line, namely the date, procedure codes, modifiers, units, amounts, diagnosis linkage, and provider.

Keep in mind, when entering a charge into Medisoft, the provider on the transaction line defaults to the assigned provider in the Case. If the provider has changed since the patient's last visit and the user is not careful to create a new Case or modify the transaction line, the charge could be billed under the wrong provider. To proof your work, patient day sheets should be run each day to match against the superbills. This will be discussed in further detail later in this chapter.

In addition to adding one charge or procedure code at a time, the user has the option to add groups of charges or procedures with a single code. This is known as the **MultiLink Code**. This is especially helpful for services where two or more procedures are always done; for example, lab work is always done when a physical is performed.

PRACTICE EXERCISE 3-1   Adding a Charge

To become familiar with Transaction Entry, we will add a few charges to Medisoft.

1   Select Activities from the menu bar at the top of Medisoft.

2   Select Enter Transactions from the drop-down menu (Figure 3-1).

3   Using the current date, add a doctor visit of 99213 to the following three patients: Dwight Again, Jay Brimley, and Sammy Catera. **Note:** The transaction screen is divided into two sections (Figure 3-2). Charges are on top and Payments/Adjustments and Comments are on the bottom. To add a new charge, simply enter the patient's chart number and click New under the Charges heading. For additional help, press the F1 key from which Transaction Entry and full detail will be given.

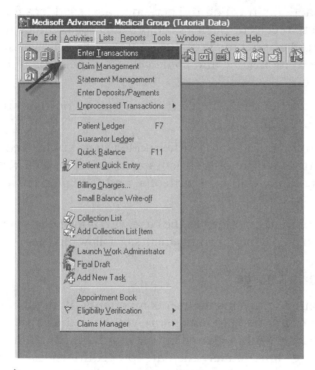

▶ Figure 3-1   Opening Transaction Entry

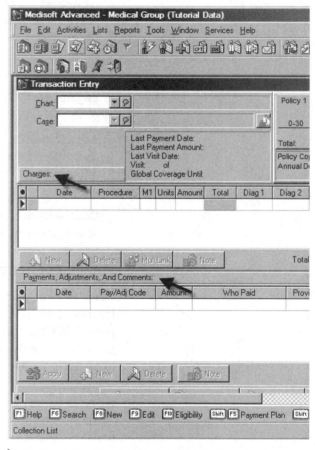

▶ Figure 3-2   Viewing Charges versus Payments, Adjustments, and Comments

The Components of a Payment

Clinics receive two types of payments: patient payments and third-party payments. Third-party payments usually come from insurance companies or government programs, but can sometimes come from churches or nonprofit or other agencies. Payments that are received from patients are posted in the Transaction Entry screen. Payments that are received from third parties are posted in the Enter Deposits/Payments screens, which are only available in Advanced and Network Professional versions designed for insurance billing. In this chapter, we review only the patient payments. Third-party payments will be reviewed in Chapter 5.

The essential components of a patient payment are the date, payment code, who has paid, description, provider, amount, check number, and unapplied.

PRACTICE EXERCISE 3-2   Posting a Payment

To become familiar with payment entry, we will now add cash payments to the patients we just entered charges for.

1   Select Activities from the menu bar at the top of Medisoft.

2   Select Enter Transactions from the drop-down menu.

3   Using the current date, add a $10.00 cash payment to the following three patients: Dwight Again, Jay Brimley, and Sammy Catera. **Note:** The transaction screen is divided into two sections: Charges on top and Payments/Adjustments and Comments on the bottom. To add a new payment, click New under the Payment/Adjustment and Comment heading. Again, if additional explanation is needed, press F1 to view the available Help.

4   Applying payments is a two-step process. After the payment detail has been entered, the payment needs to be applied to the appropriate service. Click the Apply button and post the payment to the current date of service (Figure 3-3).

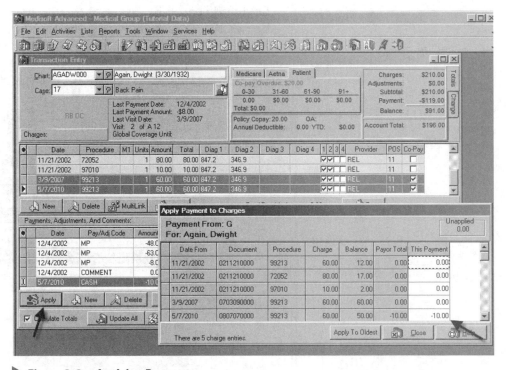

▶ Figure 3-3   Applying Payments

The Components of an Adjustment

There are three typical types of adjustments; **billing charges** (finance charges), **hardship or bad debt write-offs**, and **insurance contractual adjustments**. Billing charges are the fees assessed to the patient if the full amount due cannot be paid at the initial billing. Hardship and bad debt write-offs are adjustments made to patient accounts for those who cannot pay or those who refuse to pay when the clinic deems it acceptable to cancel the debt. Insurance contractual adjustments are write-offs to patient accounts under the contractual agreement between the healthcare provider and insurance company. Again, insurance contractual adjustments are posted in the Enter Deposits/Payments screen (available only in the Advanced and Network Professional versions designed for insurance billing). In this chapter, we review hardship and bad debt write-offs. The billing charges will be addressed in Chapter 8, and insurance adjustments will be addressed in Chapter 5.

PRACTICE EXERCISE 3-3   Posting an Adjustment

An office may adjust patient balances for many reasons. First, they may have contracts with insurance companies that require them to do so. Or, a patient may have a hardship case where arrangements have been made to make adjustments to the account. In this exercise, Sammy Catera will have $20.00 written off his account.

1   Select Activities from the menu bar at the top of Medisoft.

2   Select Enter Transactions from the drop-down menu.

3   Using the current date, make a $20.00 adjustment to Sammy Catera's account using the Write-off Welfare code. If the correct code cannot be found, select the F6 button while on the Pay/Adj Code field and search by Description (Figure 3-4). **Note:** Adjustments can be positive or negative. To deduct $20.00 from Sammy's account, make sure the adjustment is entered as a negative.

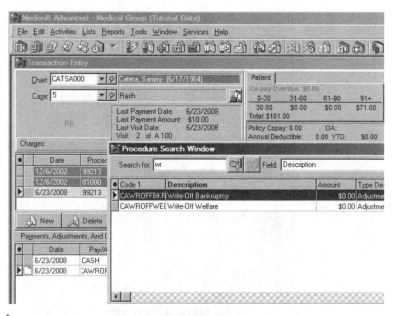

▶ **Figure 3-4   Procedure Search Window**

4 After the adjustment in entered into Medisoft, it must be applied to the appropriate date of service. Click the Apply button and proceed.

The Components of a Comment

The comment feature of Medisoft is an invaluable feature that can save users hours of time. It is used to document **internal notes**, **statement notes**, **Electronic Data Interchange (EDI)** documentation, and **Explanation of Benefits (EOB)** documentation to name a few (Figure 3-5).

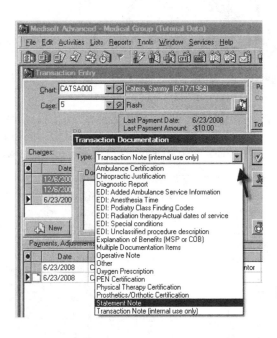

▶ **Figure 3-5** **Selecting Transaction Documentation Type**

Internal notes are comments entered into Medisoft that help the user to handle the patient and the account more effectively. It may be information that insurance coverage has changed, the patient is going to make a payment, or any number of reminders that are worthwhile to save. Statement notes are comments entered into Medisoft that will print on patient statements. **EDI comments** vary upon specialty; however, the intent is the same. They provide additional information to the insurance company as to the services provided. Finally, **EOB comments** are posted in the Enter Deposits/Payments screen as the payments and adjustments from insurance companies are entered. They contain additional information that was given by the insurance company on the EOB, such as coverage terminated, no full-time student letter received, or insurance premium not paid/coverage terminated. Again, the details of this feature will be reviewed in Chapter 5.

PRACTICE EXERCISE 3-4   Adding Notes and Comments

As discussed, Medisoft offers an exceptional tool to its users: notes and comments. Notes and comments can be added in two different ways. After adding a transaction, the user can click on the Note button either in the Charge line or Payments/Adjustments/Comments line (Figure 3-6).

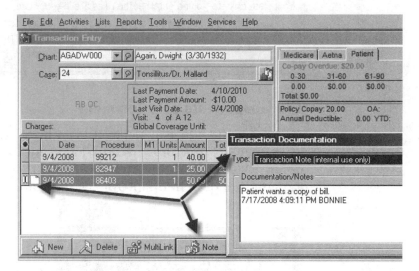

▶ Figure 3-6   Clicking on Notes

1   The hotkey to stamp the user name, date, and time of notes is Control-T. Open a note and try stamping it now. **Note:** If security has not been set up, only the date and time will be stamped on the note.

2   To create a comment separately and not attach it to any charge, click New in the Payments/Adjustments/Comments line. Add the Comment as a procedure code, then click Note and add the pertinent note (Figure 3-7).

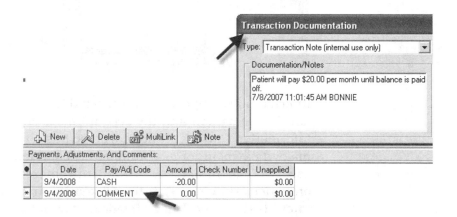

▶ Figure 3-7   New Comment Transaction

3   Notice that once a note is added to a transaction line, there is a little piece of paper next to the date (Figure 3-8). This tells the user there is more information attached to this line, and the user can hit the Note button to view the information.

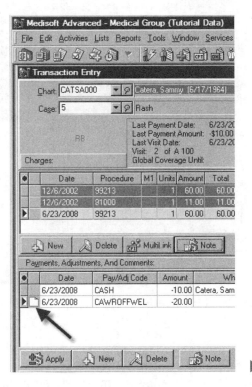

▶ Figure 3-8　Viewing a Comment

4　In addition to transaction notes, statement notes will print on the
patient statements, and EDI notes will go on the electronic claims.
Hit the down arrow next to Type in the Transaction Documentation
to view the options available to the user.

MODIFYING THE GRID COLUMNS

Each practice may have different needs when entering transactions.
Some practices are strictly cash practices and do not need modifiers on
the charge line, for example. Other practices may have a specialty that
may need multiple modifiers. So, to accommodate these various
situations, Medisoft allows the columns in Transaction Entry to be
modified. It is simple to modify the **grid columns**. Grid columns are the
fields within each Medisoft table that store data.

PRACTICE EXERCISE 3-5　**Modifying Grid Columns**

In this exercise, fields will be added, moved, and deleted from the Grid
Column view to demonstrate how this feature can increase efficiency.

1　Click on the black dot to the left of the date on the Charges line and
a box called Grid Columns will pop up. **Note:** A patient with a Case
must be in the Chart/Case fields (Figure 3-9).

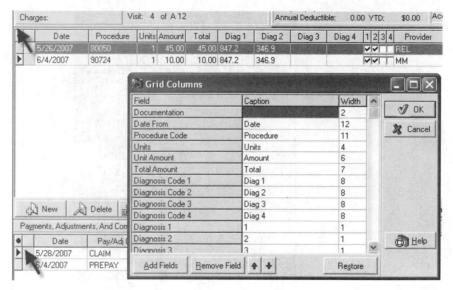

▶ **Figure 3-9   Grid Columns**

2   At the bottom of the pop-up box are Add Fields and Remove Fields buttons plus up and down arrows to adjust the field positions. Remove TOS and Allowed, move M1 so it is right below the Procedure, and add Claim Number to the displayed fields. Check your work (Figure 3-10).

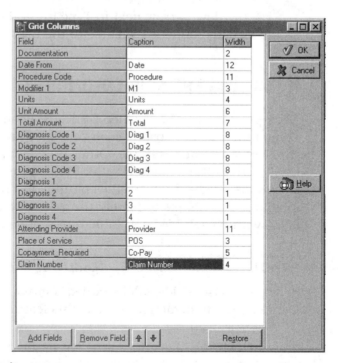

▶ **Figure 3-10   Modifying the Grid Columns: Check Your Work**

| Medisoft Quick Tip | Pertinent Versus Nonpertinent Fields |

Some of the fields in Medisoft became obsolete when the new CMS-1500 claim form was implemented. One field **TOS**, type of service, was deleted from the CMS-1500 form. Some fields may not be pertinent to a clinic. The field Allowed stands for the amount that contracted payers allow the clinic to charge for the service. If the clinic is not contracted and or is a cash practice, this field is not required. Since Medisoft has these two fields as defaults, many users prefer to remove them rather than view unused fields.

DEFINING CODING SYSTEMS

The heart of billing is a series of codes. Codes tell the insurance company what service or product the patient received (**CPT*** and **HCPCS** Codes), what was wrong with the patient (**ICD-9-CM** codes), where the service was performed (**POS**), and additional information about the service (**modifier**). Medisoft created shortcut codes, MultiLinks, that allow the user to add multiple services by just keying in one code.

CPT* and HCPCS Codes

The procedure codes that are used to identify the product or services the patient receives are CPT* (**Current Procedural Terminology**) codes and HCPCS (**Healthcare Common Procedure Coding System**) codes. CPT* codes, also called HCPCS Level 1 codes, are copyrighted by the American Medical Association (**AMA**) and are five-digit numerical codes. The AMA maintains, updates, and distributes CPT* codes each year on January 1st. HCPCS Level 2 codes are assigned by **CMS** (Centers for Medicare and Medicaid Services), start with an alpha character, are five digits long, and are a standard code set for reporting professional services, procedures, and supplies. HCPCS Level 2 codes are also updated on January 1st each year.

Each product or service a patient receives is identified to the insurance company via a CPT* or HCPCS code—very similar to the bar coding system used by stores. Proper coding is very important because it affects reimbursement. There are several ways to learn coding: books, classes, software, and schools. In addition, there are many certification and credentialing programs that allow individuals to demonstrate proficiency in coding. Typically, you will find certified coders working in hospitals and large physcian practices.

PRACTICE EXERCISE 3-6 Using Medisoft Help to Research Key Terms

One of the many benefits of Medisoft is its Help program, which provides information on not only utilizing Medisoft, but also information about medical billing. In this exercise, Help will be used to research key terms.

1 Click on Help on the top toolbar of Medisoft.

2 Select Medisoft Help from the drop-down menu (Figure 3-11).

*CPT is a registered trademark of the American Medical Association.

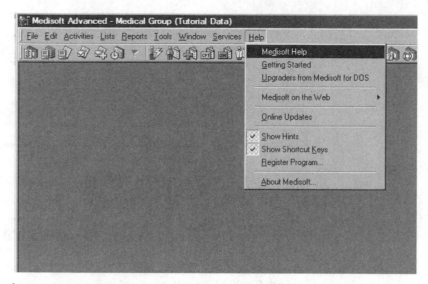

▶ Figure 3-11   Medisoft Help

3   In the Index tab, look up the following items and document your findings:

- Place of service
- Type of service
- Clickable CMS-1500 form (Figure 3-12)

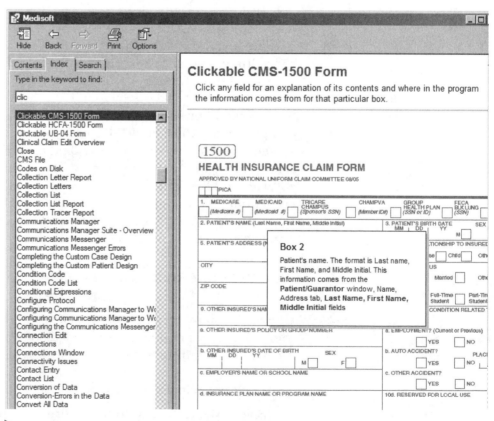

▶ Figure 3-12   Clickable CMS-1500 Form

4 Next, in the index tab, look up Place of Service codes. This will give an itemized listing of the various places a service may be performed and the correct code to use for that location. **Note:** Place of Service Codes are not unique to Medisoft but required on the CMS-1500 form and used by the entire healthcare profession. This is an example of how Medisoft offers Help on areas broader than its software (Figure 3-13).

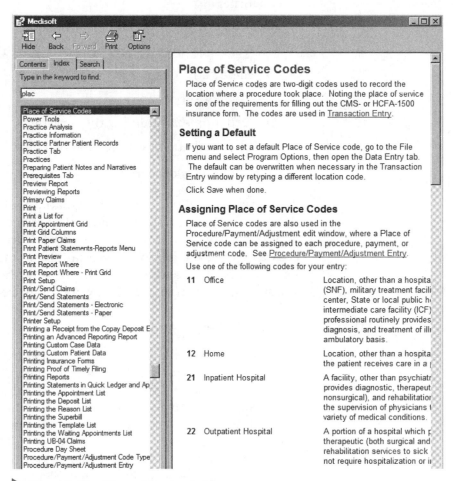

▶ **Figure 3-13   Place of Service Codes**

Modifiers

Modifiers are two-digit codes that are added to the transaction line on the claim form in box 24D. The CMS-1500 form allows up to four modifiers. Some modifiers are maintained by the AMA as part of the CPT* codes; additional modifiers are maintained by CMS as part of HCPCS Level 2 codes. Modifiers are used to give additional information to the insurance company regarding services provided, including the following:

• Only a professional or technical component of the procedure is being billed for, usually only found in laboratory and radiology, but occasionally in urology, ophthalmology, optometry, and some of the medicine procedures.

• More than one provider participated in the performance of the procedure.

• A service or procedure was increased or reduced.

*CPT is a registered trademark of the American Medical Association.

- Only part of a service or procedure was performed.
- Significant, separately identifiable evaluation and management service by the same physician the same day of a procedure or other service.
- Another related service/procedure was performed at the same time.
- Another nonrelated service/procedure was performed at the same encounter.
- A bilateral procedure was performed.
- A service or procedure was provided more than once.
- A specific body location of the procedure.
- A mandated service/procedure.
- The credentials/training of the provider.
- Condition of patient at time of anesthesia.
- Unusual events occurred.

As with many billing rules and regulations, the modifiers you will be using will vary upon the specialty of the practice in which you are billing. Again, it would be a good idea for all healthcare billing specialists to contact their local board or association to obtain the billing requirements for their specialty and to stay current with the government regulations by visiting websites and attending workshops frequently.

Diagnosis Linkage

Diagnosis linkage is the process of associating the CPT* or HCPCS code on the transaction line with the appropriate diagnosis from Box 21. The reference number of the diagnosis is entered in box 24E. Here is an example: Dwight Again is a patient with diabetes who has been seeing Dr. Mallard. While painting the house, he falls off the ladder and is seen for a possible broken hand. Upon doing the exam (CPT* 99214), Dr. Mallard orders an X-ray (CPT* 73130) and a blood glucose test (CPT* 82947). Dwight's diagnoses would be a fractured finger (diagnosis code 816.00) and diabetes (diagnosis code 250.01). To view how this looks inside the Case and on the CMS-1500 form, see Figures 3-14, and 3-15. **Note:** Box 21 shows both diagnoses that were presented by Dwight Again. On transaction line 1 box 24E, it shows that both diagnoses were linked to

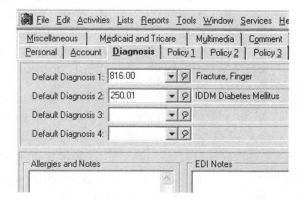

▶ **Figure 3-14   Diagnoses Inside the Case**

*CPT is a registered trademark of the American Medical Association.

1500		

HEALTH INSURANCE CLAIM FORM

APPROVED BY NATIONAL UNIFORM CLAIM COMMITTEE 08/05

MEDICARE
1111 HOHOKAM CIR
AMWATUKEE AZ 85678

☐P PICA   PICA ☐☐

1. MEDICARE MEDICAID TRICARE CHAMPUS CHAMPVA GROUP HEALTH PLAN FECA BLK LUNG OTHER	1a. INSURED'S I.D. NUMBER (For Program in Item 1)
☒ (Medicare #) ☐ (Medicaid #) ☐ (Sponsor's SSN) ☐ (Member ID#) ☐ (SSN or ID) ☐ (SSN) ☐ (ID)	0101010101

2. PATIENT'S NAME (Last Name, First Name, Middle Initial)	3. PATIENT'S BIRTH DATE MM DD YY SEX	4. INSURED'S NAME (Last Name, First Name, Middle Initial)
AGAIN DWIGHT	03 30 1932 M ☒ F ☐	AGAIN DWIGHT

5. PATIENT'S ADDRESS (No., Street)	6. PATIENT RELATIONSHIP TO INSURED	7. INSURED'S ADDRESS (No., Street)
1742 N 83RD AVE	Self ☒ Spouse ☐ Child ☐ Other ☐	1742 N 83RD AVE

CITY	STATE	8. PATIENT STATUS	CITY	STATE
PHOENIX	AZ	Single ☐ Married ☒ Other ☐	PHOENIX	AZ

ZIP CODE	TELEPHONE (Include Area Code)		ZIP CODE	TELEPHONE (Include Area Code)
85021	(555) 4345777	Employed ☒ Full-Time Student ☐ Part-Time Student ☐	85021	(555) 4345777

9. OTHER INSURED'S NAME (Last Name, First Name, Middle Initial)	10. IS PATIENT'S CONDITION RELATED TO:	11. INSURED'S POLICY GROUP OR FECA NUMBER
AGAIN DWIGHT		NONE

a. OTHER INSURED'S POLICY OR GROUP NUMBER	a. EMPLOYMENT? (Current or Previous) ☐ YES ☒ NO	a. INSURED'S DATE OF BIRTH MM DD YY SEX
		03 30 1932 M ☒ F ☐

b. OTHER INSURED'S DATE OF BIRTH MM DD YY SEX	b. AUTO ACCIDENT? PLACE (State) ☐ YES ☒ NO	b. EMPLOYER'S NAME OR SCHOOL NAME
03 30 1932 M ☒ F ☐		

c. EMPLOYER'S NAME OR SCHOOL NAME	c. OTHER ACCIDENT? ☐ YES ☒ NO	c. INSURANCE PLAN NAME OR PROGRAM NAME
REALLY USEFUL TRUCKING CO		AETNA INSURANCE

d. INSURANCE PLAN NAME OR PROGRAM NAME	10d. RESERVED FOR LOCAL USE	d. IS THERE ANOTHER HEALTH BENEFIT PLAN?
AETNA		☒ YES ☐ NO If yes, return to and complete item 9 a-d.

READ BACK OF FORM BEFORE COMPLETING & SIGNING THIS FORM.

12. PATIENT'S OR AUTHORIZED PERSON'S SIGNATURE I authorize the release of any medical or other information necessary to process this claim. I also request payment of government benefits either to myself or to the party who accepts assignment below.

SIGNED SIGNATURE ON FILE   DATE

13. INSURED'S OR AUTHORIZED PERSON'S SIGNATURE I authorize payment of medical benefits to the undersigned physician or supplier for services described below.

SIGNED SIGNATURE ON FILE

14. DATE OF CURRENT: MM DD YY ILLNESS (First symptom) OR INJURY (Accident) OR PREGNANCY(LMP)	15. IF PATIENT HAS HAD SAME OR SIMILAR ILLNESS. GIVE FIRST DATE MM DD YY	16. DATES PATIENT UNABLE TO WORK IN CURRENT OCCUPATION MM DD YY MM DD YY
09 01 2008		FROM TO

17. NAME OF REFERRING PROVIDER OR OTHER SOURCE	17a.	18. HOSPITALIZATION DATES RELATED TO CURRENT SERVICES MM DD YY MM DD YY
	17b. NPI	FROM TO

19. RESERVED FOR LOCAL USE	20. OUTSIDE LAB? $ CHARGES
	☐ YES ☒ NO

21. DIAGNOSIS OR NATURE OF ILLNESS OR INJURY (Relate Items 1, 2, 3 or 4 to Item 24E by Line)	22. MEDICAID RESUBMISSION CODE ORIGINAL REF. NO.
1. 816 . 00 3. ___ . ___	
2. 250 . 01 4. ___ . ___	23. PRIOR AUTHORIZATION NUMBER

24. A. DATE(S) OF SERVICE From MM DD YY To MM DD YY	B. PLACE OF SERVICE	C. EMG	D. PROCEDURES, SERVICES, OR SUPPLIES (Explain Unusual Circumstances) CPT/HCPCS MODIFIER	E. DIAGNOSIS POINTER	F. $ CHARGES	G. DAYS OR UNITS	H. EPSDT Family Plan	I. ID. QUAL.	J. RENDERING PROVIDER ID. #
1	09 01 08 09 01 08	11		99214	1 2	60 00	1		NPI	0123456789
2	09 01 08 09 01 08	22		73130	1	45 00	1		NPI	0123456789
3	09 01 08 09 01 08	11		82947	2	10 00	1		NPI	0123456789
4									NPI	
5									NPI	
6									NPI	

25. FEDERAL TAX I.D. NUMBER SSN EIN	26. PATIENT'S ACCOUNT NO.	27. ACCEPT ASSIGNMENT? (For govt. claims, see back)	28. TOTAL CHARGE	29. AMOUNT PAID	30. BALANCE DUE
123456789 ☒	AGADW000	☒ YES ☐ NO	$ 115 00	$	$ 115 00

31. SIGNATURE OF PHYSICIAN OR SUPPLIER INCLUDING DEGREES OR CREDENTIALS (I certify that the statements on the reverse apply to this bill and are made a part thereof.)	32. SERVICE FACILITY LOCATION INFORMATION	33. BILLING PROVIDER INFO & PH # (800) 3334747
JD Mallard MD 07/07/07 SIGNED DATE	DESERT VALLEY HOSPITAL 1200 S SOUTHERN AVE MESA AZ 85202 a. 3123456789 b.	JD MALLARD MD 5222 E BASELINE RD GILBERT AZ 58234 a. 1123456789 b.

NUCC Instruction Manual available at: www.nucc.org   **PLEASE PRINT OR TYPE**   APPROVED OMB-0938-0999 FORM CMS-1500 (08-05)

▶ **Figure 3-15 Diagnoses on the CMS-1500 Form**

the exam charge. On transaction line 2 box 24E, it shows that only the fractured finger diagnosis was linked to the X-ray, and on transaction line 3 box 24E, the diabetes diagnosis was linked to the blood glucose test. The reason this is so important is that a service needs to meet medical criteria in order for the insurance to cover the service. If transaction lines 2 and 3 were wrong, the services would be denied. Having diabetes does not substantiate the need for an X-ray of the patient.

Place of Service (POS) Codes

Place of service (POS) codes are entered in box 24B on the CMS-1500 form. The POS is a two-digit code that identifies where the service was rendered. It is significant because insurance coverage can vary depending on location. For example, a patient may have insurance coverage if a chiropractic visit is done at the office (POS 11), but there may be no coverage if it is done at home (POS 12). It is also important to be sure the POS for each service is consistent with the description of the service. For example, if the physician visits a patient in the hospital (CPT* 99221), the POS should be 21, Inpatient Hospital. Currently, there are 82 possible different POS codes, but the one used most frequently in medical offices is POS 11. A list of POS codes can be found in the front of the CPT* manual.

MultiLink Codes

MultiLink codes are a Medisoft feature that can save users hundreds of hours of time over the course of a year. The MultiLink function groups commonly used CPT* codes together under one access code. This saves not only data entry time, but also reduces errors. An example of this is created in the Tutorial practice in the Diabetes Screening. You can view this in your data by going to Lists and MultiLink Codes, then Edit the code named Diabetes Screening (Figure 3-16). In Transaction Entry, we can enter one MultiLink code that will add all the procedure codes listed in the profile group. In later exercises, we will enter charges using MultiLink codes.

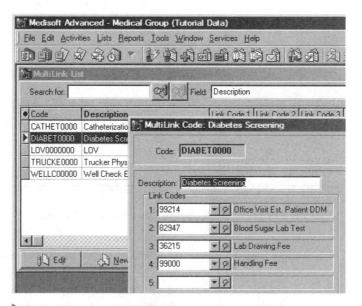

▶ **Figure 3-16   MultiLink Codes**

*CPT is a registered trademark of the American Medical Association.

PRACTICE EXERCISE 3-7 **Entering Charges, Payments, Adjustments and Comments**

Each day prior to seeing patients, superbills are printed for patients and charts are pulled and given to the doctor to document the visit. You may review how to print superbills in Chapter 1. Then, for the purpose of this exercise, refer to the patient superbills in Appendix C. These source documents will be used to enter the charges, payments, adjustments, and comments for this exercise.

1 Go to Activities and Transaction Entry. In this screen, we will enter all four transaction types. To add a new charge, click New on the top portion of the screen. To add a payment, click New on the bottom portion of the screen.

2 Enter the transactions for superbills 1024 to 1046. Each superbill contains the patient's name, date of service, doctor code, procedure codes, diagnosis and linkage, and co-pay amount. There are 23 superbills in all.

3 Print preview the superbills for 9/4/08 and see that you have the same number. You should have three new patients from the previous exercises.

4 Pay particular attention to date of service, procedure codes or MultiLink codes, modifiers, diagnosis linkage, and attending provider.

5 Make sure that each case is assigned to the correct provider and diagnosis and both are listed in the description. This may cause you to copy or create new cases.

Note: The three new patients have new patient exams, and the existing patients have established patient exams.

6 If you find a CPT* code that is not in the system, create a new one by hitting F8. Charge $50.00 for any new service. If, after hitting F8, you have questions, select Help to walk you through the procedure.

7 If the payment amount shows a check number, use the code CHECK to post the payment and enter the check number. Otherwise, use the code CASH to apply the patient payments and apply the payments. To apply the payments, click Apply and enter the amount in the first line item (Figure 3-17). **Note:** Insurance companies apply the co-payment to the first service on the claim form. This is because if the patient only had one service, he or she still would have a co-pay applied to the visit. Hence, you should apply all the co-payments for the superbills to the first service entered.

*CPT is a registered trademark of the American Medical Association.

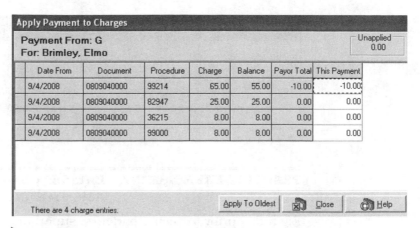

▶ Figure 3-17 **Payment Application**

8 To create a MultiLink code, click MultiLink instead of New and the code and date. Then press Create Transactions (Figure 3-18).

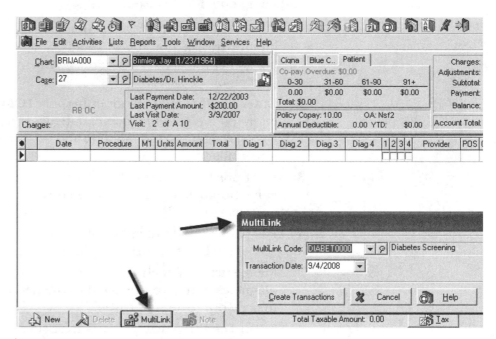

▶ Figure 3-18 **Creating MultiLink Transactions**

If a patient does not have a case, create a Cash Case. Remember to check the Cash Case option in the Personal tab.

Medisoft Quick Tip   Apply to Oldest Feature

When applying payments, you have the option to select Apply to Oldest. This works well for patient payments received via the mail on older balances. However, for patient co-pays made on the date of service, it is better to apply the payment to the charge for that date. This is because patients will remember making these payments and will later associate them to their visit. So, to sum up patient payment application, if payment is made during a patient visit, apply it to that visit. If it's made via the mail, apply it to the oldest outstanding balance.

PRACTICE EXERCISE 3-8   Checks and Balances: Patient Day Sheet

After all of the superbills have been entered into the computer, the final step is to run a **Patient Day Sheet** to proof your work.

1   Go to Reports, Day Sheets, and Patient Day Sheets (Figure 3-19).

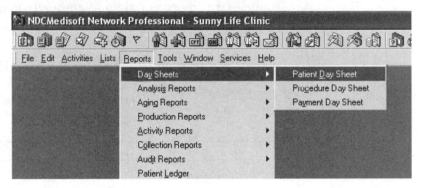

▶ Figure 3-19   **Patient Day Sheet**

2   Next, we can filter the data by using Data Selection Questions. The Date Created is the date the charge or payment was put into the computer. The Date From is the date the charge was incurred or payment was made. We want to make the Date Created either the date you entered the charges or payments or a broad span to include the dates. Then, the Date From should be the date of service you are auditing, 9/4/2008 in this case (Figure 3-20).

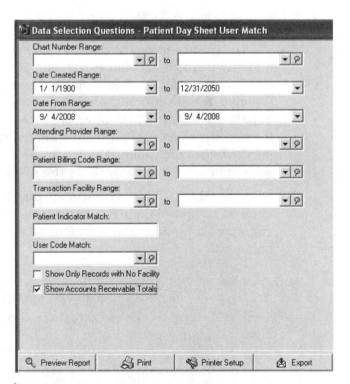

▶ Figure 3-20   **Data Selection Questions on the Patient Day Sheet**

3 We could apply many other filters to this report, such as for a certain provider, facility, or user, but we are going to leave those blank for now. However, depending upon the practice size, these could be very useful.

4 At the bottom of the report, we have the option to check Show Accounts Receivables Totals. This option provides for a good safeguard to protect against embezzlement. We will review this in detail in Chapter 9. For now, check this box to become familiar with information that it provides.

5 Now, let's preview the report (Figure 3-21).

Patient Day Sheet User Match
July 08, 2007
9/4/2008

Entry	Date	Document	POS	Description	Provider	Code	Modifiers	Amount
AGADW000	**Again, Dwight**							
109	9/4/2008	0809040000	11	Office Visit Est. Patient FFS	JM	99212		40.00
110	9/4/2008	0809040000	11	Blood Sugar Lab Test	JM	82947		25.00
111	9/4/2008	0809040000	11	Strep Screen	JM	86403		50.00
112	9/4/2008	0809040000	11	Cash Payment--Thank You!	JM	CASH		-20.00

Patient's Charges	Patient's Receipts	Insurance Receipts	Adjustments	Patient Balance
$115.00	-$20.00	$0.00	$0.00	$426.00

Entry	Date	Document	POS	Description	Provider	Code	Modifiers	Amount
AUSAN000	**Austin, Andrew**							
113	9/4/2008	0809040000	11	Office Visit Est. Patient FFS	REL	99212		40.00
114	9/4/2008	0809040000	11	X-Ray, Chest, 2 Views	REL	71020		53.00
115	9/4/2008	0809040000	11	Cash Payment--Thank You!	REL	CASH		-10.00

Patient's Charges	Patient's Receipts	Insurance Receipts	Adjustments	Patient Balance
$93.00	-$10.00	$0.00	$0.00	$48.00

▶ **Figure 3-21** **Patient Day Sheet Report**

The report shows the patient's name, date of service, and charges and payments. It also tallies the total of each under the charges and payments for each patient. Finally, at the end of the report, it summarizes the entire day for the clinic—everything from the number of patients seen to the number of procedures performed. In addition, it categorizes charges, payments, and adjustments and gives a net effect on the receivables. Finally, at the bottom of the report, we can see the Practice Totals for the entire history of the practice.

6 Now, run the Patient Day Sheet for the charges and payments you entered and proof them against your superbills. Fix any errors that you may have and make sure your charge and receipts amounts balance.

Billing Insight Watching for Embezzlement

It has been discovered that when funds are embezzled, an employee may take the cash received today and delete past posted payments. This way, the patient payments for today may balance, but not the overall payments for the practice. It is important for an audit person at each clinic to keep a running total of the accounts receivable for the practice. In addition, it is useful to know how much is outstanding for the practice. As a healthcare collector, you develop a system to try and get this number as low as possible and the payments as high as possible.

CHAPTER REVIEW

Multiple Choice

1. Which transaction type is a billing charge?
   a. Adjustment
   b. Payment
   c. Charge
   d. Comment

2. Which transaction type is a contracted insurance write-off?
   a. Adjustment
   b. Comment
   c. Payment
   d. Charge

3. Which code is used to define the product or service received?
   a. Diagnosis
   b. CPT*
   c. Modifier
   d. ICD-9-CM

4. Which code is used to define the injury or illness of the patient?
   a. CPT*
   b. Diagnosis
   c. Modifier
   d. HCPCS

5. Who owns the trademark on CPT* codes?
   a. CMS
   b. All insurance companies
   c. AMA
   d. NPI

6. What does a MultiLink code group together?
   a. Procedure codes
   b. Diagnosis codes
   c. Modifiers
   d. Payments

7. Who is responsible for HCPCS codes?
   a. CMS
   b. AMA
   c. Insurance companies
   d. Doctors

8. Which POS is most commonly used by medical offices?
   a. 11
   b. 12
   c. 82
   d. 69

*CPT is a registered trademark of the American Medical Association.

9. Where is a MultiLink code created initially?
   a. List and MultiLink
   b. Transaction Entry
   c. Both a and b
   d. Help feature

10. How often should billing rules and regulations be researched?
    a. Never
    b. Once per year
    c. At least once per month
    d. After insurance denials are received

11. Why should you show the total Accounts Receivable Totals?
    a. To protect against embezzlement
    b. To show the total outstanding to the practice
    c. Both a and b
    d. To know the total charges billed

12. When do you select the option Cash Case?
    a. When there is no insurance coverage
    b. When you want the patient to pay cash
    c. When you want the to patient to pay prior to his or her visit
    d. When you received cash from the patient prior to billing the insurance

13. To select diagnosis linkage for box 24E you should
    a. only put the proper diagnosis in the case.
    b. click the proper diagnosis on the charge line.
    c. both a and b.
    d. type the correct diagnosis in the charge line.

14. The report to run to proof charges and payment is the
    a. procedure day sheet.
    b. patient day sheet.
    c. charge and payment day sheet.
    d. procedure patient day sheet.

15. Which date should you put in for the Date From?
    a. The date the patient was charged or payment received
    b. The date the charge and payment were entered
    c. Either a or b
    d. The date you expect to receive payment

True/False

Identify each of the following statements as true or false.

1. Medisoft users should always watch which diagnosis is linked to each charge and make sure the proper diagnosis box is checked.

2. The user should create a new case if the patient's diagnosis or provider changes.

3. Modifiers are used to tell what is wrong with the patient.

4. Billing charges are adjustments.

5. The diagnosis tells what is wrong with the patient.

6. The CPT* code tells what is wrong with the patient.

7. Modifiers give additional information to the insurance company about was service was provided to the patient.

8. HCPCS codes are usually for supplies and are maintained by CMS.

9. CPT* codes tell an insurance company what was provided to the patient.

10. Grid columns allow the Medisoft user to add more fields to the CMS-1500 form.

Short Answer

1. List the various types of adjustments a clinic could make to a patient's account and how you would manage these in Medisoft.

2. Describe the different places you might obtain billing rules and regulations; give at least five examples.

3. Explain how diagnosis codes are linked to the procedure codes in a case.

Resources

Any time you need to get a list of codes such as modifiers or place of service (POS) codes, you generally can find ample examples of codes by going to your favorite search engine on the web, for example, **www.google.com** or **www.yahoo.com**

This site offers a list of place of service codes for professional claims. **www.cms.hhs.gov/PlaceofServiceCodes/Downloads/POSDataBase.pdf**

Besides newsletters from insurance carriers, boards, and associates, there are many billing associations that keep members up to date on current legislation and vital healthcare changes. One reputable association is the Healthcare Billing and Management Association. Visit its website at **www.hbma.org**.

*CPT is a registered trademark of the American Medical Association.

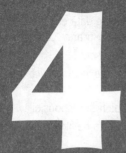

Chapter Four

Claim Management

Learning Objectives

After completing this chapter, you should be able to:

♦ Define and spell the key terms in this chapter.

♦ Understand and define the components of Claim Management.

♦ Explain how to create claims.

♦ Demonstrate how to print paper claims and transmit electronic claims.

♦ Discuss the differences between primary, secondary, and tertiary claims.

♦ Identify various ways to manage claims in Claim Management.

♦ List and define each of the eight different claim statuses.

♦ Describe how the claim statuses change from one category to another.

♦ Demonstrate three different ways to find claims.

♦ Explain how to view claim detail and identify the purpose of each tab.

♦ Demonstrate how to rebill claims.

♦ Discuss how to align the claim form.

Key Terms

Alert a claim status used to indicate that there are special circumstances surrounding the claim and the office is monitoring the progress.

birthday rule determines which insurance is primary when two policies are valid for a child. The plan of the parent whose birthday comes first in the calendar year is usually primary.

Challenge a claim status used to indicate that the insurance company has processed the claim and the office intends to dispute it.

claim name for a bill that is sent to the insurance company.

Claim Management the utility inside of Medisoft that allows the user to submit primary, secondary, or tertiary claims to insurance companies, along with tracking the status of each claim.

Claims Manager a separate, add-on program sold by Medisoft to manage electronic transactions.

claim status explains the current position of a claim, i.e., sent, paid, or rejected.

clearinghouse a company that receives claims from multiple providers, evaluates them, and batches them for electronic submission to multiple insurance carriers.

create claims   the process used within Claim Management to search for transactions that have not been billed and create claims for them.

Done   a claim status used to indicate the insurance has completed processing the claim.

Electronic Data Interchange (EDI)   the process of exchanging data electronically between healthcare covered entities: the clinic, the clearinghouse, and the insurance company.

Hold   a claim status used to indicate the claim is not ready to be sent.

Pending   a claim status used to indicate the claim is waiting at the insurance company for additional information.

primary claim   a claim sent to the patient's insurance that has first responsibility.

Ready to Send   a claim status used to indicate the claim needs to be filed either on paper or electronically.

Rejected   a claim status used to indicate that the claim was transmitted electronically and an electronic reject was posted to the comment tab inside the claim details.

secondary claim   a claim sent to the patient's insurance that has secondary responsibility.

Sent   a claim status used to indicate the claim has been sent to the insurance carrier.

tertiary claim   a claim sent to the patient's insurance that has responsibility after the secondary insurance.

Abbreviations

ANSI   American National Standards Institute
CMS   Centers for Medicare and Medicaid Services
EDI   Electronic Data Interchange
MSP   Medicare Secondary Payer
NSF   National Standard Format
NUCC   National Uniform Claim Committee
OCR   optical character reader

■ ■ ■ ■

INTRODUCTION

After all of the patients and charges have been entered into Medisoft and the work has been proofed for the day, it is time to bill the insurance companies. The billing process initiates payments by the insurance companies to the medical office. In the billing industry, the bill that is sent to the insurance company is called a **claim**. **Claim Management** is the tool inside of Medisoft that allows the user to create and process the claims that need to be filed to the insurance companies on either paper CMS-1500 forms (see Figure 1-10) or electronically through **Electronic Data Interchange (EDI)**. **CMS** stands for Centers for Medicare and Medicaid Services and is the government agency responsible for overseeing healthcare services given to the elderly, disabled and indigent. In addition to creating claims, Claim Management allows the user to track paid and unpaid **primary**, **secondary**, and **tertiary claims**. Patients often have more than one insurance paying on their claims. The insurance that is responsible to pay first is called the primary insurance. Hence, the insurance responsible to pay second is the secondary insurance, and the third payer would be the tertiary insurance.

OVERVIEW OF CLAIM MANAGEMENT

There are two ways to access Claim Management in Medisoft. The first way is to go to Activities and select Claim Management (Figure 4-1), and the second option is to click on the Claim Management icon on the toolbar (Figure 4-2).

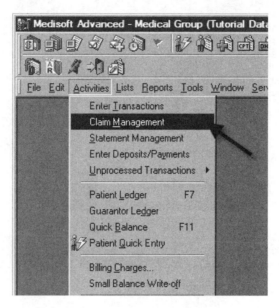

▶ Figure 4-1 Accessing Claim Management Through Activities

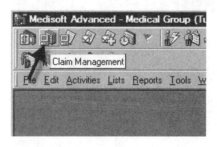

▶ Figure 4-2 Accessing Claim Management Through the Toolbar

Creating Claims

Each day after the transactions have been entered and proofed, the claims need to be created. To **create claims**, open Claim Management, then click on the Create Claims button on the bottom toolbar (Figure 4-3). You have the option to filter your claims by several data fields from transaction dates to insurance companies to amounts. In most situations, it is best to leave the filters empty and click Create. This causes Medisoft to search for all the transactions that have not been billed yet and create new claims for them. After the claims are created, they will be listed as **Ready to Send** (Figure 4-4).

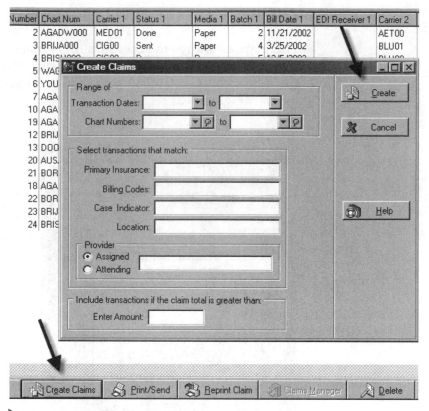

Number	Chart Num	Carrier 1	Status 1	Media 1	Batch 1	Bill Date 1	EDI Receiver 1	Carrier 2
2	AGADW000	MED01	Done	Paper	2	11/21/2002		AET00
3	BRIJA000	CIG00	Sent	Paper	4	3/25/2002		BLU01
4	BRISU000	CIG00	D	P	5	12/15/2002		BLU00

Create Claims

Range of
Transaction Dates: [ ] to [ ]
Chart Numbers: [ ] to [ ]

Select transactions that match:
Primary Insurance: [ ]
Billing Codes: [ ]
Case Indicator: [ ]
Location: [ ]

Provider
● Assigned
○ Attending [ ]

Include transactions if the claim total is greater than:
Enter Amount: [ ]

Create
Cancel
Help

Create Claims | Print/Send | Reprint Claim | Claims Manager | Delete

▶ Figure 4-3   **Creating Claims**

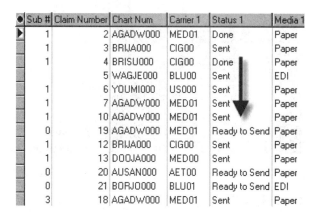

●	Sub #	Claim Number	Chart Num	Carrier 1	Status 1	Media 1
▶	1	2	AGADW000	MED01	Done	Paper
	1	3	BRIJA000	CIG00	Sent	Paper
	1	4	BRISU000	CIG00	Done	Paper
		5	WAGJE000	BLU00	Sent	EDI
	1	6	YOUMI000	US000	Sent	Paper
	1	7	AGADW000	MED01	Sent	Paper
	1	10	AGADW000	MED01	Sent	Paper
	0	19	AGADW000	MED01	Ready to Send	Paper
	1	12	BRIJA000	CIG00	Sent	Paper
	1	13	DOOJA000	MED00	Sent	Paper
	0	20	AUSAN000	AET00	Ready to Send	Paper
	0	21	BORJO000	BLU01	Ready to Send	EDI
	3	18	AGADW000	MED01	Sent	Paper

▶ Figure 4-4   **Ready to Send Claims**

PRACTICE EXERCISE 4-1   Creating Claims

There are two essential steps to printing and sending claims within Medisoft. The first step is to create claims, and the second is to print or send them electronically. When initiating Create Claims, the program searches all transactions and creates claims for any accounts that have both insurance and unbilled charges. Take the following steps to create claims:

1   First, open Claims Management.

2   Select Create Claims from the bottom toolbar.

3 Select Create again from the pop-up box and notice the new claims that are generated.

Printing and/or Transmitting Claims

After the claims are created, they must be either printed to paper or transmitted electronically. Newly created claims appear on the list with the status Ready to Send, and they do not have a bill date.

Paper Claims

To print the paper claims that are Ready to Send, first click on the Print/Send button (Figure 4-5), click on Paper radio button, and click OK. Next, select the applicable claim form to print your claims. For primary insurance, select CMS-1500 Primary, then click OK. The next option allows the user to preview the claims, print the claims, or export them to a file. For this example, select preview, then press Start. In order to print the claims, the printer option would be selected either prior to previewing or after the preview is open.

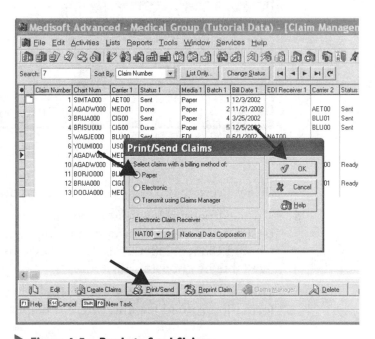

▶ **Figure 4-5   Ready to Send Claims**

PRACTICE EXERCISE 4-2   Printing Claims

After claims are created, they need to be printed to the CMS-1500 form. In this exercise, we will print claims.

1   Inside Claim Management, click on the Print/Send button.

2   Next, select Paper claims and click OK. **Note:** Medisoft also gives the option to send claims electronically or using **Claims Manager**. Claims Manager is a special add-on program sold separately by Medisoft that initiates electronic transactions.

3   Select the Laser CMS (Primary) W/Form and select OK (Figure 4-6). **Note:** There are numerous forms available to choose. As discussed earlier, primary means the first insurance responsible to pay. Each day the primary insurance companies should be billed. Secondary and tertiary insurance companies are billed as needed and if there is a balance remaining.

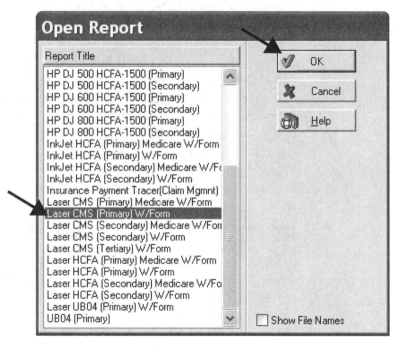

▶ Figure 4-6   **Laser CMS (Primary) W/Form**

4   Select Preview the report on the screen and Start.

5   The next pop-up box that appears allows for claims to be filtered based upon a variety of options ranging from Chart Numbers to Unpaid Claims Older Than Days. Let's display all the claims available by choosing OK.

6   Take a moment to review the CMS-1500 forms. Note some of the information you added and where it displays on the form.

Electronic Claims

To transmit electronic claims that are Ready to Send, first click on the Print/Send button, click on the Electronic radio button, and select the Electronic Claim Receiver, then click OK (Figure 4-7). This will open the NDC Electronic Claims processing module. Next, choose Send Primary Claims. The program will then give you a list of filters. Most clinics send all the claims that are Ready to Send, but be aware that options are available to filter the claims to be sent. Next, Medisoft gives the option to print or preview a verification report. After approval, select Yes to continue with the transmission. Medisoft will now batch the claims and transmit via the Internet to the clearinghouse.

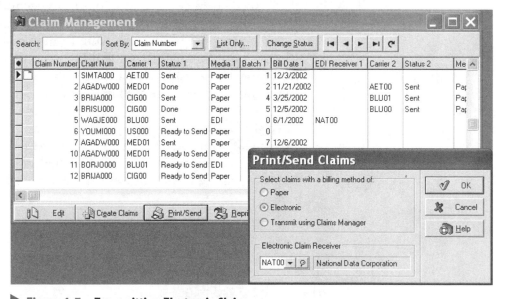

▶ **Figure 4-7   Transmitting Electronic Claims**

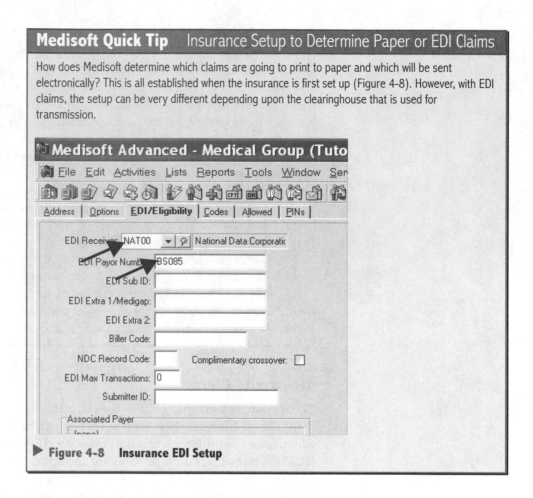

Medisoft Quick Tip Insurance Setup to Determine Paper or EDI Claims

How does Medisoft determine which claims are going to print to paper and which will be sent electronically? This is all established when the insurance is first set up (Figure 4-8). However, with EDI claims, the setup can be very different depending upon the clearinghouse that is used for transmission.

▶ Figure 4-8 **Insurance EDI Setup**

Primary, Secondary, and Tertiary Claims

Many patients have more than one insurance company that covers their visits. The insurance company that pays first on behalf of its beneficiary is called the primary insurance, and the primary claim form that will be selected to print the claims is called the CMS-1500 (Primary) (Figure 4-9). An insurance company that pays second after the primary insurance has paid is called the secondary insurance, and the form used to print the secondary claim form is called the CMS-1500 (Secondary). Finally, if a patient is fortunate enough to have three insurances, the insurance that pays after the primary and secondary insurance is called the tertiary insurance. To print a tertiary claim, select CMS-1500 (Tertiary). Note that when you are selecting these claims, you have the option to choose the claim forms that end in Medicare Century. These claim forms are for submitting to Medicare carriers that require an eight-digit date format along with other small changes in the form. Medicare claim form requirements can vary state to state.

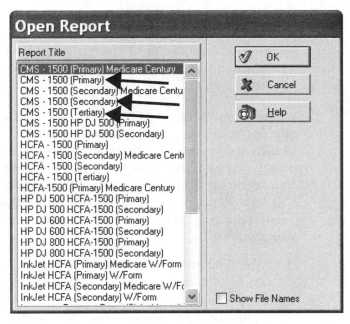

▶ Figure 4-9 **Primary, Secondary, and Tertiary Claim Forms**

Determining Order of Coverage

When a patient has more than one insurance plan, the order of coverage must be determined. Technically the patient and/or insured is responsible for notifying the providers of the proper order of their insurance coverage, but they do not always do that or are too confused themselves to be able to do so. In addition, there are established rules to determine the order of coverage; the choice of primary vs. secondary policy is not the patient's choice. It is determined by industry-wide rules adopted by state insurance commissioners.

The following are general guidelines to determine the order of coverage:

1. Any time a patient is seen who has been injured, the clinic must find out how the injury occurred. If it is auto accident or workers' compensation related, the accident insurance is usually primary. If the patient fell or was injured on a third-party property, the insurance for that property may be primary.

2. If the visit is not accident-related and the patient is an adult with two insurances, find out who the insured person is in each policy. If it is the patient and his or her spouse, then the patient's own insurance is primary.

3. If the patient is a child with two insurances and the insureds on the policies are the patient's parents, then the **birthday rule** applies. This rule says that the insurance of whichever insured's birthday falls first in the calendar year is the primary insurance. (Be careful: This does not mean the oldest insured; the birthday rule goes strictly by the position of birthday in the calendar year.)

4. If the patient is a child with two insurances, the visit is not an injury, and the coverage is not under two parents, most likely the coverage is through one parent's employer and Medical Assistance from the state in which the patient resides. The employer insurance would be the first payer.

When billing Medicare, CMS requires the office to make a good faith attempt at determining primary, secondary, or tertiary coverage. Medicare does this to protect the funds that pay Medicare claims. The proper acronym for Medicare Secondary Payer is **MSP**. CMS has excellent documents at www.cms.gov to assist the office personnel in determining coverage (Figures 4-10 and 4-11). Acquaint yourselves with these documents now. MSP guidelines include the following common situations:

5. If the patient is an adult over 65 years old, the visit is not an injury, and they have two insurances, most likely the patient has Medicare and possibly a supplement to Medicare. Medicare is primary. Supplement policies are secondary and generally pick up the deductible, coinsurance and certain other items not paid by Medicare.

6. Some Medicare beneficiaries participate in Medicare Part C, in which they assign their Medicare benefits to a managed care plan. Part C often gives the patient better benefits at the same or lower cost as traditional Medicare, but the choice of providers is usually limited and other restrictions may apply. In this scenario, the claims are sent to the Part C managed care provider, not Medicare.

7. If a Medicare recipient is still working or has a working spouse with insurance through the employer, that insurance is usually primary over Medicare if the employer has 20 or more employees. If a retiree has a full group health policy through the employer (not a supplemental policy), the retiree policy is always secondary to Medicare. Be careful to distinguish between a patient with traditional Medicare and a supplemental plan, a patient with Part C, a patient over 65 covered by an employer group policy, and a patient with Medicare as well as a retiree group health policy.

8. If a patient has both Medicare and Medical Assistance, Medicare is primary. Medical Assistance is always the payer of last resort and the patient is always the insured.

9. For Medicare coverage, the patient is always the insured.

These are general outlines to follow. It is recommended that coverage is always verified with the patient and/or payers.

Medicare Secondary Payer Fact Sheet

for Provider, Physician, and Other Supplier Billing Staff

Background

Maintaining the viability and integrity of the Medicare Trust Fund becomes critical as the Medicare Program matures and the "baby boomer" generation moves toward retirement. Providers, physicians, and other suppliers can contribute to the appropriate use of Medicare by complying with all Medicare requirements, including those applicable to the Medicare Secondary Payer (MSP) provisions. The purpose of this Fact Sheet is to provide a general overview of the MSP provisions for individuals involved in the admission and billing procedures at provider, physician, and other supplier settings.

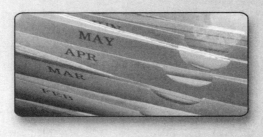

What is Medicare Secondary Payer (MSP)?

Since 1980, the Medicare Secondary Payer (MSP) provisions have protected Medicare funds by ensuring that Medicare does not pay for services and items that certain health insurance or coverage has primary responsibilities for paying. The MSP provisions apply to situations when Medicare is not the beneficiary's primary insurance. It provides the following benefits for both the Medicare program and providers, physicians, and other suppliers:

- National program savings - Medicare saves more than $4.5 billion annually on claims processed by insurers that are primary to Medicare.

- Increased provider, physician, and other supplier revenue - Providers, physicians, and other suppliers that bill a liability insurer *before* billing Medicare may receive more favorable payment rates. Providers, physicians, and other suppliers can also reduce administrative costs when health insurance or coverage is properly coordinated.

- Avoidance of Medicare recovery efforts - Providers, physicians, and other suppliers that file claims correctly the first time may prevent future Medicare recovery efforts on that claim.

To realize these benefits, providers, physicians, and other suppliers must have access to accurate, up-to-date information about all health insurance or coverage that Medicare beneficiaries may have. Current law and regulations require that all entities that bill Medicare for services or items rendered to Medicare beneficiaries must determine whether Medicare is the primary payer for those services or items.

When Does Medicare Pay First?

Primary payers are those that have the primary responsibility for paying a claim. Medicare remains the primary payer for beneficiaries who are not covered by other types of health insurance or coverage. Medicare is also the primary payer in other instances, provided several conditions are met. Table 1 lists some common situations when Medicare may be the primary or secondary payer for a patient's claims:

1

▶ Figure 4-10   **MSP Fact Sheet**

Medicare Secondary Payer Fact Sheet

IF THE PATIENT...	AND THIS CONDITION EXISTS...	THEN THIS PROGRAM PAYS FIRST...	AND THIS PROGRAM PAYS SECOND
Is age 65 or older, and is covered by a Group Health Plan through current employment or spouse's current employment...	The employer has less than 20 employees...	Medicare	Group Health Plan
	The employer has 20 or more employees, or at least one employer is a multi-employer group that employs 20 or more individuals...	Group Health Plan	Medicare
Has an employer retirement plan and is age 65 or older or disabled and age 65 or older...	The patient is entitled to Medicare...	Medicare	Retiree coverage
Is disabled and covered by a Large Group Health Plan through his or her own current employment or through a family member's current employment	The employer has less than 100 employees...	Medicare	Large Group Health Plan
	The employer has 100 or more employees, or at least one employer is a multi-employer group that employs 100 or more individuals...	Large Group Health Plan	Medicare
Has End Stage Renal Disease and Group Health Plan Coverage...	Is in the first 30 months of eligibility or entitlement to Medicare...	Group Health Plan	Medicare
	After 30 months...	Medicare	Group Health Plan
Has End Stage Renal Disease and COBRA coverage...	Is in the first 30 months of eligibility or entitlement to Medicare...	COBRA	Medicare
	After 30 months...	Medicare	COBRA
Is covered under Workers' Compensation because of a job-related illness or injury...	The patient is entitled to Medicare...	Workers' Compensation (for health care items or services related to job-related illness or injury). Payment may be made from a Workers' Compensation Medicare Set-aside Arrangement.	Medicare
Has been in an accident or other situation where no-fault or liability insurance is involved...	The patient is entitled to Medicare...	No-fault or liability insurance for accident or other situation related health care services	Medicare
Is age 65 or older OR is disabled and covered by Medicare and COBRA...	The patient is entitled to Medicare...	Medicare	COBRA

Table 1. List of Common Situations When Medicare May Pay First or Second

2

▶ **Figure 4-10   MSP Fact Sheet (*continued*)**

Are There Any Exceptions to the MSP Requirements?

In most cases, Federal law takes precedence over state laws and private contracts. Even if a state law or insurance policy states that they are a secondary payer to Medicare, the MSP provisions should be followed when billing for services.

What Happens if the Primary Payer Denies a Claim?

In the following situations, Medicare *may* make payment assuming the services are covered and a proper claim has been filed.

- The GHP denies payment for services because the beneficiary is not covered by the health plan;

- The no-fault or liability insurer does not pay, or denies the medical bill; or

- The WC program denies payment, as in situations where WC is not required to pay for a given medical condition.

- The Workers' Compensation Medicare Set-aside Arrangement (WCMSA) is exhausted.

In these situations, providers, physicians, and other suppliers should include documentation from the primary payer stating that the claim has been denied and/or benefits have been exhausted when submitting the claim to Medicare.

When Will Medicare Make a Conditional Payment?

Medicare will make a conditional payment for Medicare covered services in liability, no-fault, and WC situations where another payer is responsible for payment and the claim is not expected to be paid within the "promptly" period. Medicare makes conditional payments to prevent the beneficiary from using his or her own money to pay the claim. However, Medicare has the right to recover any conditional payments.

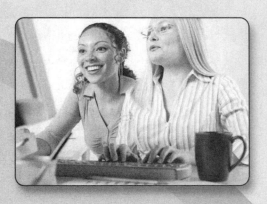

How Is Beneficiary Health Insurance or Coverage Information Collected and Coordinated?

The Centers for Medicare & Medicaid Services (CMS) established the Coordination of Benefits (COB) Contractor to collect, manage, and maintain information on Medicare's Common Working File (CWF) regarding other health insurance or coverage for Medicare beneficiaries. Providers, physicians, and other suppliers must collect accurate MSP beneficiary information for the COB Contractor to coordinate the information.

To support the goals of the MSP provisions, the COB Contractor manages several data gathering programs. These programs were implemented in three phases, as discussed in the next section.

What Are Some of the Activities Managed by the COB Contractor?

The COB Contractor implemented the first two phases of the contract in April 2000:

- **Initial Enrollment Questionnaire (IEQ)** - The COB Contractor sends out the IEQ approximately three months before an individual is eligible for Medicare. This

3

▶ **Figure 4-10   MSP Fact Sheet (*continued*)**

Medicare Secondary Payer Fact Sheet

questionnaire asks the beneficiary if he or she has other health insurance or coverage (including prescription drug coverage) that may be primary to Medicare.

- **Internal Revenue Service/Social Security Administration/CMS (IRS/SSA/CMS) Data Match Project Coordination** - The Omnibus Budget Reconciliation Act of 1989 requires each agency to share information it has regarding employment of Medicare beneficiaries or their spouses. This information helps determine whether a beneficiary may be covered by a Group Health Plan (GHP) that pays primary to Medicare. This information is sent to the COB Contractor, which coordinates the Data Match Project.

- **As part of the Data Match Project,** the Voluntary Data Sharing Agreement (VDSA) program allows for the electronic data exchange of GHP eligibility and Medicare information between CMS, employers, and various insurers (including prescription drug plans). Employers, to meet the mandatory reporting requirements, can sign a VDSA in lieu of completing and submitting the IRS/SSA/CMS Data Match questionnaire.

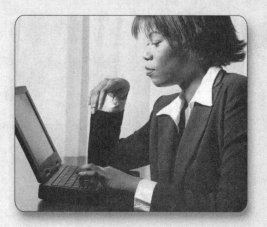

CMS has also developed a new data exchange, similar to the VDSA program, for Supplemental Drug Plans [Non-Qualified State Pharmaceutical Assistance Programs (SPAPs)] to coordinate with Medicare Part D.

In January 2001, an additional phase of the COB contract was implemented:

- **MSP Claims Investigation Process** - The COB Contractor assumed responsibility for all initial MSP development activities previously performed by Intermediaries and Carriers. The COB Contractor provides a one-stop customer service approach for all MSP-related inquiries. However, the COB Contractor does not process claims, nor does it handle any mistaken payment recoveries or claim-specific inquiries. Each provider, physician, or other supplier should continue to call the Medicare contractor that processes their claims regarding specific claim-based issues.

What Is the Provider's, Physician's, or Other Supplier's Role in the MSP Provisions?

Providers, physicians, and other suppliers must aid in the collection and coordination of beneficiary health insurance or coverage information by:

- Asking the patient or his/her representative questions concerning the patient's MSP status. A suggested method is to incorporate a MSP questionnaire into all patient health records.

- Billing the primary payer before billing Medicare, as required by the Social Security Act.

How Do Providers, Physicians, and Other Suppliers Gather Accurate Data from the Beneficiary?

Providers, physicians, and other suppliers can save time and money by collecting patient health insurance or coverage information at *each* patient visit. Some suggested questions that providers,

4

▶ **Figure 4-10   MSP Fact Sheet (*continued*)**

physicians, and other suppliers should ask include, but are not limited to:

- Is the patient covered by any GHP through his or her current or former employment? If so, how many employees work for the employer providing coverage?

- Is the patient covered by a GHP through his or her spouse or other family member's current or former employment? If so, how many employees work for the employer providing the GHP?

- Is the patient receiving Workers Compensation (WC) benefits?

- Does the patient have a WCMSA?

- Is the patient covered under no-fault insurance or liability insurance?

- Is the patient being treated for an injury or illness for which another party could be held liable?

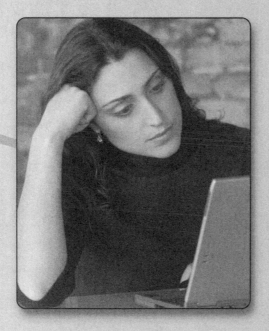

Providers, physicians, and other suppliers may also use a model questionnaire published by CMS to collect patient information. This tool is available online in the MSP Manual in chapter 3, section 20.2.1 at *http://www.cms.hhs.gov/manuals/downloads/msp105c03.pdf* on the CMS website.

If the provider, physician, or other supplier does not furnish Medicare with a record of other health insurance or coverage that may be primary to Medicare on any claim and there is an indication of possible MSP considerations, the COB Contractor may request that the provider, physician, or other supplier complete a Development Questionnaire.

Why Gather Additional Beneficiary Health Insurance or Coverage Information?

The goal of MSP information-gathering activities is to quickly identify possible MSP situations, thus ensuring correct primary and secondary payments by the responsible parties. This effort may require that providers, physicians, and other suppliers complete Development Questionnaires to collect accurate beneficiary health insurance or coverage information. Many of the questions on the Development Questionnaires are similar to the questions that providers, physicians, and other suppliers might ask a beneficiary during a routine visit. This similarity provides another good reason to routinely ask patients about their health insurance or coverage. If a provider, physician, or other supplier gathers information about a beneficiary's other health insurance or coverage and uses that information to complete the claim properly, a Development Questionnaire may not be necessary. Accurate submittal of claims may accelerate the processing of the provider's, physician's, or other supplier's claim.

The COB Contractor may submit a Secondary Claim Development (SCD) Questionnaire to providers, physicians, and other suppliers.

What Is a Secondary Claim Development (SCD) Questionnaire?

An SCD Questionnaire may be sent to the provider, physician, or other supplier when a claim is submitted with an Explanation of Benefits (EOB)

5

▶ **Figure 4-10   MSP Fact Sheet** (*continued*)

Medicare Secondary Payer Fact Sheet

attached from an insurer other than Medicare, and relevant information was not submitted to properly adjudicate the submitted claim. The COB Contractor provides the names and Health Insurance Claim Number (HICN) of each individual for which the provider, physician, or other supplier must complete an SCD Questionnaire. The provider, physician, or other supplier must complete and submit the SCD Questionnaire to the COB Contractor.

What Happens if the Provider, Physician, or Other Supplier Submits a Claim to Medicare Without Providing the Other Insurer's Information?

The claim may be paid if it meets all Medicare requirements, including Medicare coverage and medical necessity guidelines. However, if the beneficiary's Medicare record indicates that another insurer should have paid primary to Medicare, the claim will be either returned unprocessed to the provider or denied or suspended for development. If the Medicare contractor has enough information, they may forward the information to the COBC and the COBC may send the provider, physician, or other supplier a Secondary Claim Development

Questionnaire to complete for additional information if they were the informant. Medicare will review the information on the questionnaire and determine the proper action to take.

What Happens if the Provider, Physician, or Other Supplier Fails to File Correct and Accurate Claims with Medicare?

Federal law permits Medicare to recover its conditional payments. Providers, physicians, and other suppliers can be fined up to $2,000 for knowingly, willfully, and repeatedly providing inaccurate information relating to the existence of other health insurance or coverage.

How Does the Provider, Physician, or Other Supplier Contact the COB Contractor?

Providers, physicians, and other suppliers may contact the COB Contractor at 1-800-999-1118 (TTY/TDD: 1-800-318-8782), Monday - Friday, 8 a.m. to 8 p.m. Eastern Time (excluding holidays). Providers, physicians, and other suppliers may contact the COB Contractor to:

- Report potential MSP situations;
- Report incorrect insurance information; or
- Address general MSP questions/concerns.

Specific claim-based issues (including claim processing) should still be addressed to the provider's, physician's, or other supplier's Medicare claims processing contractor[1].

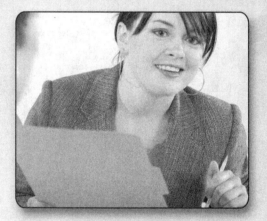

Medicare Contracting Reform (MCR) Update - Section 911 of the Medicare Prescription Drug, Improvement, and Modernization Act of 2003 (MMA) Congress mandated that the Secretary of the Department of Health and Human Services replace the current contracting authority under Title XVIII of the Social Security Act with the new Medicare Administrative Contractor (MAC) authority. This mandate is referred to as Medicare Contracting Reform. Medicare Contracting Reform is intended to improve Medicare's administrative services to beneficiaries and health care providers. Currently, there are four Durable Medical Equipment (DME) MACs that handle the processing of DME claims and three A/B MACs (Jurisdiction 3, Jurisdiction 4, and Jurisdiction 5) to handle the processing of both Part A and Part B claims for those beneficiaries located within the states included in Jurisdiction 3, Jurisdiction 4, and Jurisdiction 5. All Medicare work performed by Fiscal Intermediaries and Carriers will be replaced by the new A/B MACs by 2011. Providers may access the most current MCR information to determine the impact of these changes at *http://www.cms.hhs.gov/MedicareContractingReform/* on the CMS website.

6

▶ **Figure 4-10   MSP Fact Sheet (*continued*)**

Are There Any Other Contractors That Identify MSP Situations?

In addition to the COB Contract, Medicare has a demonstration project in place to assist with the identification of claims that should have had an alternate primary payer. The Medicare Prescription Drug Improvement and Modernization Act of 2003 (MMA) mandated a 3-year project to demonstrate the use of Recovery Audit Contractors (RACs) in identifying underpayments, overpayments, and Medicare Secondary Payer situations for Medicare claims.

The RAC Demonstration Project consists of two different types of audit contractors: Claim RACs and MSP RACs. The Claim RACs are tasked with identifying underpayments and overpayments made on Medicare claims, while the MSP RACs are responsible for identifying claims where Medicare was not the primary payer. The RAC Demonstration is currently operating in three states with the highest rate of Medicare utilization: California, Florida, and New York.

For more information about the RAC demonstration, including MLN Matters articles on the topic, and a Frequently Asked Questions list, please visit *http://www.cms.hhs.gov/RAC/* on the CMS website.

Where Can I Find More Information on the Provider's, Physician's, or Other Supplier's Role in MSP and COB?

CMS offers several online references for information about MSP, COB, and the Medicare Program:

- **The Medicare Learning Network Home Page**

  The Medicare Learning Network (MLN) is the brand name for official CMS educational products and information for

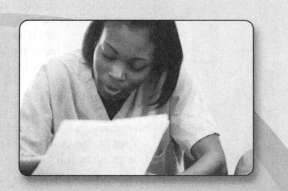

Medicare fee-for-service providers. For additional information visit the Medicare Learning Network's web page at *http://www.cms.hhs.gov/MLNGenInfo* on the CMS website.

- **The Medicare Coordination of Benefits Home Page**

  http://www.cms.hhs.gov/COBGeneral Information/

  The Medicare Coordination of Benefits Home Page features materials related to the MSP provisions.

- **The Contacting the COB Contractor Web Page**

  http://www.cms.hhs.gov/COBGeneral Information/03_ContactingtheCOBContractor .asp

  The Contacting the COB Contractor Web Page contains the contact information and specific addresses for submitting COB Contractor-requested materials.

7

▶ **Figure 4-10   MSP Fact Sheet (*continued*)**

COB Fact Sheets: MSP Claims Investigation Fact Sheet for Providers

The Coordination of Benefits Contractor (COBC) initiates a Medicare Secondary Payer (MSP) investigation when it learns that a beneficiary has other insurance. The purpose of this investigation is to determine whether Medicare or the other insurance has primary responsibility for meeting the beneficiary's health care costs. This process involves developing additional information related to the beneficiary's health benefit coverage and resolving any conflicts in the information to ensure Medicare pays only what it is obligated to pay.

The goal of these MSP information-gathering activities is to identify MSP situations rapidly, thus ensuring correct primary and secondary payments by the responsible parties. Providers, physicians, and other suppliers benefit from these activities because the total payments received for services provided to Medicare beneficiaries are greater when Medicare is a secondary payer to a group health plan (GHP) than when Medicare is the primary payer.

MSP Claims Investigation

Trauma Development
Trauma/injury diagnosis codes submitted on a Medicare claim or information received will alert the COBC that an accident or traumatic injury may have occurred, and the possibility of an MSP situation warrants development. This process is known as **Trauma Development (TD)**.

In situations where the medical services are related to a workers' compensation injury, automobile accident, or other liability, another payer has the primary responsibility for payment of medical claims related to the injury. When the possibility of a liability situation arises to the extent that payment has been made or can reasonably be expected to be made by another liable party, and the Medicare claim submitted does not contain pertinent information about the other payer, a development questionnaire is issued. Payment may not be made under Medicare when payment has been made or can reasonably be expected to be made promptly (120 days) for covered items or services under any no-fault insurance (including a self-insured plan). Medicare is secondary to no-fault insurance even if state law or a private contract of insurance stipulates that its benefits are secondary to Medicare benefits or otherwise limits its payments to Medicare beneficiaries. If Medicare payments have been made but should not have been, or if the payments were made on a conditional basis, they are subject to recovery. If an MSP liability situation is identified after the Medicare claim is paid primary, you may be required to reimburse Medicare. The claim may be reprocessed or adjusted to reflect Medicare as the secondary payer.

A properly filed claim prevents the need for follow-up development and expedites the payment process. In these situations, it is important to include the date of incident and the insurance carrier's name, address, and policy number on the Medicare claim.

▶ Figure 4-11 **MSP Questionnaire**

The Provider's Role in Data Gathering

Prior to billing Medicare, providers must ensure that they are billing the correct primary payer. A few minutes during each visit can later save time and money. When collecting this data, the provider must indicate if the health care coverage is due to retirement and a supplemental policy.

A sample of the kind of questions a provider should ask are listed below:

- Does the patient have any group health plan (GHP) coverage based upon his/her current employment? (Medigap coverage should not be indicated.)
- Does the patient have any GHP coverage based upon his/her former employment?
- How many employees, including the patient, work for the employer from whom the patient has health insurance?
- Does the patient have any GHP coverage based upon his/her spouse's or another family member's current employment?
- Does the patient have any GHP coverage based upon his/her spouse's or another family member's former employment?
- How many employees, including the patient's spouse or other family members, work for the employer from whom the patient has health insurance?
- Is the patient receiving Black Lung benefits?
- Is the patient receiving workers' compensation benefits?
- Is the patient receiving treatment for an injury or illness for which another party could be held liable or is covered under automobile no-fault insurance?

The answers to these questions will assist you with completing a beneficiary's claim and submitting it to the correct primary payer. It is important that the questionnaire be completed in its entirety and in the exact format of the questionnaire.

Contacting the COBC

Questions regarding the First Claim Development process and all other MSP Claims Investigation processes should be directed to the COBC. Please call the COBC's Customer Service Department toll-free at 1-800-999-1118 or TTY/TDD: 1-800-318-8782 for the hearing and speech impaired. Customer Service Representatives are available to assist you from 8 a.m. to 8 p.m., Monday through Friday, Eastern Time, except holidays. Providers must identify themselves by supplying the representative with a valid UPIN, OSCAR, or NSC number. This ensures the privacy of the beneficiary's information. The mailing address for written inquiries is indicated below. Please visit the COBC's Web site at http://cms.hhs.gov/medicare/cob for more information regarding the COBC and the MSP Claims Investigation Project.

Medicare - COB
MSP Claims Investigation Project
P.O. Box 5041
New York, NY 10274-5041

▶ **Figure 4-11 MSP Questionnaire (*continued*)**

▶ **Test Your Knowledge 4-1**

After reviewing the MSP Fact Sheet and MSP Questionnaire in Figures 4-10 and 4-11, read the examples below and write the name of the primary insurance in the space that follows.

1. A 45-year-old patient comes in with coverage under two insurance policies; one is Medicare and one is Medical Assistance. Which is primary?

_____

2. A 12-year-old patient comes in with a broken leg from a car accident, and the father has insurance coverage through his work. What kind of insurance would likely be responsible?

_____

3. A 55-year-old patient is seen who has Blue Shield and Mutual of Omaha. The Mutual of Omaha policy is under her husband's employer, and the Blue Shield policy is under her own employer. Which is primary?

_____

4. A 15-year-old patient is seen who has Aetna and Prime Mutual Insurance. The Aetna is through her mother, whose birthdate is 03/15/60, and the Prime Mutual Insurance is through her father, whose birthdate is 10/14/58. Is her mother or father's insurance primary?

_____

5. A 67-year-old man comes in with Medicare and Blue Shield coverage. The Blue Shield coverage is through the wife's employer. Which is primary?

_____

Billing Insight   The Standard Electronic Claim Format

When electronic claims originally started, there was no standard format in which all parties—provider, payer and clearinghouse—exchanged information. Then, the National Standard Format (**NSF**) was developed. NSF was a set of defined specifications that insurance companies, clearinghouses and providers used to communicate claim information. Unfortunately, each entity started modifying the specifications and quickly, there were over 400 NSF formats for claims everyone was trying to manage. This was very cumbersome for all parties involved. (A comparison would be if vacuum cleaners had 400 possible types of plug-ins. It would be difficult to get one that worked.) So, the American National Standards Institute (**ANSI**) became involved to create a standard electronic claim format; the common name for clinics is the ANSI 837P.

MANAGING CLAIMS IN CLAIM MANAGEMENT

Clinics depend upon getting the insurance companies to pay claims, and the faster the claims are paid, the better. In the healthcare industry, the 80/20 principal applies to claims. In general 80 percent of the claims get processed the first time, but the 20 percent that do not get processed take 80 percent of the office's time. This time can be reduced by properly utilizing the Claim Management features. Medisoft provides features in Claim Management that assist in follow-up, such as claims status, claim grid, list only, search and sort, and claim details. These tools will be discussed individually next (Figure 4-12).

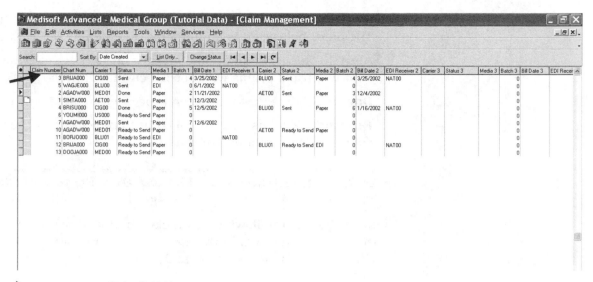

Medisoft Advanced - Medical Group (Tutorial Data) - [Claim Management]

Claim Number	Chart Num	Carrier 1	Status 1	Media 1	Batch 1	Bill Date 1	EDI Receiver 1	Carrier 2	Status 2	Media 2	Batch 2	Bill Date 2	EDI Receiver 2	Carrier 3	Status 3	Media 3	Batch 3	Bill Date 3	EDI Recei
3	BRIJA000	CIG00	Sent	Paper	4	3/25/2002		BLU01	Sent	Paper	4	3/25/2002	NAT00				0		
5	WAGJE000	BLU00	Sent	EDI	0	6/1/2002	NAT00				0						0		
2	AGADW000	MED01	Done	Paper	2	11/21/2002		AET00	Sent	Paper	3	12/4/2002					0		
1	SIMTA000	AET00	Sent	Paper	1	12/3/2002					0						0		
4	BRISU000	CIG00	Done	Paper	5	12/5/2002		BLU00	Sent	Paper	6	1/16/2002	NAT00				0		
6	YOUMI000	US000	Ready to Send	Paper	0						0						0		
7	AGADW000	MED01	Sent	Paper	7	12/6/2002					0						0		
10	AGADW000	MED01	Ready to Send	Paper	0			AET00	Ready to Send	Paper	0						0		
11	BORJO000	BLU01	Ready to Send	EDI	0		NAT00				0						0		
12	BRIJA000	CIG00	Ready to Send	Paper	0			BLU01	Ready to Send	EDI	0		NAT00				0		
13	DOOJA000	MED00	Ready to Send	Paper	0						0						0		

▶ **Figure 4-12** **Claim Grid Line**

Defining Claim Status

Once the Ready to Send claims have been processed either by paper or electronically, you will see that the status of the claims will be changed to Sent. Medisoft has incorporated in Claim Management a way for users to track the status of primary, secondary, and tertiary claims at a glance (Figure 4-13). The following are the types and meanings of claim statuses in Medisoft:

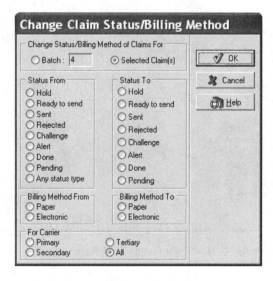

▶ **Figure 4-13** **Claim Status**

Hold: Claims that the user has put on hold so they will not be printed. (Usually, the claims are missing information, or additional information such as medical records needs to be sent with them.)

Ready to Send: Claims that are ready to print to paper or transmit electronically.

Sent: Claims that have been sent to the insurance companies.

Rejected: Claims that have been transmitted electronically and have been rejected. The reason can be found inside the claim in the Comment tab.

Challenge: Claims the office has noted the insurance has denied. The office believes it is an inappropriate denial and wants to appeal it.

Alert: This is an additional **claim status** that gives the user the ability to track claims with special circumstances.

Done: Claims that have been processed by the insurance company.

Pending: Claims that are billed but are waiting at the insurance company for additional information.

PRACTICE EXERCISE 4-3 **The List Only Feature of Claim Management**

When rebilling or following up on claims, it is very useful to view only the specific claims needed. In this exercise, we are going to view claims that are in the Sent status for Dwight Again.

1 Once inside Claim Management, select the List Only button at the top of the grid columns. Notice in the pop-up box that appears there are several criteria available to sort claims. Hit the Help button to the right to view the definitions of each criterion (Figure 4-14).

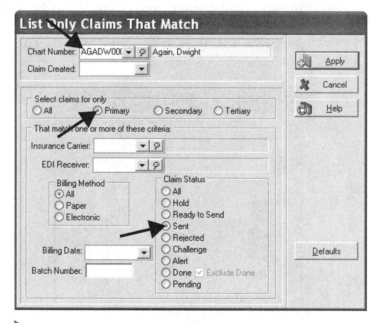

▶ Figure 4-14 **List Only Claims That Match**

2 To view the outstanding claims for Dwight Again, enter the Chart number for Dwight, select Exclude Done, and press Apply.

3 Write a quick synopsis of the claims for Dwight that are still outstanding, including the dates of service and the payer(s) still needing to process the claims.

Automatic Versus Manual Claim Status

It can be useful to differentiate claims statuses that are automated by the software from the ones manually changed by the user for tracking purposes. Let's break down the two categories for a closer look into Claim Management.

Category 1: Ready to Send, Sent, Rejected, and Done. These claim status types can be generated automatically by the computer or manually by the user.

Category 2: Hold, Challenge, Alert, and Pending. These claim status types are generated only by the user. We have already reviewed some suggested uses.

Managing Claims by the Claims Grid, Search and Sort, and List Only

Once claims are printed and sent or transmitted electronically to the insurance companies, Claims Management is utilized to follow up on unpaid claims. There are many ways to find a claim for a patient or insurance company. First, we can sort the columns in the grid by clicking on any column header. Next, we can select the item we want to sort and type the applicable item in the search box. Finally, we perform multiple searches to filter the claims by clicking on List Only. Each option is described in detail in the following section.

The Claims Grid

To sort the information on the Claims Grid, simply point and click on any column header (Figure 4-15). The most popular items to sort by are

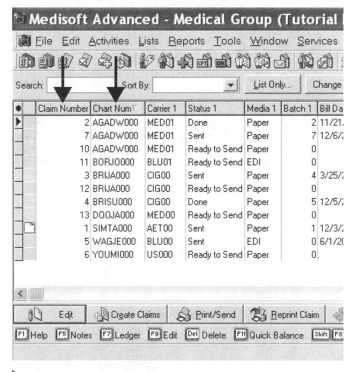

▶ Figure 4-15 Sorting Claims

the first two options: claim number and chart number. Questions often come from patients and insurance companies that require finding a specific claim to obtain crucial information such as the date the claim was billed, the method in which it was billed (paper or electronically), or additional information in the comment tab, to name a few. To locate a claim, office staff must first go to the patient's ledger and look up the patient's chart number and claim number. The claim number is set to appear automatically in the ledger, but not in transaction entry. As we reviewed in previous chapters, the grid columns in these areas may be modified to display additional information, and many users modify the transaction entry screen to display the claim number.

PRACTICE EXERCISE 4-4   Finding Claims

In this exercise, finding claims in Claim Management will be demonstrated in three unique ways: changing the view of the claims grid, Search and Sort, and List Only. This skill is imperative in claim follow-up. In all three examples, we will use the same claim number and chart number that we did in the previous sections of this chapter, claim 7 for Dwight Again and chart number AGADW000.

1   Find claim number 7 for chart number AGADW000 by sorting the grid columns first by claim number and then by chart number. To do this, click on the top of each column and watch Medisoft sort the columns. Then, visually find the appropriate item.

2   Use the Search and Sort options toward the top of the Claim Management screen. To do this, change the drop-down Sort arrow to Claim Number; then type claim 7 in the Search field. Next, change the drop-down Sort arrow to Chart Number; then type AGADW000 in the Search Field (Figure 4-16). Notice in each example there will be a black arrow to the left of the gridline pointing to the appropriate claim.

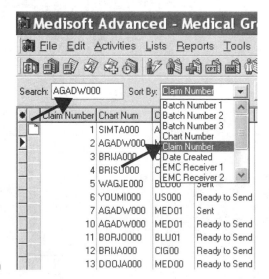

▶ **Figure 4-16   Drop-down Sort Button**

3 Use the List Only option to sort for all of Dwight Again's claims. Notice in this example that you do not have the option to sort by Claim Number. However, because we are changing the view to see only Dwight's claims, this is not an issue. Click on List Only at the top of the Claim Management screen, type Dwight's chart number, AGADW000 into the Chart Number area, and click Apply. This will display only the claims for Dwight Again (Figure 4-17).

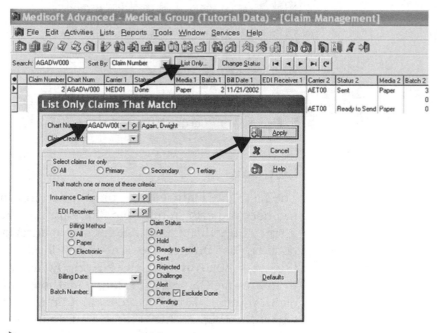

▶ **Figure 4-17   List Only Option**

Search and Sort

Another option for finding claim 7 for Dwight Again is the search and sort option. This option can be performed by first entering the claim number in the search field and changing the sort drop-down arrow to Claim Number (Figure 4-18). Or, we could enter Dwight's chart number (AGADW000) in the search and change the sort field to chart number (Figure 4-19).

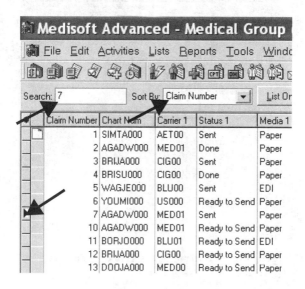

▶ **Figure 4-18   Sorting by Claim Number**

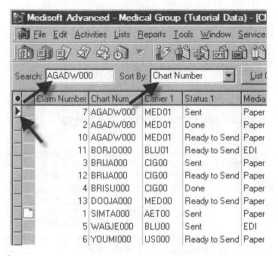

▶ Figure 4-19 **Sorting by Chart Number**

List Only

The List Only feature is the only option in Claim Management that allows the user to perform multiple filters on the claims at the same time and to display only the claims meeting those criteria. Using the same example, click on List Only and look at the options available to filter the claims (Figure 4-20). **Note**: We can search by many options from Chart Number to Insurance Company to Billing Method, but we cannot sort by a specific claim number. However, this is not an issue because by filtering by the Chart Number, AGADW000, we minimize our view to the claims for Dwight Again. Then, if needed, the Claim Number column can be clicked on to sort the claims for Dwight.

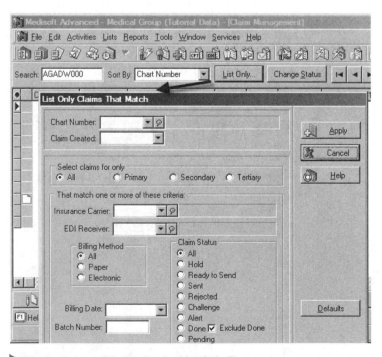

▶ Figure 4-20 **Sorting by the List Only Feature**

Medisoft Quick Tip — Mass Rebilling Insurance Companies

Occasionally in the medical billing field it becomes necessary to resend all of the unpaid claims for a particular insurance company—e.g., Medicare, Blue Shield, or an HMO. This occurs for a variety of reasons—for example, changed billing regulations or changed provider numbers and contracts or rebilling electronic claims. The List Only feature is very useful for this. First, you can filter the particular insurance in the List Only feature. Next, you can highlight all the claims and choose Change Status (Figure 4-21). The Change Status button allows you to change all the claims from a particular status (most likely Sent) to another status (Ready to Send allows us to resend).

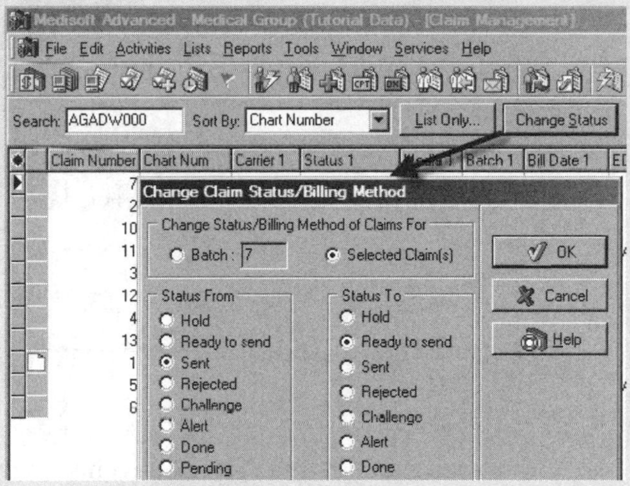

▶ **Figure 4-21 Changing Claim Status**

Viewing Claim Detail

Claim Management offers another important tool, viewing claim details. To view the claim details, double-click on any claim to bring up the detail window (Figure 4-22). At the top of the claim detail, four items are displayed: Claim Number, Chart Number, Claim Creation Date, and Case Number. Inside the detail window, there are five tabs: Carrier 1, Carrier 2, Carrier 3, Transactions, and Comment. The following is a list of the information contained in each tab.

Carrier 1: Gives the claim status, billing method, initial billing date, batch number, submission count, last billing date, insurance billed, and EMC receiver used of the primary insurance.

Carrier 2: Gives the claim status, billing method, initial billing date batch number, submission count, last billing date, insurance billed, and EMC receiver used of the secondary insurance.

Carrier 3: Gives the claim status, billing method, initial billing date batch number, submission count, last billing date, insurance billed and EMC receiver used of the tertiary insurance.

Transactions: Gives transaction detail for this claim including the date(s) of service, document number(s), procedure code(s), charge amount, and insurance companies billed.

Comment: Two types of comments are stored in the claim detail, automatic and manual comments. Automatic comments are recorded

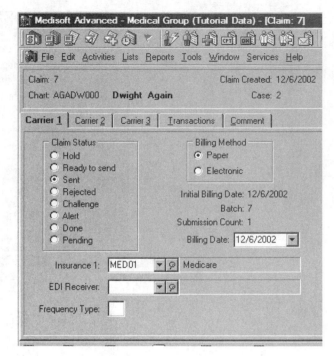

▶ Figure 4-22   Claim Details

when a claim is rejected electronically by Medisoft's clearinghouse. A manual comment is added by the user to track claim events.

Rebilling Claims

Occasionally, claims need to be resent to insurance companies. Once a claim has been billed, it cannot be printed again by hitting the Print/Sent button. Several ways to reprint claims are shown in the following list (Figure 4-23).

Reprint One Claim: To reprint one claim, either right-click on the claim and select Reprint, or hit Reprint Claim on the bottom toolbar and follow the previous directions for printing claims.

Reprint Several Claims: To reprint several claims at once, the control key can be held down as the claims are selected. Then, right-click on the claims and select Reprint or click the Reprint Claims on the bottom menu and follow the previous directions for printing claims.

Reprint a Group of Claims: To print a group of claims, click the first claim in the group while holding the shift key down and clicking the last claim in the group. **Note:** The claims will all be highlighted. Then, right-click on the claims and select Reprint or click the Reprint Claims on the bottom menu bar and follow the previous directions for printing claims.

Unfortunately, in the billing world, about 20 percent of the claims billed do not get paid the first time, hence rebilling claims is necessary. There are three ways you can rebill claims: one at a time, selected multiple claims, or groups of claims.

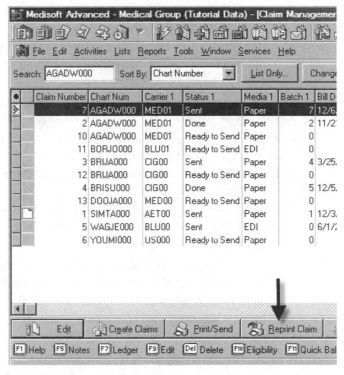

▶ Figure 4-23   Reprinting Claims

PRACTICE EXERCISE 4-5   Rebilling Claims One at a Time

In this exercise, rebilling claims one at a time will be reviewed.

1   Rebilling one claim at a time is quite simple. First, find the claim that needs to be rebilled through the sorting processes discussed previously.

2   Next, highlight the claim.

3   Click Reprint Claim on the bottom toolbar or right-click on the highlighted claim and choose Reprint Claim from the drop-down menu (Figure 4-24). This will bring up the Open Report box and printing options discussed previously.

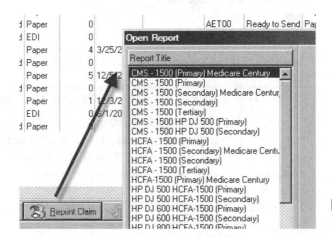

▶ Figure 4-24   Reprinting Claims/Open Report Box

4 Select the appropriate claim form and Preview it to the screen. **Note**: If the form fails to appear, it is because the claim form selected does not match the criteria for printing the claim. Example: An EDI claim is selected to print as a Paper claim or a secondary claim form is chosen to print a primary claim.

PRACTICE EXERCISE 4-6   Rebilling Claims by Selection

Occasionally, it becomes necessary to selectively pick and choose claims. This can be done by holding the Control key down on the keyboard and pointing and clicking on desired claims. Let's practice.

1 While holding the Control key down, point to three or four claims in the Claim Management grid. After the claims are selected, they will be highlighted in blue.

2 There are two options for printing the claim: Either click on the Reprint Claim button on the bottom toolbar or right-click on one of the selected claims, then choose Reprint Claims on the drop-down menu (Figure 4-25). This will bring up the Open Report box and printing options discussed previously.

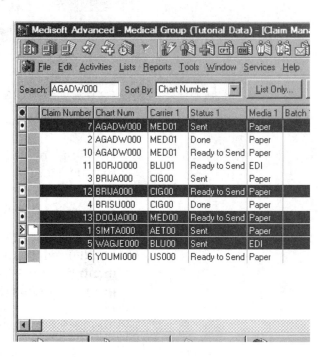

▶ **Figure 4-25   Selecting Multiple Claims**

3 Select the appropriate claim form to preview the claims.

PRACTICE EXERCISE 4-7   Rebilling Claims in a Group

Finally, billers often find themselves rebilling entire groups of claims either for a particular patient or insurance company. The most effortless way to accomplish this is to first filter the claims for the patient or insurance company as discussed in previous exercises.

1 After opening Claim Management, select List Only from above the grid columns.

2 In the Insurance Carrier filter, enter MED01 to filter the Medicare claims and then hit Apply.

3 Next, hold the shift key down while pointing to the first claim and then the last claim in the group (Figure 4-26). Notice all the selected claims will turn blue.

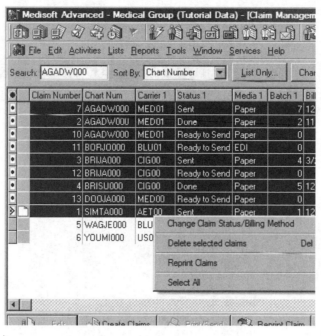

▶ **Figure 4-26** **Reprinting Groups of Claims**

4 Again, there are two options to printing the claim: Either click on the Reprint Claim button on the bottom toolbar or right-click on one of the selected claims, then choose Reprint Claims on the drop-down menu. This will bring up the Open Report box and printing options discussed previously.

5 Display and view the claims.

ALIGNING THE CLAIM FORM

One of the most frustrating problems a user encounters in Claim Management is when the CMS-1500 form does not align properly. The CMS-1500 is printed in a specific shade of red so that optical character readers **(OCR)** ignore the red color and scan the printed information. The gridlines on the claim form serve as a guide for offices to know where the data must be printed in ordered to be picked up by the OCR. If the data is outside of the appropriate box, the claim may be returned to the office as unable to be processed. The only way to fix the layout is to go to Design Custom Reports and Bills. To open Design Custom Reports and Bills, go to Reports on the main menu, and then Design Custom Reports and Bills at the bottom of the list. Once inside this feature, you will notice that it looks very similar to any word processing software. Go to File on the main menu and Open. For this example, choose to open the CMS–1500 Primary form (Figure 4-27). If the claim form has only several fields that need to be adjusted, it is easy to drop and drag the fields on the displaying page. If the claim form has numerous fields misaligned, hours of time could be saved by changing the band widths. To explore the details of Design Custom Reports and Bills, click on the Help icon or hit F1 once inside the program. All the fine points of designing will be explained.

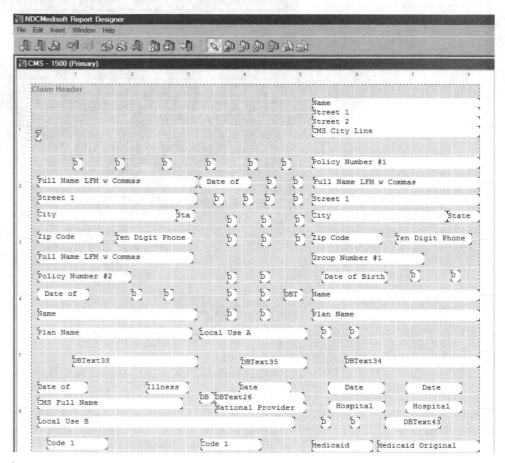

▶ Figure 4-27 **Design Custom Reports and Bills**

PRACTICE EXERCISE 4-8   A Final Review of Creating, Filtering, and Printing Claims

In this comprehensive exercise, claims will be created, filtered, and printed. Creating claims is the first step when sending claims to the insurance company to be processed. Complete the following steps to perform this process.

1   Familiarize yourself with opening Claim Management. Remember, there are two options to arrive at Claim Management. First, from the menu bar located at the top of Medisoft, select Activities, then Claim Management. Second, open Claim Management by selecting the icon that has a red claim form on it on the upper toolbar. Notice as you point to the different icons on the toolbar, pop-up messages will tell you which Medisoft process you are accessing. Open Claim Management using both options now.

2 Next, after you are in Claim Management, click on the Create Claims button on the bottom toolbar (Figure 4-28). A pop-up screen will appear. This screen shows the available filters to apply to the claims. Click on the Help button in this screen and review the meaning of each filter.

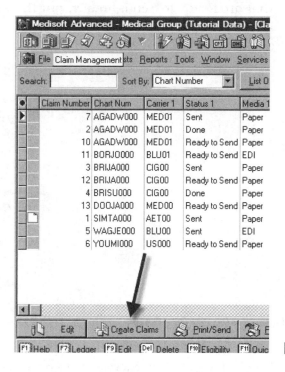

▶ **Figure 4-28   Create Claims**

3 Close the Help screen and click the Create button in the upper right corner of the box (Figure 4-29). Medisoft will now review all the transactions in the database that have insurance and have not been placed on a claim and will create claims for each.

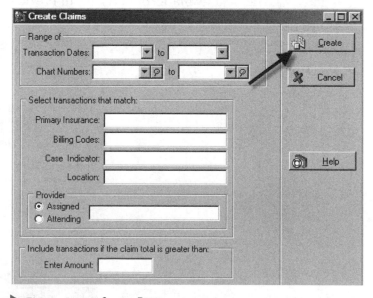

▶ **Figure 4-29   Create Button**

4 Next, filter the claims to first show the Ready to Send, then the Sent claims, then back to the Ready to Send claims. This is done by hitting the List Only button (Figure 4-30). In List Only, select Primary and Ready to Send. This will show you the Primary Claims that are ready to print to paper or transmit electronically. This same procedure can be run again to show the Secondary or Tertiary claims that are Ready to Send. Finally, put the view back to the Primary claims that are Ready to Send.

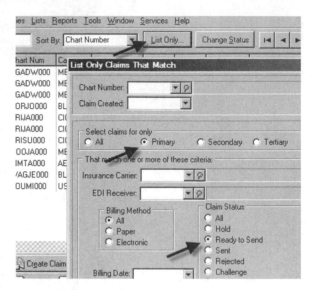

▶ **Figure 4-30   List Only Button**

5 The last step in this exercise is to Print/Send the claims. Click on the Print/Send button (Figure 4-31). This brings up the option to send on paper, electronically, or through Claims Manager. Claims Manager is a new service provided by Medisoft and will not be covered in this chapter. Select the paper radio button and then OK. Next, the Open Report option will pop up. Remember, we are going to print the primary claims, pick the CMS-1500 (Primary) form and then hit OK. The next available options are to Preview, Print, or Export; select

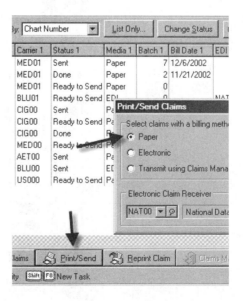

▶ **Figure 4-31   Print/Send Button**

Preview and Start. Now, the filter options appear, but we want to preview all available claims, so select OK. This will display all the paper claims that are Ready to Send. At this point, please check with your instructor to see if you have the option to print to a printer, PDF, or MDI file. If so, do that now. You can watch the Ready to Send paper claims change to Sent automatically by Medisoft.

6   To send electronic claims, click Print/Send and choose the Electronic radio button and hit OK (Figure 4-32). This should bring up the NDC Electronic Claims Processing module. (If a prompt appears to register the program, select Register Later.) In this module, primary and secondary claims can be billed as well as other options. To view the complete information on the options available, click on Help. Next, to transmit the primary claims, click Send Primary Claims, and the filter box pops up. We will send all available electronic claims, so click OK. The next pop-up will ask if you want to view the Verification report. This report gives detailed information on the claims that are ready to transmit, so click Yes. Note on the report that the cover sheet shows the filter options, the last page gives the totals of the number of claims that will be sent and the dollar amount, and the pages in between show the details of the claims that will be sent. Now, click the Close button on the top toolbar. It will ask if you want to continue with the transmission since the system isn't set up to transmit, click No.

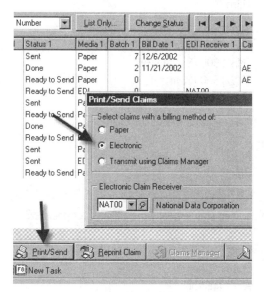

▶ **Figure 4-32   NDC Electronic Claims Processing Module**

CHAPTER REVIEW

Multiple Choice

1. What is the name for the bill sent to insurance companies?
   a. Claim Management
   b. Claim
   c. Bill
   d. All of the above

2. What is the process used to search for transactions not billed and create claims?
   a. Ready to Send
   b. Create Claims
   c. Claim Management
   d. EDI

3. What are the two ways to send claims?
   a. Paper and EDI
   b. Primary and secondary
   c. Create Claims and Ready to Send
   d. All of the above

4. If a patient has three insurances, what is the third insurance called?
   a. Secondary
   b. Primary
   c. Tertiary
   d. Third

5. What claim form is used to bill secondary insurance?
   a. Secondary form
   b. CMS-1500 (Secondary)
   c. CMS-1500 (Primary)
   d. CMS (Secondary)

6. Which claim status means the claim is paid?
   a. Sent
   b. Done
   c. Hold
   d. Pending

7. Which claim status means the claim is not paid yet?
   a. Sent
   b. Hold
   c. Pending
   d. All of the above

8. Which claim status means the insurance processed the claim but the clinic does not agree with the outcome?
   a. Alert
   b. Pending
   c. Hold
   d. Challenge

9. Which claim status means the claim has not been sent yet because additional information is needed?
   a. Ready to Send
   b. Hold
   c. Alert
   d. Pending

10. What can you find in the Comment tab of the claim detail?
    a. EDI rejected information
    b. Notes from the biller
    c. Both a and b
    d. Comments from the insurance

11. What are two examples of claim statuses automatically generated by Medisoft?
    a. Alert and Ready to Send
    b. Ready to Send and Pending
    c. Ready to Send and Hold
    d. Ready to Send and Sent

12. What is the name of the utility used to align the claim form?
    a. Claim Form Aligner
    b. Correct Claim Form
    c. Align Claim Management Form
    d. Design Custom Reports and Bills

13. How would a Medisoft user reprint a single claim?
    a. Open the claim and click Reprint
    b. Highlight the claim and click the Reprint Claim on bottom toolbar
    c. Right-click and choose Reprint Claim
    d. Both b and c

14. To sort for a single claim number, which is the correct option?
    a. Click on Claim Number at the top of the Grid and find claim in list
    b. Select the claim number in the Sort By field and type the claim number in the search box
    c. Click on List Only and enter the Chart Number associated with the Claim and the click Apply
    d. All of the above

15. Which of the following is an example of why claims may need to be filtered?
    a. To only bill certain dates
    b. To only bill certain procedure codes
    c. To only bill certain policy numbers
    d. To only bill diagnoses

True/False

Idenfity each of the following statements as true or false.

1. After claims are created in Claim Management, the claim status is marked Sent.

2. After claims are printed or transmitted, they are marked Sent in Claim Management.

3. Claims are marked Pending automatically by the system.

4. To print a paper claim for the primary insurance, select the CMS-1500 form (Primary).

5. There are six tabs in the claim detail.

6. In claim detail, the number of submissions for primary, secondary, and tertiary submissions can be found.

7. In the Comment tab of the claim detail, the date and time the claim was sent to the insurance is recorded.

8. The claim detail tells whether the insurance was sent on paper or EDI for each insurance company.

9. Claims are automatically marked Sent by the system.

10. Claims that are marked Done are sent but not paid.

11. Claims that are marked Challenged are not processed yet by the insurance.

Short Answer

1. List and define three ways to sort claims in Claim Management.

2. Describe the typical process of sending paper and EDI claims.

3. List and define each of the eight claim statuses.

4. Define clearinghouse.

Resources

American National Standards Institute (ANSI): **www.ansi.org**

ANSI is an organization that oversees the development of standards for numerous agencies including products, services, systems, and personnel. The standard for the electronic claim format is the ANSI ASC X12N 837.

Centers for Medicare and Medicaid Service (CMS): **www.cms.gov**

The CMS website provides tools to both providers and beneficiaries on the Medicare and Medicaid programs.

National Uniform Claim Committee (NUCC): **www.nucc.org**

NUCC is a voluntary organization that assisted in creating the CMS-1500 form. On the website, NUCC offers a free downloadable claim form manual.

Washington Publishing Company (WPC): **www.wpc-edi.com**

WPC offers a comprehensive website to assist with Electronic Data Interchange standard transactions.

5

Posting Mail Payments and Balancing the Day

Learning Objectives

After completing this chapter, you should be able to:

- ◆ Define and spell the key terminology in this chapter.
- ◆ Understand and define the components of Enter Deposits/Payments.
- ◆ Explain how to open, prepare, and process the mail.
- ◆ Demonstrate how to post insurance and patient payments in the Deposit List.
- ◆ Identify and describe the differences in creating deposits for patient, insurance, and capitation payments.
- ◆ Describe how to apply patient, insurance, and capitation payments.
- ◆ Create and print a Deposit List.
- ◆ Create and print a Patient Day Sheet.
- ◆ Explain how to balance the daily deposits.

Key Terms

Adjustment Code   a code used in deposit/payment entry to post a write-off amount on a patient's account; may be insurance- or patient-related adjustments.

capitation plan   contract that a provider signs with a carrier agreeing to treat a certain number of members in the carrier's plan. The carrier then pays the provider based on a designated fee each month for each member in that plan.

Copayment Code   a Medisoft code used in deposit/payment entry to apply a patient co-pay to a patient's account.

Deductible Code   the Medisoft code used to record the deductible transaction into the patient's account.

Deposit Code   a code assigned in Medisoft to each deposit that allows the deposit report to be sorted by the desired code.

Deposit List   the utility in Medisoft Advanced and Network Professional that allows the user to record payments, adjustments, and comments; also referred to as Enter Deposits/Payments.

Deposit Report   report inside of Enter Deposit/Payments that prints the deposits for a range of dates allowing filters for different payment options.

Enter Deposits/Payments   the utility inside of Medisoft that allows the user to post deposits and apply payments.

initial balance tape   an adding tape that is initially created by adding up the receipts of the day and used to balance the deposits and payments.

Insurance Code   the five-digit code assigned to the insurance by Medisoft when it is initially created.

Patient Day Sheet   Medisoft report used to proof daily transactions, showing all transactions posted on patient accounts for the selected time frame.

Payment Code   a Medisoft code used in deposit/payment entry to apply the payment to a patient's account.

Rejection Code   a Medisoft code that indicates the reason the insurance rejected the charge.

remittance advice (RA)   term that is used interchangeably with the term explanation of benefits.

Take Back Code   a Medisoft code used in deposit/payment entry to record the amount the insurance deducts from a payment to compensate for a previous overpayment.

Withhold Code   a Medisoft code used in deposit/payment entry to record the amount a contracted insurance company deducts from the provider's payment and may be paid back to the provider at the end of the fiscal period.

Abbreviations

BCBS   Blue Cross Blue Shield
RA   Remittance Advice

■ ■ ■ ■

INTRODUCTION

Clinics, like all businesses, need a cash flow to operate. There are two ways clinics receive revenue: as in-person payments and as mail payments. In Chapter 3, the correct procedure to apply payments received in person was demonstrated. This chapter will examine how to properly post payments and denials received via mail into Medisoft. Payments received via the mail may come from insurance companies, patients, or guarantors.

OVERVIEW OF POSTING MAIL PAYMENTS

Let's review our daily processes of inputting data into Medisoft and then add posting the mail. First, patients will call and schedule appointments. The office staff enters the appointment into Medisoft. Next, when the patient arrives at the clinic, he or she may complete patient information forms for the first time or update existing forms. The office staff enters the new or updated information in the system. Third, the patient is seen by the doctor and may make a payment prior to leaving the office. The office staff adds charges and patient same-day payments to the system. Finally, the mail will arrive and the office staff will process insurance payments and adjustments, insurance deductibles and denials, and patient payments and other inquiries. In this chapter, our focus will be on how to process the daily mail. In particular, Medisoft handles this process through a utility called **Enter Deposits/Payments**.

Accessing Enter Deposit/Payments

There are two ways to access Enter Deposit/Payments in Medisoft. The first is to go to Activities and select Enter Deposit/Payments (Figure 5-1); the second option is to click on the Enter Deposit/Payments icon on the toolbar (Figure 5-2). **Note:** Once inside this area, Medisoft refers to this as the **Deposit List**.

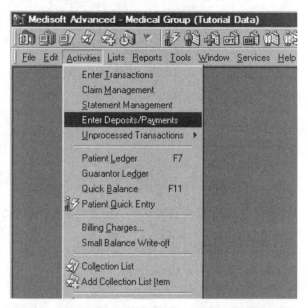

▶ **Figure 5-1** **Accessing Deposits/Payments Through Activities**

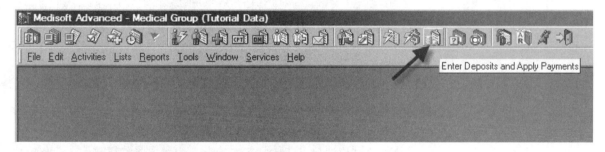

▶ **Figure 5-2** **Accessing Deposits/Payments Through the Toolbar**

PRACTICE EXERCISE 5-1 Viewing Deposits in the Deposit List

In this exercise, readers will become familiar with viewing and displaying deposits in the Deposit List. Both applied and unapplied payments will be viewed.

1 Open Enter Deposits/Payments or the Deposit List.

2 Click on Show All Deposits to view all the deposits that have been made in the system. **Note:** Some of the deposits have been applied and some are unapplied (Figure 5-3). Now, highlight a deposit that has been applied and click on Detail to view how the deposit was posted (Figure 5-4).

3 Finally, select the Show Unapplied Only button found directly below the Show All Deposits. This will display the deposits that have not yet been completed. At the completion of each day, this area should be empty and all deposits should have been applied.

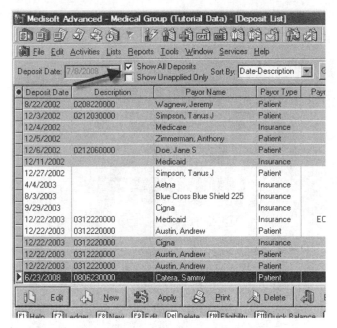

▶ **Figure 5-3 Show All Deposits**

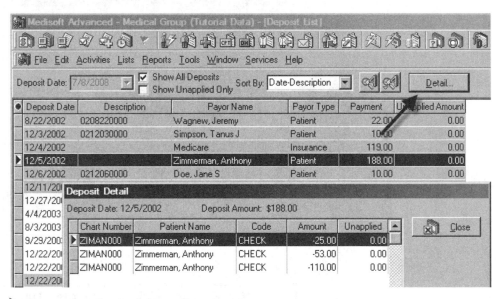

▶ **Figure 5-4 Detail of a Deposit**

Opening and Preparing to Process the Mail

Each day when the mail arrives, it should be opened and sorted. There will be numerous categories of mail including junk mail, bills to pay, and mail pertaining to the patient accounts, such as payments, denials, and requests for information. This chapter addresses the mail pertaining to patient accounts. The clinic will sort the mail associated with the patient accounts into one pile and add up the mail payments received. This amount is added to the same-day payments received from patients in the office. Together, these amounts create the **initial balance tape**, which should be run twice in order to assure its accuracy. The medical biller's task will be to process this portion of the mail into the Deposit List. When finished, a **Deposit Report** (Figure 5-5) will be printed and used as deposit slip for the bank. The Deposit Report needs to equal the initial balance tape and the payments on the **Patient Day Sheet**. The Patient Day Sheet, as discussed in Chapter 3, will assist the office in proofing and balancing the daily transactions.

Happy Valley Medical Clinic
Deposit Report
7/8/2008

Description	Check No.	Payor	Checks	Cash	Credit Card	Electronic	Totals
Thursday - September 4, 2008							
0809040000		Again, Dwight		20.00			20.00
0809040000		Austin, Andrew		10.00			10.00
0809040000	463	Brimley, Elmo	10.00				10.00
0809040000	553	Brimley, Susan	10.00				10.00
0809040000		Clinger, Wallace		15.00			15.00
0809040000		Gooding, Charles		10.00			10.00
0809040000	56510	Jacks, Theodore	5.00				5.00
0809040000		Jasper, Stephanie L		15.00			15.00
0809040000	60011	Johnson, William J	20.00				20.00
0809040000		Jones, Suzy Q		10.00			10.00
0809040000	126	Karvel, Jessica C	10.00				10.00
0809040000		Lyle, David F		15.00			15.00
0809040000		Peters, Anthony		5.00			5.00
0809040000	967	Peters, Zach	5.50				5.50
0809040000		Shepherd, Jarem		10.00			10.00
0809040000		Simpson, Tanus J		10.75			10.75
0809040000		Palmdale, Timothy		10.00			10.00
9/4/2008 Items: 17			$60.50	$130.75	$0.00	$0.00	$191.25
Total Deposit Items: 17		Report Totals:	$60.50	$130.75	$0.00	$0.00	$191.25

▶ Figure 5-5   **Deposit Report**

Billing Insights   Items in the Mail

Many items received in the mail do not include payments; however, they are very important to the patient's account. Examples of these items include EOBs with charges applied to deductibles, denials for no coverage, or requests for medical records. Believe it or not, processing these pieces of mail is just as important as processing the payments. By processing the nonpayments, accounts move one step closer to getting paid.

Creating a New Deposit

Posting payments in the Deposit List entails two steps. The first step is to create a new deposit and the second step is to apply the deposit to the proper account. Applying the deposit to the patient's account is what creates transactions in the patient's ledger. Completing the new deposit varies depending upon the payer type. There are three payer types: patient, insurance, and **capitation**. Capitation plans are contracts that a provider signs with a carrier agreeing to treat a certain number of members in the carrier's plan. The carrier then pays the provider based on a designated fee each month for each member in that plan. This gives the insurance company or large group a maximum amount it will have to pay for any given contract. The healthcare provider then assumes the risk. The healthcare provider may not provide as many services as anticipated and therefore realize a gain. Or, the healthcare provider may provide more services than expected and realize a loss. Capitation by design transfers risk from one entity to another.

Creating Deposits for Patient Payments

Three types of payments may be entered into Enter Deposits/Payments: patient payments, insurance payments, and capitation payments. The first payer type reviewed will be the patient payment. Let's review how to create deposits for patient payments by first opening the Deposit List. Next, click on New on the bottom toolbar. This will cause a pop-up window to appear (Figure 5-6). The following are the options you need to understand and complete:

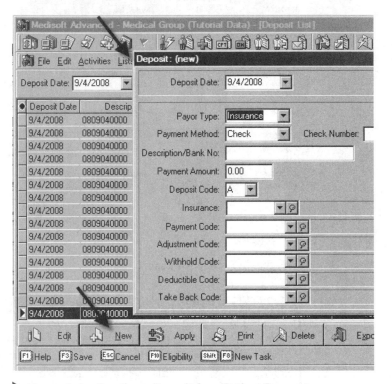

▶ **Figure 5-6 Creating a Deposit for a Patient Payment**

Date: Enter the date of the deposit. (Usually, it is the current day. Only if a past day of deposits is being posted would it be different.)

Payer Type: Select Patient for patient payments (*Patient* means payments from the patient, *Insurance* means payments or denials from the insurance, and *Capitation* means payments from a capitated plan.)

Payment Method: Enter Check, Cash, Credit Card, or Electronic.

Check Number: If applicable, enter the check number.

Description/Bank No.: This field allows the user to enter the bank name and account number so the Deposit Report will double as a deposit slip.

Payment Amount: Enter payment amount.

Deposit Code: This field allows the user to sort deposits by an assigned code. There are 26 available alpha categories and nine numerical categories. (Some clinics assign each employee a deposit code to balance out receipts. Other clinics use this to identify certain types of receipts such as patient versus insurance or one insurance type versus another.)

Chart Number: Enter the patient's Chart Number.

Payment Code: Enter the appropriate payment code.

Adjustment Code: Enter the appropriate adjustment code. The most common adjustment offices allow their patients are cash discounts for payments made at the time of service.

Copayment Code: If the patient payment is related to a co-pay, enter the appropriate copayment code. (A co-pay is the patient's responsibility for each visit prior to the insurance payment.)

Applying Deposits for Patient Payments

Once a new patient deposit has been created, the next step is to apply the payment. This is first done by highlighting the deposit in the list and clicking Apply on the bottom toolbar. This will bring up a pop-up window for the associated patient. In this pop-up box, there are many buttons and options; click F1 (Help) once the pop-up box appears and each will be explained in detail. The following are the options you should be most concerned with:

For: Chart number the payment will be applied to.

Unapplied Amount: Amount of the deposit that remains to be applied.

Apply to Oldest: Automatically applies the payment to the oldest charges.

Apply to Co-Pay: Applies the payment to any co-pay amount owed.

Save Payments/Adjustments: Saves the payments applied.

Close: Closes the pop-up window for this patient.

PRACTICE EXERCISE 5-2   Creating a Patient Payment Deposit

In this exercise, a self-pay payment of $10.00 will be posted to Dwight Again using the current date. First, a new deposit will be created and second, the payment will be applied to the patient account.

1   Open Enter Deposits/Payments.

2   Click on New at the lower portion of the Deposit List.

3   Complete each option using the information provided in Figure 5-7 and press Save. If needed, press F1 for Help to get further clarification of each field.

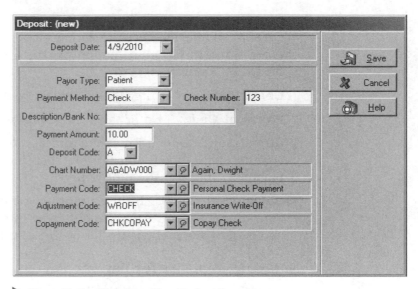

▶ Figure 5-7 **Creating a New Patient Deposit**

4 Next, click on Apply at the bottom of the screen and a pop-up box will be initiated.

5 If insurance has not paid on an account yet, the balance will not automatically appear for the payment to be posted. Hence, the Show Remainder Only needs to be unchecked in order to apply the payment. Apply the payment to the oldest balance (Figure 5-8).

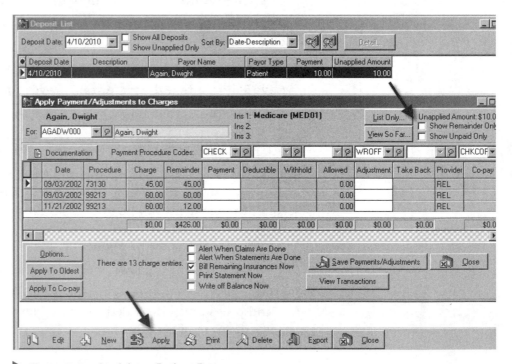

▶ Figure 5-8 **Applying a Patient Payment**

6 Click Save Payments/Adjustments and Close.

Creating Deposits for Insurance Payments

The second payer type reviewed will be the insurance payment. Again, this payment application begins by first opening the Deposit List. Next, click on New on the bottom toolbar, which will cause a pop-up window to appear. The following are the options that need to be understood and completed:

Date: Enter the date of the deposit. (Generally, it is the current day. Only if a day of deposits was missed and past days are being posted would it be different.)

Payer Type: Select Insurance (Again, *Patient* means payments from the patient, *Insurance* means payments or denials from the insurance, and *Capitation* means payments from a capitated plan.)

Payment Method: Enter Check, Cash, Credit Card, or Electronic.

Check Number: If applicable, enter check number.

Description/Bank No.: Allows the user to enter the bank name and account number so the Deposit Report will double as a deposit slip.

Payment Amount: Enter payment amount.

Deposit Code: Allows the user to sort deposits by an assigned code. There are 26 available categories. (Some clinics assign each employee a deposit code to balance out receipts. Other clinics use this to identify certain types of receipts such as patient versus insurance or one insurance type versus another.)

Insurance Code: Enter the code associated to the insurance making the payment.

Payment Code: Enter the appropriate payment code.

Adjustment Code: Enter the appropriate adjustment code for the insurance write-off. The adjustment code is used to record the difference between the billed amount and the contracted rate.

Withhold Code: Enter the withhold code associated with the insurance. A withhold amount is an amount in the contracted insurance holds out of the provider's payment and will possibly pay as a bonus at the end of the fiscal period.

Deductible Code: Enter the code to apply any insurance deductible amount. (Deductibles are the amount the insurance requires the policy holder to pay before the insurance starts to pay.)

Take Back Code: Enter the appropriate code to record an insurance take back. (Insurance companies sometimes pay in error and then later take back the payment out of their insurance checks.)

Applying Deposits for Insurance Payments

Once a new insurance deposit has been created, the next step is to apply the payment(s). This is first done by highlighting the deposit in the list and clicking Apply on the bottom toolbar. This will bring up a pop-up window for the associated deposit. In this pop-up box, there are many buttons and options; click F1 (Help) once the pop-up box appears and each will be explained in detail. Notice that the fields that appear in this window look like a spreadsheet. We will apply the payments/deductibles/denials in a method very similar to typing into a spreadsheet. The following are the options you should be most concerned with:

For: Chart number the payment will be applied to.

Unapplied Amount: The amount of the deposit that remains to be applied.

Payment: Amount paid by the insurance.

Deductible: Amount that insurance applies to the patient's deductible.

Withhold: Amount the insurance deducts from the provider's check according to the contractual agreement. The provider may recoup some of the withheld funds when the activity is reviewed at the end of the fiscal period.

Allowed: Refers to the amount the insurance will approve for service.

Adjustment: Amount the provider needs to adjust off of the patient's bill according to the contractual agreement with the insurance company.

Take Back: Occasionally, insurance companies pay in error and later recoup the payment from another check. This field is used for that purpose.

Complete: Used to indicate the payer has completed processing this charge. Medisoft then marks the claim done for that payer and moves the remaining amount due to the next responsible party.

Rejection: A code that indicates the reason for an insurance denial. The rejection code is initially created under Lists and Claim Rejection Messages.

Documentation: A pop-up box appears after clicking this box that allows the user to enter additional information regarding the transaction. Once inside of the pop-up area, the type of documentation can be created. If Statement Note is selected, the message typed will also appear on the patient's statement. This is specifically helpful if the office staff wants to convey to the patient why the balance is due from the patient.

PRACTICE EXERCISE 5-3   Creating an Insurance Deposit

In this exercise, an insurance payment of $20.00 will be applied to Tanus Simpson after $376.00 is applied to her deductible for date of service 12/3/2002. First, a new deposit will be created, and second, the deductible and payment will be applied to the patient's account.

1   Open Enter Deposits/Payments.

2   Click on New at the lower portion of the Deposit List.

3   Complete each option as shown in Figure 5-9 and press Save. If needed, press F1 for Help to get further clarification of each field.

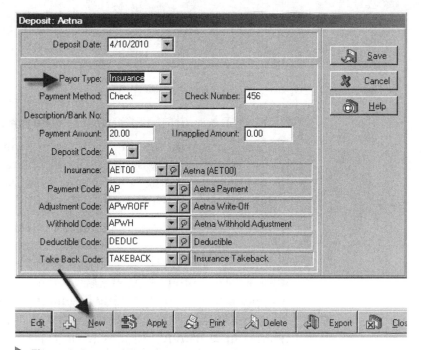

▶ Figure 5-9   **Creating a New Insurance Deposit**

4   Next, click on Apply at the bottom of the screen and a pop-up box will be initiated.

5   Look at the dates of service for 12/3/2002. The first three will be processed entirely against the patient's deductible, and $20.00 of the last charge was paid after $40.00 was applied toward the deductible. Post the deductible and payments now (Figure 5-10).

6   Click Save Payments/Adjustments and Close.

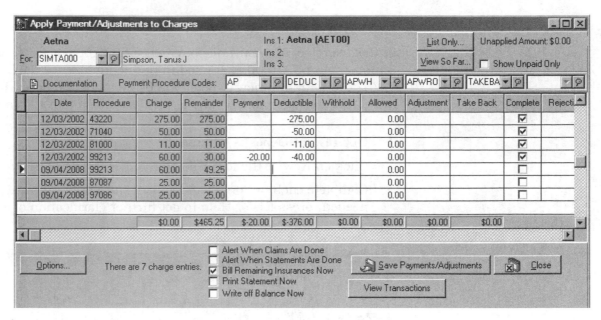

▶ Figure 5-10 **Applying an Insurance Payment**

Creating Deposits for Capitation Payments

The third payer type reviewed will be the capitation payment. Begin this payment application by opening Deposit List. Next, click on New on the bottom toolbar. This will cause a pop-up window to appear. The following are the options you need to understand and complete:

Date: Enter the date of the deposit. (Generally, it is the current day. Only if a day of deposits was missed and past days are being posted would it be different.)

Payer Type: Select Capitation (Again, *Patient* means payments from the patient, *Insurance* means payments or denials from the insurance, and *Capitation* means payments from a capitated plan.)

Payment Method: Enter Check, Cash, Credit Card, or Electronic.

Check Number: If applicable, enter check number.

Description/Bank No.:   Allows the user to enter the bank name and account number so the Deposit Report will double as a deposit slip.

Payment Amount: Enter payment amount.

Deposit Code: Allows the user to sort deposits by an assigned code. There are 26 available categories. (Some clinics assign each employee a deposit code to balance out receipts. Other clinics use this to identify certain types of receipts such as patient versus insurance or one insurance type versus another.)

Insurance Code: Enter the code associated with the insurance making the payment.

Applying Payments/Adjustments to Charges

After a deposit has been created in the Deposit List, the money is to be applied to the proper account if the deposit is a patient or insurance payment. However, if the payment is a capitation payment, it will not be applied. Capitation payments are flat payments that cover a group of people, not specifically any one patient.

PRACTICE EXERCISE 5-4   Creating a Capitation Deposit

In this exercise, a capitation payment of $50,000.00 will be posted. Unlike insurance and patient payments, capitation payment application contains only one step.

1 Open Enter Deposits/Payments.

2 Click on New at the lower portion of the Deposit List.

3 Complete each option as shown in Figure 5-11 and press Save. If needed, press F1 for Help to get further clarification of each field.

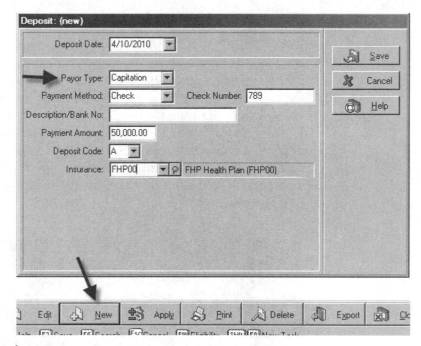

▶ **Figure 5-11   Creating a New Capitation Deposit**

4 After Save has been done, look at the list of deposits. They have all been applied (Figure 5-12). Capitation payments are not applied to a specific patient's account. The clinic receives a flat sum to provide unlimited contracted services to a group.

5 Click Save Payments/Adjustments and Close.

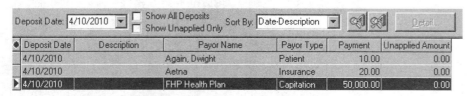

Deposit Date	Description	Payor Name	Payor Type	Payment	Unapplied Amount
4/10/2010		Again, Dwight	Patient	10.00	0.00
4/10/2010		Aetna	Insurance	20.00	0.00
4/10/2010		FHP Health Plan	Capitation	50,000.00	0.00

▶ **Figure 5-12   Viewing the Deposits**

Medisoft Quick Tip   Copayments

Copayments are the amount a patient owes each visit before the insurance begins paying. This amount is logged into the patient's case information in Medisoft, and the payments can be tracked for each visit. This can be a big time saver for the office staff.

Healthcare providers will contract with insurance companies to provide services at a reduced rate. The most common contracted payers are Medicare, Medicaid, and Blue Cross Blue Shield (**BCBS**). The providers bill all insurance companies for services at the same rate; however, when the payment arrives, the amount over and above the contracted rate is written off as an adjustment. Occasionally, noncontract insurance companies will modify their **remittance advice** (**RA**) to show an amount over the usual and customary billed rate. Since there is no contractual obligation, the provider is not obligated to write off those amounts. The office staff needs to be certain which insurance companies are contracted payers so only the appropriate charges are adjusted.

Printing the Deposit Report

After all the deposits have been entered and the payments applied, it is time to print the Deposit Report. Printing the Deposit Report is done inside of the Deposit List. First, click Print on the bottom toolbar and then choose the options to preview, print, or export to a file. Finally, select the date range for the Deposit Report that needs to be printed (Figure 5-13). The report can also be filtered by Deposit Code and type of deposit, i.e., cash, check, insurance, etc. The total of this report must match the total of the initial balance tape that was created after the mail was opened. If it does not, the entries need to be compared to the tape to find the discrepancy.

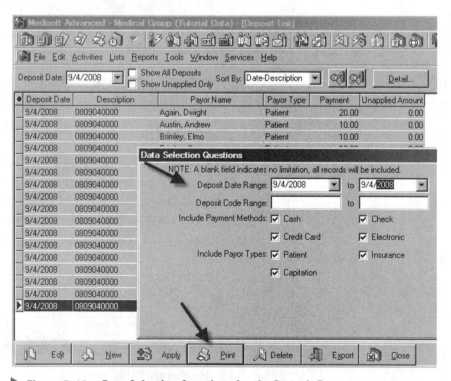

▶ Figure 5-13   **Data Selection Questions for the Deposit Report**

Printing the Patient Day Sheet and Balancing the Day

Once it is verified that the total of the Deposit Report equals the total of the initial balance tape, it is time to run the Patient Day Sheet. The Patient Day Sheet shows all the transactions that affected the patient's accounts for a designated time period. In Chapter 3, we reviewed printing the Patient Day Sheet to proof our charges and payments made at the time of service. In practice, the Patient Day Sheet would be printed after the charges, same-day payments, and mail payments are posted. To print the Patient Day Sheet, go to Reports on the main menu, then Day Sheets and Patient Day Sheet (Figure 5-14). This will bring up the data selection window for the report (Figure 5-15). This portion of the program can be a little tricky. The two areas of concern are the Date Created Range and the Date From Range. The Date Created Range is the dates the transactions

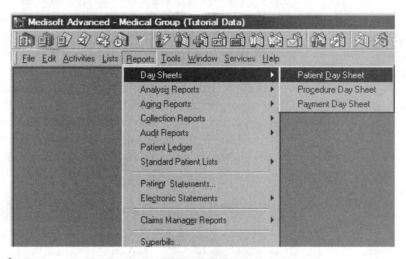

▶ Figure 5-14   **Printing the Patient Day Sheet**

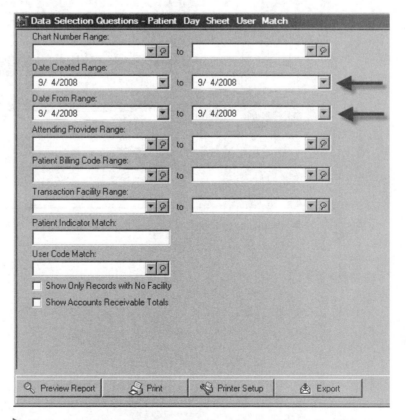

▶ Figure 5-15   **Data Selection Questions for the Patient Day Sheet**

were entered into the system, and the Date From Range is the dates the transactions actually occurred. For example, if the patient was seen on 03/11/2010 and the biller entered the charges and payments on 03/12/2010, the Date From Range would be 03/11/2010 while the Date Created Range would be 03/12/2010. **Note:** Medisoft defaults the Date Created Range to be the current date and the Date From Range to be a broad span of 150 years. If the report is being run the same date as the entries, the Date Created Range can be left alone. Otherwise, it needs to be changed to the span of dates the transactions were created. The Date From Range will always need to be changed to the date on the Deposit Report. To review a complete description of all the data selection questions, press F1. Next, choose the option to preview, print or export to a file on the bottom tool bar. This report will display the transactions posted to patient accounts. Since the capitated payments are not applied to the patient accounts, the capitated payments need to be added manually to this report and it needs to be verified that it equals the Deposit Report and the initial balance tape. If there is a discrepancy, the transactions on the Patient Day Sheet need to be compared to the Deposit List. If needed, the detail of each deposit can be displayed by highlighting the deposit and clicking Detail on the upper tool bar. (Figure 5-16)

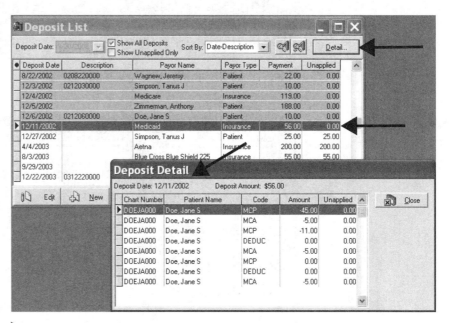

▶ Figure 5-16   **Displaying the Detail of a Deposit**

Medisoft Quick Tip One of Medisoft's Little Known Secrets

Medisoft has a little known secret that can be found inside of Apply Payment/Adjustments to Charges (Figure 5-17). The tool can be found by right-clicking any place on the transaction grid and a drop-down box will appear. Everything from viewing transaction detail to changing the claim status can be done from this box. This feature can save hours of time and contributes to more effective follow-up.

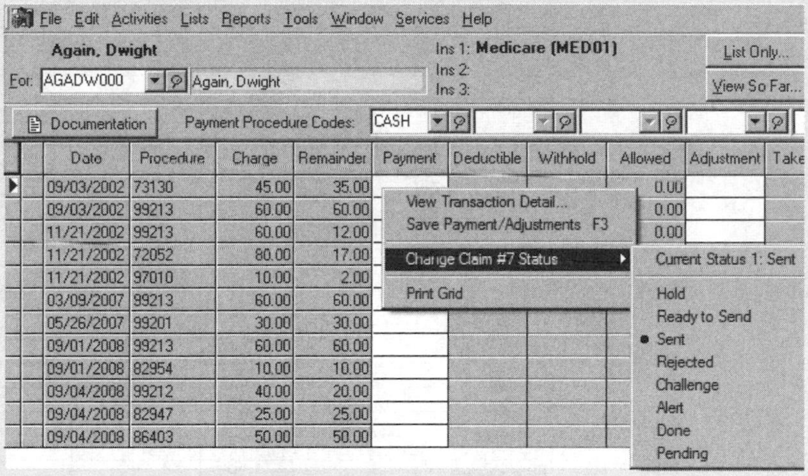

▶ **Figure 5-17 One of Medisoft's Little Known Secrets**

▶ Test Your Knowledge 5-1

Imagine you are the person responsible for posting the receipts for a large clinic. Explain a good checks-and-balance system that you have implemented to proof your work.

PRACTICE EXERCISE 5-5 Entering New Deposits: Additional Practice

For the purpose of this exercise, imagine the mail has arrived, has been sorted, and an initial balance tape has been created. Generally, the mail would include many different types of documents from different insurance companies and patients. For the purpose of this exercise, the insurance and patient payments have been condensed to a spreadsheet (Refer to Figure 5-18). Take the following steps to enter the deposits:

1 Open Enter Deposits/Payments.

2 Create a new deposit for the each of the items on the spreadsheet, identifying the following items (Figure 5-19):

a Date

b Payer Type

c Payment Method

d Check Number (if applicable)

e Payment Amount

f Insurance or Chart

g Codes as applicable (i.e., Payment, Adjustment, etc.)

3 Once the deposits are entered into the Enter Deposits/Payments, print a Deposit report to make sure it balances with the spreadsheet.

Sunny Life Clinic
Payment Journal - 03/11/2010

Payer Source		Amount Billed	Ins/Pt Payment	Insurance Adjustment
Aetna - re: Tanus J. Simpson - Ck #112		$396.00	$200.00	$0.00
Cigna - re: Jay Brimley - Ck #8721		$95.00	$50.00	$20.00
Medicare - re: Dwight Again - Ck #9078		$105.00	$80.00	$5.00
John Borden - Ck #896		$106.00	$20.00	
Susan Brimley - Cash		$12.00	$12.00	
Sammy Catera - Ck #2783		$71.00	$71.00	
			$433.00	
Insurance Application				
Tanus Simpson - Aetna	CPT*	Billed	Insurance Pmt	Adjustment
DOS: 12/03/2002	43220	$275.00	$89.00	$0.00
	71040	$50.00	$50.00	$0.00
	81000	$11.00	$11.00	$0.00
	99213	$60.00	$50.00	$0.00
Dwight Again - Medicare				
DOS: 09/03/2002	CPT*			
	73120	$45.00	$32.00	$5.00
	99213	$60.00	$48.00	
Jay Brimley - Cigna				
Payer Source	CPT*			
	99214	$65.00	$20.00	$0.00
	97260	$30.00	$30.00	$0.00

▶ Figure 5-18   Payment Journal for Medical Group

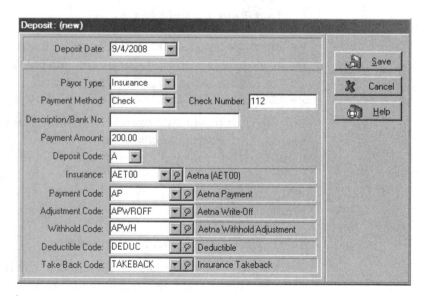

▶ Figure 5-19   Creating Deposits

PRACTICE EXERCISE 5-6   Applying Deposits: Additional Practice

Now that the deposits are created in Enter Deposits/Payments, we must apply the payments to the patient accounts. (Remember, if we had a payment from a capitated plan, it is not applied to the patient account.)

1   Open Enter Deposits/Payments.

*CPT is a registered trademark of the American Medical Association.

2 Highlight the first deposit in the list and click Apply.

3 Look at the Insurance Application of the Payment Journal and apply the payments accordingly. With insurance payments, make sure to apply the contract adjustments if applicable and with patient payments apply the payment via the Apply to Oldest option. Some accounts may need the Show Remainder Only or Show Unpaid Only check box unchecked to apply the payment.

4 Repeat until all payments have been applied.

PRACTICE EXERCISE 5-7   Balancing the Day: Additional Practice

After the deposits have been created and the payments applied, it is time to balance the day and make sure everything is in order. This will be done by printing the Deposit Report and the Patient Day Sheet.

1 Open Enter Deposit/Payments and click Print on the bottom toolbar. Follow the prompts to either display or print the report.

2 Next, run the Patient Day Sheet by going to Reports, Day Sheets, Patient Day Sheet, following the prompts to either display or print the report. If the Deposit Report and the Patient Day Sheet are created and the totals do not match, compare the details of the Deposit Report, Patient Day Sheet, and payment journal/spreadsheet to find the discrepancy. Fix the error and reprocess the reports until the day is balanced.

CHAPTER REVIEW

Multiple Choice

1. What is the name of the code assigned to a deposit and used to sort the deposits?
   a. Deposit Code
   b. Deductible Code
   c. Adjustment Code
   d. All of the above

2. What is the name of the code used to report the amount of money the insurance company withholds from an insurance check due to a previous incorrect payment?
   a. Withhold Code
   b. Take Back Code
   c. Payment Return Code
   d. All of the above

3. Which type of payment(s) are included in the Deposit List?
   a. Patient
   b. Insurance
   c. Capitation
   d. All of the above

4. Which type of payment(s) are not included on the Patient Day Sheet?
   a. Patient
   b. Insurance
   c. Capitation
   d. All of the above

5. Which type of payment(s) are included in the Deposit Report?
   a. Patient
   b. Insurance
   c. Capitation
   d. All of the above

6. Where are insurance payments posted?
   a. Transaction Entry
   b. Insurance Deposit
   c. Enter Deposits/Payments
   d. All of the above

7. Where are patient payments posted?
   a. Transaction Entry
   b. Payment Deposit
   c. Enter Deposits/Payments
   d. Both a and b

8. What is the name of an insurance plan that pays a flat fee for its members?
   a. Flat fee insurance
   b. Capitated plan
   c. Max fee insurance
   d. Capitated fee insurance

9. Capitated plan payments show up on which reports?
   a. Deposit Report
   b. Patient Day Sheet
   c. Both a and b
   d. Capitated Report

10. When creating an insurance deposit, which code is selected to indicate the payer?
    a. Payment Code
    b. Insurance Code
    c. Adjustment Code
    d. Procedure Code

11. Which adjustments are providers obligated to take?
    a. Patient write-offs
    b. Noncontract payers
    c. Contract payers
    d. None of the above

12. Which note type should be selected for reject notices to print on a patient statement?
    a. Patient Note
    b. Transaction Note
    c. Statement Note
    d. All of the above

13. Which report only shows insurance payments?
    a. Deposit Report
    b. Insurance Payment Report
    c. Patient Day Sheet
    d. None of the above

14. Which of the following reports is run to proof charges and payments?
    a. Procedure Day Sheet
    b. Patient Day Sheet
    c. Charge and Payment Day Sheet
    d. Procedure Patient Day Sheet

15. Which receipts are not included in the Patient Day Sheet?
    a. Patient receipts
    b. Contract insurance receipts
    c. Noncontract insurance receipts
    d. Capitated plan receipts

True/False

Identify each of the following statements as true or false.

1. There are two ways a clinic receives payments: in person and in the mail.

2. There are two types of payments: insurance and patient payments.

3. Clinics need a cash flow to operate.

4. An adjustment code is used when the clinic writes off an amount of the charge per its contract with the insurance company and may receive some of the money back at the end of the contract fiscal period.

5. Anytime an insurance company lists an adjustment amount on the explanation of benefits, the clinic needs to write off that amount.

6. Every type of Medisoft has the Enter Deposit/Payment screen.

7. Clinics write off the adjustment amounts listed by noncontract insurance companies.

8. The payment amount on the Deposit Report and Patient Day Sheet should balance.

9. The Deposit Report only shows insurance payments.

10. The initial balance tape includes only patient payments initially made.

Short Answer

1. Explain the differences between patient, insurance and capitation payments.

2. Describe how to create a new deposit and apply it for all three payment types.

3. Document the proper procedure to close and balance a day of receipts.

Resources

Blue Cross Blue Shield (BCBS) Association: **www.bcbs.com**

This website is a great resource on insurance information for consumers and providers. An interactive explanation of benefits can be reviewed at: www.bcbs.com/blueresources/anti-fraud/explanation-of-benefits.html

6

Statement Management

Learning Objectives

After completing this chapter, you should be able to:

♦ Define and spell the key terms in this chapter.
♦ Understand and define the activities of Statement Management.
♦ Identify the two ways to access Statement Management.
♦ Explain how to filter and create new statements.
♦ Demonstrate how to filter and print statements.
♦ Identify and describe ways to sort, locate, and modify statements.
♦ Describe a follow-up policy for self-pay accounts.
♦ Identify two ways to create customized statements.
♦ Explain cycle billing.

Key Terms

Billing Code   a unique identifying code created by the user inside the Chart to identify a patient for the purpose of filtering statements, claims, and reports.

Case Indicator   a unique identifying code created by the user inside the Case to identify a patient for the purpose of filtering statements, claims, and reports.

electronic statements   statements sent electronically to a clearinghouse to be printed, stuffed, stamped, and mailed by the clearinghouse.

guarantor balance   the balance due from the person responsible for the patient's account; i.e., the parent of a minor child.

paper statements   statements printed, stuffed, and stamped by the office.

patient balance   the balance due from the patient/guarantor after all insurance sources have paid.

remainder statements   statements that print only for balances due from the patient.

self-pay balance   the balance due from the patient/guarantor.

standard statements   statements that print for all patients that have a balance, regardless of who owes the balance, insurance or guarantor.

Statement Management   the utility inside of Medisoft used to process and track statements.

Abbreviation

POS   place of service

■ ■ ■ ■

INTRODUCTION

Businesses like to be paid for their services on the day they were performed, so, ideally this chapter would not be necessary. However, in healthcare, many patients and guarantors do not pay their portion of the medical bill without being billed a time or two. This chapter will cover how to handle balances due from patients/guarantors.

OVERVIEW OF STATEMENT MANAGEMENT

Statements are the forms used to bill the patient/guarantor. There are two types of statements in Medisoft: **standard statements** and **remainder statements.** Standard statements are used when the clinic wants to print statements for all patients who have balances regardless if the balance is due from the insurance or the patient. Remainder statements are used when the practice wants to print statements only when the balance is due from the patient/guarantor, meaning all of the payer sources (insurances) have completed processing the charges on the patient's account.

In medical billing, the term **patient balance** is used loosely. If all payer sources (mostly insurance companies) have been exhausted and the balance remaining is owed by the patient, clinics often call it **self-pay balance** or patient balance. However, the real person responsible for the bill is the guarantor, who might not be the patient. This example is most commonly seen in parent/child relationships. The patient may be a child, who is not legally liable for the bill; the parent (guarantor) is. Going forth, the terms patient and **guarantor balance** or self-pay will be used interchangeably and refer to the person legally liable for the bill. In addition, some clinics bill statements once per month, and some clinics break their statements into a cycle and bill a set number of statements each day. This chapter will first cover how to create and print statements and then how to break them into a cycle.

Accessing Statement Management

The tool used inside of Medisoft to process and track statements is called **Statement Management.** There are two ways to open Statement Management. The first option is to click on the menu bar on Activities, then Statement Management (Figure 6-1). Or, on the toolbar click the Statement Management icon (Figure 6-2).

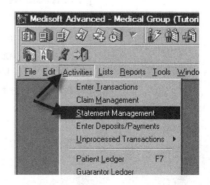

▶ Figure 6-1   Accessing Statement Management Through Activities

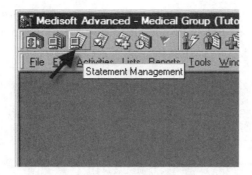

▶ Figure 6-2　Accessing Statement
Management Through the Toolbar

Medisoft Quick Tip　Printing Statements from Reports on the Menu Bar

Medisoft Basic users do not have the option to print statements using Statement Manager. So, there is a third way to print statements; this option is under Reports on the menu bar and then Patient Statements (Figure 6-3). This option does not offer the clinic staff the ability to track paid versus unpaid statements or to visually see the transactions or other details related to the patient statement. In addition, Medisoft Basic does not allow the user to print remainder statements. Since Basic was designed for cash practices, this is not a big issue because all the statements sent should be due from the patient. However, if a clinic processes a fair volume of statements each month, the Advanced or Network Professional programs should be used. The additional cost will be quickly absorbed by the time saved in Statement Management.

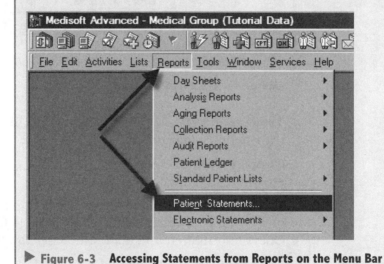

▶ Figure 6-3　**Accessing Statements from Reports on the Menu Bar**

Creating Statements

The first step to printing statements is to create them. This is done by first accessing Statement Management, then clicking on the Create Statements button at the bottom of the screen (Figure 6-4). This will give the user a pop-up menu to filter the statements that are to be created. When Create is selected, Medisoft will by default search for all statements that need to be sent out unless a filter is placed on the creation to restrict some statements from being created. Filters can be used to customize statement creation. They can be used to create statements for specific patients, transaction dates, chart numbers, billing codes, insurance company, statement type, or transactions that exceed a specific dollar amount. The following are the options for filtering statements. If the user chooses to enter a filter(s), Medisoft will create statements only for accounts that match the desired filters. If none of the filters are utilized, Medisoft will create all statements available in the system.

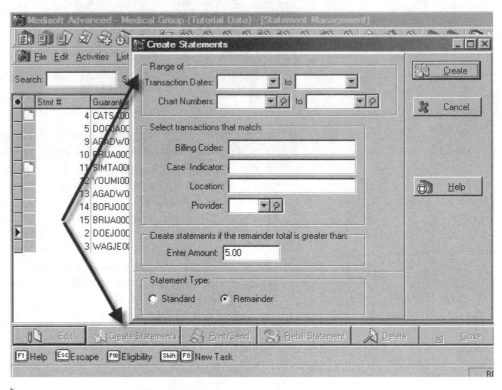

▶ **Figure 6-4 Creating Statements**

Transaction Dates: Allow the user to filter statements only for the transaction range entered.

Chart Numbers: Allow the user to filter for certain guarantors to receive a statement.

Billing Codes: Unique identifiers created by the user for the purpose of filtering guarantors. This billing code is found in the guarantor Chart information and allows the user to filter by this field.

Case Indicator: Unique identifiers, found in the Case, created by the user to filter Cases.

Location: Two-digit place of service (**POS**) code entered into Transaction Entry. For example, an office visit has a POS of 11 and a home visit has a POS of 12. This field allows the user to filter by visit type.

Provider: Allows the user to filter by transactions assigned to a certain provider.

Statement Amount: Allows the user to enter a threshold amount to not print statements below the amount listed. If an amount is not listed, the program will ask if the user wants to print statements with negative balances. If an amount is listed, the program will remember that amount each time until it is changed by the user.

Statement Type: Allows the user to create Standard Statements or Remainder Statements as defined previously in this chapter.

Printing Statements

The next step to printing statements is just that, printing them. This is done inside Statement Management by clicking on the Print/Send button at the bottom of the screen (Figure 6-5). This will give the user a pop-up menu to choose between **paper statements** and **electronic statements.** Paper statements will be printed at the office site to be stuffed, stamped, and mailed, whereas electronic statements will be printed and processed at a clearinghouse. For the purpose of this example, we will review printing paper statements. However, keep in mind that having a third party process bulk volumes of statements can save a practice a lot of time and money. Clearinghouses may offer this as an optional service.

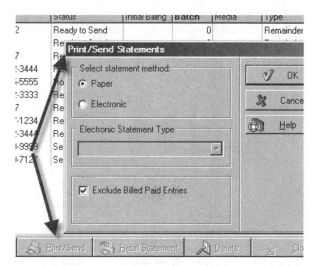

▶ **Figure 6-5**   **Printing Statements**

After selecting Print/Send and the option for Paper and OK, an Open Report box will appear (Figure 6-6). This gives the user the option to print statements in a variety of pre-defined formats. Users can also create their own statements in Design a Custom Report and add such items as logos or customize other data. All available statements, Medisoft or user-created, will appear in the Open Report box. The statements that have the word "remainder" in them will print remainder statements. All other statements will print standard statements. Again, standard statements bill the patient whether the balance is due from the insurance or the patient, and remainder statements bill the patient when the balance remaining is due from the patient.

Next, select one of the statements and OK, then Preview and Start, and a pop-up box will appear with another list of filters (Figure 6-7). One might

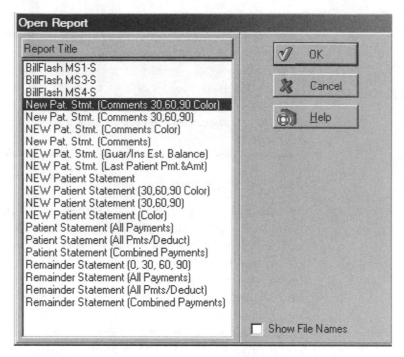

▶ Figure 6-6　**Choosing the Appropriate Statement**

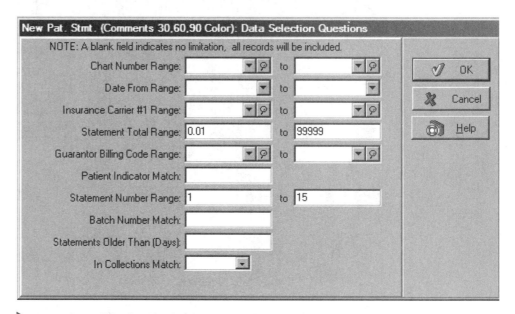

▶ Figure 6-7　**Filtering the Statements**

filter statement selections for a certain group of patients or statements within a certain date range. For example, for those clinics that use cycle billing, patients are divided into groups and statements are printed and mailed at different times throughout the month. These clinics would use Chart Number Range to send out batches of statements weekly based upon patients' last names. For those clinics that send large volumes of statements at certain times of the month to specific carriers, such as Medicare, Insurance Carrier #1 Range would be used. **Note:** Wherever you see options in Medisoft, use the Help button to define the options. The following are some options for printing statements:

Chart Number Range: Allows the user to filter statements by the guarantors' Chart numbers. This is used often by clinics that want to send out batches of statements weekly based upon last name. This helps to even the workload for statement processing and phone calls.

Date From Range: Allows the user to filter statements by transaction dates.

Insurance Carrier #1 Range: Allows the user to filter statements by the primary insurance code. This is especially helpful if the office wants to send large volumes of statements, for example, Medicare, at certain times of the month.

Statement Total Range: Allows the user to filter statements by statement balances. An example is that many clinics send statements only if the patient owes $5.00 or more; other clinics want to filter larger statements, say over $500.00, to do extra collection work and secure a payment plan.

Guarantor Billing Code Range: Allows the user to filter by the billing code that is listed for the guarantor. Remember, the guarantor code is listed on the Personal tab of the Case and is a unique code created by the user.

Patient Indicator Match: Allows the user to filter by the Patient Indicator. The Patient Indicator is a unique code created by the user.

Statement Number Range: Allows the user to print statements in a certain numerical range which is assigned by Medisoft. This is helpful if the printer jams up and only a few statements need to be reprinted, or if the clinic wants to print a certain volume of statements per day.

Batch Number Match: Allows the user to print statements by Medisoft batch number. The same reasons that apply to the Statement Number Range apply to Batch Number Match.

Statements Older Than (Days): Allows the clinic to print statements over a certain number of days old. This is particularly helpful if the clinic wants to send warning or collection statements to patients that have been billed previously.

In Collection Match: Looks at an activity in Medisoft called the Collection List that can be found under Activities. There are two possibilities, True or False. If the patient is in collections, the True filter will apply. Clinics use this to send customized collection statements to the appropriate patients.

After the applicable filters are applied, OK is selected and the statements are previewed to give the user the number of statements to be printed and to allow a chance to proof the statements prior to their printing (Figure 6-8). Finally, after the statements have been reviewed, they may be printed in this same window by selecting the printer button at the top.

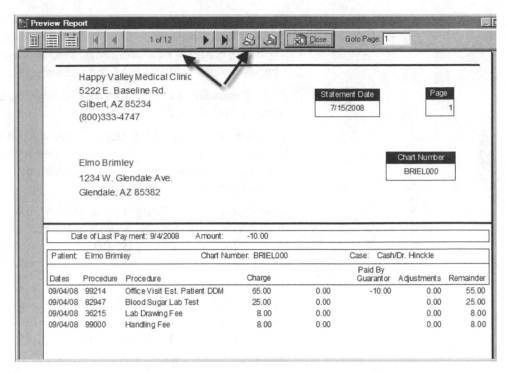

▶ Figure 6-8   Proofing and Printing the Statements

PRACTICE EXERCISE 6-1   Creating and Printing Statements

Creating statements is your first step in sending statements either on paper or electronically. Complete the following steps to complete this practice exercise.

1   Familiarize yourself with opening Statement Management. Remember, there are two ways to get to Statement Management. First, from the menu bar at the top select Activities, then Statement Management, or open Statement Management by selecting the icon that has a blue computer and statement on it. Notice as you point to the different icons on the toolbar, pop-up messages will tell you which tool you are accessing. Practice opening Statement Management using both options now.

2   Next, after you are in Statement Management, click on the Create Statements button on the bottom toolbar. A pop-up screen will appear. This screen shows the available filters to apply to the claims. Click on the Help button in this screen and review what each filter will apply.

3   Close the Help screen, select Standard for the Statement Type and click the Create button in the upper right corner of the box. Medisoft will then review all the transactions that have a balance and have not been put on a statement and will create statements for each. Note how many statements are created.

4   Next, display statements by selecting Print/Send. Remember, the statement chosen in the list must match the Statement Type created. The statements that say Remainder next to them will only print Remainder statements. The other statements print the standard statements. Display each of the statements available for the Standard Statement Type.

5 Next, mass delete the batch of statements just created and recreate statements using Remainder for the Statement Type. Note how many statements are created. Compare your previous count.

Medisoft Quick Tip   Statement Customizing Options

Medisoft offers two options to customizing statements: Design Custom Reports and Bills (DCRB) and Statement Wizard. Design Custom Reports and Bills can be found in the Reports menu, and Statement Wizard can be found under the Tools menu. To get acquainted with the features in these two options, open each item and hit the F1 for Help. Complete details will be displayed. One of the differences is Design Custom Reports and Bills allows the user to add logos, whereas Statement Wizard allows the user to customize electronic statements. DCRB is discussed in detail in chapter 10.

Tracking Statements

Once statements are created, printed and sent; the next task is to track the statements. The following list describes the columns that are on the Statement Management grid (Figure 6-9).

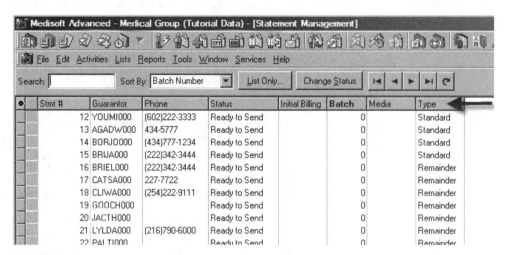

▶ **Figure 6-9   Tracking Statements**

Stmt #:   Gives the number assigned to the statement. Statement numbers are useful because they can be found in the transaction entry and in the patient ledger and assist the user in tracking the dates of service included in a statement. It also allows the user to filter or sort by the statement number.

Guarantor: Shows the Chart number of the guarantor that will receive/has received the statement. The guarantor may owe for more than one family member. If this is the case, the balances will be included in the same statement. However, the statement identifies the patient's name and chart number and portion due for each person. This feature helps the office and the guarantor reconcile balances due, as well as reducing the amount of paper that needs to be printed and statements that need to be sent.

Phone: The phone number listed is for the guarantor. This is handy for staff members who are calling on balances due.

Status: Shows the clinic at a glance what has happened with the statement. The following is a list of the status descriptions:

Hold: The office can use this status to stop statements from printing.

Ready to Send: Ready to Send statements are ones that are just created and have not been printed, or statements that the user has changed the status of to reprint.

Sent: Statements that are marked Sent have been printed or transmitted electronically.

Failed: Failed statements are those that failed to transmit electronically.

Done: Done statements have been paid in full.

Challenge: Allows the user to create a unique designation for the meaning and thereby create another way to track statements.

Initial Billing: Date the statement was initially printed or transmitted.

Batch: Each time statements are created, whether there is one statement or one hundred, Medisoft assigns the new creation a batch number. This is helpful to reprint or transmit an entire batch if there were difficulties.

Media: Shows whether the claims were printed on paper or transmitted electronically.

Type: Shows whether the statement created is a standard statement (showing all transactions due from either insurance or patient) or a remainder statement (showing only the transactions where the remainder is due from the patient).

PRACTICE EXERCISE 6-2   Tracking Statements

This exercise will familiarize the user on how to locate and find statements. This is particularly helpful in answering statement questions and performing follow-up on unpaid balances. Perform the following steps to complete this practice exercise.

1   Familiarize yourself with opening the Statement Management grid by clicking on each header of the grid. Watch the items sort by each field.

2   Next, add a field to the grid. Select the Date Created field to add.

3   Sort the Date Created field and find the oldest and newest claim created.

4   Finally, sort by the appropriate column to find the statements for Sammy Catera. Find out how many statements he has and the dates they were created.

Sorting and Filtering Statements

Frequently it is necessary to view the statements in Statement Management in a particular way. This can be done using one of two methods. As noted earlier, the user can simply click on a grid header to sort the statements based on that field. The user can still view all of the statements, but they are in a designated order. Alternatively, the user can choose to filter the statements according to selected criteria, and then will view only the statements that meet those criteria. This is accomplished by clicking on the List Only button at the top of Statement Management which causes a pop-up box to appear (Figure 6-10). The following is a list of options in the List Only pop-up box to filter the statements.

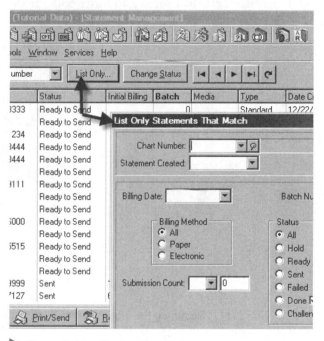

▶ Figure 6-10 Sorting Statements

Chart Number: Allows the user to view statements only for a particular guarantor.

Statement Created: Allows statements to be filtered by creation date.

Billing Date: Allows the user to view all statements billed on a date. This includes statements initially billed and statements rebilled on that date.

Batch Number: Allows the user to only view statements in a particular batch.

Billing Method: Allows the user to view statements sent on paper, transmitted electronically, or sent by both methods.

Status: Allows the user to sort statements in a particular status category. The status categories were reviewed previously.

Submission Count: Provides a very useful option for collection. Clinics often send one or two statements before a warning statement is sent. This feature allows the user to view only those statements sent a certain number of times, for example, two or more.

Modifying the Statement Management Grid

Wherever there is a grid in Medisoft, the items that display in the grid can be easily modified by clicking on the black button in the upper left corner of the grid (Figure 6-11). Grids are found in Claims Management, Transaction Entry, and under each of the List items, to name a few, and Statement Management is no exception. By modifying the grid, the work that needs to be done can be streamlined. In Statement Management, it is very useful to add the field Submission Count to the grid. This allows the user to see how many times the guarantor was billed and to sort by this number, and thereby to start collection activity if necessary.

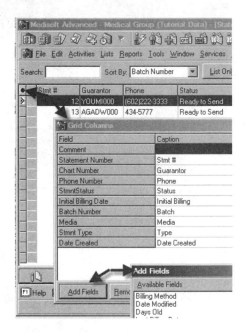

▶ **Figure 6-11   Modifying the Statement Management Grid**

▶ Test Your Knowledge 6-1

Imagine you are in charge of calling guarantors who have been billed twice but have not paid their account in full. How would you use Statement Management to quickly view guarantors meeting these criteria?

Billing Insight   Developing Clinic Policies for Self-Pay Accounts

When collecting money, it is important to have written and consistent policies. For example; after billing the guarantor, if payment is not received, how does the clinic handle the accounts at 30, 60, and 90 days? The clinic should handle all accounts consistently. Plus, by deciding on a policy, it gives staff clear direction on how to proceed. Of the clinics with one doctor or no doctors, fewer than half have verbal or written policies. Here is an example of a follow-up policy that is common:

Level One Account: The guarantor is billed the first of each month and makes payments each month.

Level Two Account: The guarantor has missed a payment and is sent a friendly reminder statement. If the guarantor makes a payment, the account will stay at a level two as long as consistent monthly payments are received.

Level Three Account: The guarantor has missed another payment. A collection letter is sent, and the guarantor is given 10 days to pay or go to collection. If payment is received, the

---

> account remains at a level three account. If payments stop, the account is promptly turned to collection.
>
> **Collection Account:** The account is written off the books as bad debt, the account flagged in Medisoft as a collection account, and the balance is turned over to a licensed collection agency. By writing the account off the books, accounts receivable integrity is retained with a true picture of collectible accounts. In addition, the clinic is able to track the amount of bad debt easily by printing a report of the bad debt procedure code.

▶ Test Your Knowledge 6-2

With the knowledge you have acquired for proofing your daily transactions, explain how you would proof the accounts turned over to collection and the amount turned over to collection.

PRACTICE EXERCISE 6-3   Creating Clinic Self-Pay Policies

In this exercise, pretend your job at a large clinic is to develop the clinic collection policies and manage patient balances. Conceptualize the clinic policies you would develop to define the collection process and how you would utilize Statement Management to adhere to the policies.

1   Outline the clinic policies for collecting patient balances, including when the first statement would be sent until when the account would be turned over to collection if it is not paid. Make sure the policy includes payment expectations—i.e., Does the account need to be paid in full? Does the patient need to set up payment plans? or Is it enough for the patient to make any kind of payment?

2   Create a detailed plan on how Statement Management would be used to accomplish the collection policies you have defined for the clinic.

Statement Management Tool Bar Options

There are some other time-saving tools that can be found in Statement Management. Let's take a look at the top and bottom toolbars in Statement Management (Figure 6-12).

The Top Toolbar

Search: Used with the next field, Sort By. For example, if you need to find a particular Batch Number or Chart Number, select the appropriate field in Sort By and enter the desired information in the Search Field (Figure 6-13).

Sort By: Gives multiple options to sort data. By selecting the appropriate item to sort, the user can either look at all the data in the sort or locate selected data by entering the item in the Search box.

List Only: Reviewed earlier in the chapter. List Only gives the user the option to display only those statements matching the criteria entered.

Change Status: Allows the user to change either a single statement or a group of statements from one status type to another. This is particularly helpful in reprinting or resending failed batches (Figure 6-14).

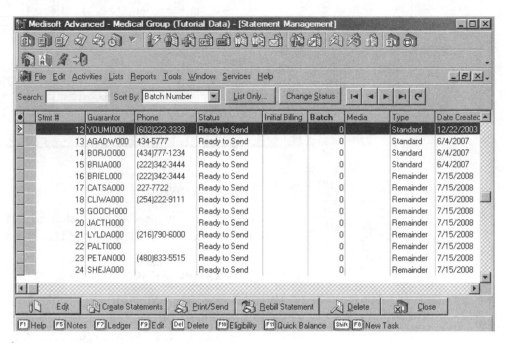

▶ Figure 6-12 **Top and Bottom Toolbars**

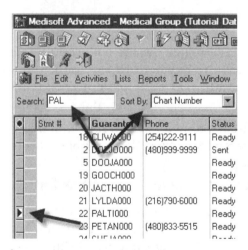

▶ Figure 6-13 **Sorting Statements**

Arrows: Used to move quickly through the statements. The first arrow jumps to the very first statement in the list. The second arrow moves up one statement in the list. The third arrow moves down one statement in the list. The fourth arrow moves to the last statement in the list, and the fifth arrow refreshes the view.

The Bottom Toolbar

Edit: By selecting a statement and clicking on Edit, allows the user to edit the status, billing method, billing date, transactions contained on the statement and to add comments for the office. The comments section is very useful to document conversations with the guarantor involving questions on the statement and payment commitments (Figure 6-15).

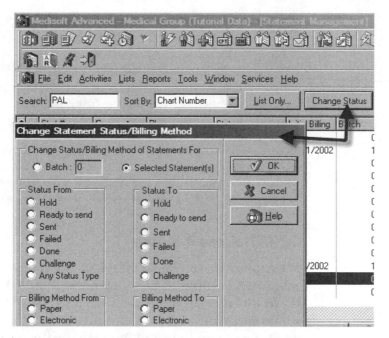

► Figure 6-14 **Change Statement Status/Billing Method**

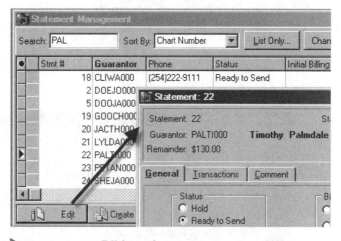

► Figure 6-15 **Editing a Statement**

Create Statements: As reviewed previously, allows the user to create statements.

Print/Send: As reviewed previously, allows the user to print or transmit statements.

Rebill Statement: Allows the user to select a statement and, by clicking on this button, rebill a single statement or a group of statements that are in the Sent Status.

Delete: By clicking this option, allows the user to delete a statement or a group of statements.

Close: Closes the Statement Management utility.

Cycle Statement Billing

Many offices, even small offices, send 300 or more statements per month. This can be a huge job done on one day, or it can be broken down into smaller jobs done over a period of time. In addition to the time it takes to print and mail the statements, the clinic also needs to handle all of the phone calls and inquiries related to those statements. It is evident that by sending statements in smaller batches, the clinic can better manage its work flow. With Medisoft, it is possible to set the program to divide the statements into batches. Here is how the user can set this up to happen.

1. Go to File and Program Options and click on the Billing tab (Figure 6-16).

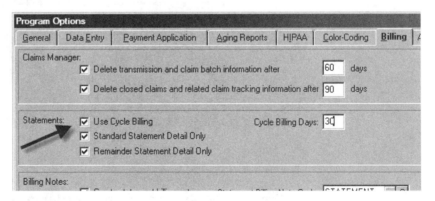

▶ Figure 6-16 **Setting Up Cycle Billing**

2. Under the Billing tab, locate the Statements section.

3. To start cycle billing, put a check mark in the Use Cycle Billing box and enter the number of days in the clinic's billing cycle. This is usually 30.

4. If the clinic wants the standard or remainder statements to show all detail for the previous balances, check the next two boxes as well. Otherwise, the statements will have a balance forward listed on them for amounts included in previous statements.

5. Statements are then created and printed in Statement Management using the same methodology, except the user does this each business day rather than once per month.

PRACTICE EXERCISE 6-4   Implementing Cycle Billing

After reviewing the option for cycle billing versus monthly billing, consider how each option would affect aspects of the business, from cash flow to work flow. Pretend you are employed at a clinic that does monthly billing, and you want to convince your superior that cycle billing should be implemented.

1   Review the clinic policies you created in Practice Exercise 6-3 and modify them to utilize cycle billing.

2   Write a presentation you could give to your superior to convince him or her of the benefits the clinic would receive by converting to cycle billing.

3   Write the step-by-step process for the changes you would make in Medisoft to start cycle billing.

PRACTICE EXERCISE 6-5   Sorting Statements and Adding Comments

Part of the daily task for medical billers is finding information such as statements, claims, and notes. Practice finding a statement for James Doogan by completing the following steps:

1   Since statements are listed by the guarantor name (not patient name), step one is to find the Chart number for James Doogan. And, since the guarantor's name is listed in the patient's Case, it can be looked up either in Transaction Entry or Patient Entry under List of the menu bar.

2   Once the Chart number is obtained, practice finding the statement for James Doogan in three different ways: first, by sorting the grid; second, by searching in the top toolbar; and third, by List Only in the top toolbar of Statement Management.

3   Once the statement is found, select the claim and edit it by hitting the Edit button on the bottom toolbar.

4   Once the statement is open, add a comment to the statement noting that "Jim has lost his job and will not be able to make a payment this month." Now, save the modified statement.

5   View the statement in Statement Management and see the note icon on the gridline (Figure 6-17).

6   Notes can be added in two other ways. Highlight any statement and right-click to see the available options. See that F5 is the shortcut key for Note. Go to Note and add a comment.

7   Highlight another statement and press F5. Add a note and view the note icons in Statement Management.

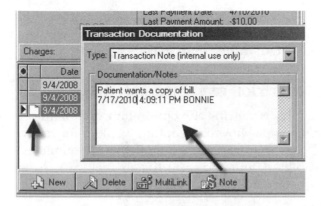

▶ Figure 6-17   Viewing the Statement Note Icon

CHAPTER REVIEW

Multiple Choice

1. On a remainder statement, who owes the balance?
   a. Patient
   b. Guarantor
   c. Insurance
   d. a or b

2. On a standard statement, who owes the balance?
   a. Patient
   b. Guarantor
   c. Insurance
   d. Guarantor and/or insurance

3. What must be done first when processing statements?
   a. Create statements
   b. Print statements
   c. Process statements
   d. None of the above

4. Where is the billing code used to filter statements found?
   a. In the patient's chart
   b. In the patient's case
   c. In the guarantor's chart
   d. In the guarantor's case

5. Who administers court orders for payment of a minor's bill?
   a. Guarantor
   b. Insurance
   c. Patient
   d. Court

6. Which grid item is useful for collections?
   a. Chart Numbers
   b. Media
   c. Submission Count
   d. Statement Number

7. Where is Cycle Billing setup?
   a. Tools, Options, Cycle Billing
   b. Activities, Cycle Billing, Options
   c. File, Program Options, Billing Tab
   d. File, Cycle Billing, Billing Tab

8. How do you select a group of statements?
   a. Hold the shift key and click on the first and last statements
   b. Hold the control key and click the first and last statements
   c. Click on the first and last statements
   d. Hold F2 and click on the first and last statements

9. How do you change selected statements from Sent to Ready to Send?
   a. Right-click on the highlighted statements and go to Change Statement Status/Billing Method
   b. Left-click on the highlighted statements and go to Change Statement Status/Billing Method
   c. Click on Change Status on the top toolbar and select the desired option
   d. Both a and c

10. To sort statements, the user can
    a. click on the desired grid column.
    b. click on the desired Sort By field in the top toolbar.
    c. enter the desired information in the Search Field and make the Sort By field match the appropriate search criteria.
    d. all of the above.

11. Which button on the bottom toolbar allows the user to reprint or resend a statement?
    a. Create
    b. Print/Send
    c. Rebill Statement
    d. Resend Statement

12. To add a note to a statement, the user should
    a. click on Note on the top toolbar.
    b. right-click on the statement and go to Note.
    c. highlight the statement and press F5.
    d. both b and c.

13. To modify the grid in Statement Management, the user should
    a. go to File, Program Option, and Modify Grid.
    b. go to Activities and Modify Grid.
    c. both a and b.
    d. click on the black dot in the upper left hand corner in Statement Management.

14. What appears on the Initial Billing Date on the grid column?
    a. The first time the statement was sent
    b. The last time the statement was sent
    c. The first time the insurance was billed
    d. None of the above

15. Which grid column shows if a Standard or Remainder statement was sent?
    a. Media
    b. Statement Type
    c. Type
    d. All of the above

True/False

Identify each of the following statements as true or false.

1. Standard Statements show balances due by both guarantors and insurances.

2. Remainder Statements only show balances due by guarantors.

3. Statements that are printed have statuses of Done.

4. Statements that are ready to Create are marked Ready to Send.

5. Cycle Billing is done once per month.

6. The List Only feature is found on the bottom toolbar.

7. If the user decides to do cycle billing rather than monthly billing, statements are created each business day.

8. As long as the office is sending statements at least monthly, they do not need to have a defined collection policy.

9. Create Statements is on the bottom toolbar.

10. The user can create statements for those with balances over $50.00.

Short Answer

1. After comparing how many statements are created for the Standard versus Remainder Statement types in Practice Exercise 6-1, explain the reason for the variances.

2. Describe how to filter statements by location code or provider.

3. Write a self-pay collection policy for an office and explain how Statement Management would be used to manage the policy.

Resources

As noted in previous chapters, three free resources come with Medisoft. View the articles available in each resource: Help within Medisoft, Knowledge Base online, and the Manual on the Installation CD.

Help Within Medisoft This is found inside of Medisoft in the upper right hand corner. After clicking on Help, select the first option Medisoft Help and note there are three tabs: Contents, Index, and Search. All three tabs will give you access to statement information.

Knowledge Base The Knowledge Base is found on the web at **www.medisoft.com**. First, click on Support on the left column, then Knowledge Base. Inside the Knowledge Base, articles on Statement Management and statements are available.

Manual on Installation CD Every Medisoft CD contains a manual in an Adobe PDF format. The CD also contains the free Acrobat Reader software to install to enable the user to open the manual if Acrobat Reader isn't already installed on the computer. Open the manual and search for the articles on Statement Management and statements. This can be done by looking at the index in the beginning of the manual or by clicking Edit and Search inside the manual and typing the information requested in the search box.

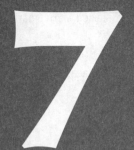

Chapter Seven

Data Backup
and Data Maintenance

Learning Objectives

After completing this chapter, you should be able to:

◆ Define and spell the key terms in this chapter.

◆ Understand and define a Backup and File Maintenance strategy.

◆ Explain the various Medisoft utilities, including Backup, Restore, and File Maintenance.

◆ Demonstrate how to create a Backup.

◆ Describe how multiple practices affect the Backup and File Maintenance utilities.

◆ Describe how to add processes to the Task Scheduler.

◆ Explain the difference between Backup Data and Backup Root Data.

◆ Demonstrate how to use the View Backup Disks utility.

◆ Explain the three forms of Medisoft help included with the program.

Key Terms

Backup Data   the Medisoft process of creating a duplicate copy of a dataset.

backup mediums   any form of data storage device such as RW-CDs, zip disks, flash drives, and external hard drives.

Backup Root Data   the process of creating a duplicate copy of the Medisoft shared files and registration files.

daily backup   backup made each day Medisoft is used.

File Maintenance   the utility in Medisoft that optimizes the performance of the system, including the processes to purge data, rebuild indexes, pack data, and recalculate balances.

off-site   refers to storing the backups at a location other than the office.

registration   the process whereby registration is created when the Medisoft program is initially installed. The sequence of the clinic's name and serial number creates the registration code.

Restore Data   the process of replacing the existing practice data with a backup copy.

Restore Root Data   the process of replacing the existing root data with a backup copy of the root data.

root data   data that is stored in the Medidata folder and shared by all practices in the folder.

Task Scheduler utility that allows the user to schedule tasks such as backups, reports, file maintenance, or eligibility verification to be performed after hours.

View Backup Disks a function that allows the user to view existing backups stored on various types of media; it gives the file name, date, and size of each file contained within a particular backup.

Abbreviations

KB Kilobytes, a storage unit used to define computer hard drive space.

■ ■ ■ ■

INTRODUCTION

An adage in the technology industry states that it is not a matter of if your computer fails, just when your computer will fail. When computers are compared with other mechanical items such as cars, washing machines, dryers or TVs, it is simple to see that all mechanical items (as well as people) do eventually fail. With that in mind, it is easy to see why data backups and maintenance are essential.

OVERVIEW OF BACKING UP MEDISOFT

There are three critical parts to backing up Medisoft: making a **daily backup**, rotating the **backup mediums**, and keeping backups **off-site** in a safe place. All three parts are indispensable. Making a daily backup is critical so the most recent changes to the data are stored. Rotating the backup media is important because media can deteriorate or be destroyed, and multiple copies add security. Finally, keeping the backup copies off-site adds protection if the office and/or computers are destroyed or stolen. The following is a list of the backup and restore features available in Medisoft and their descriptions (Figure 7-1):

Backup Data: The process of creating a duplicate copy of the Medisoft data contained inside the Medidata folder and practice folder.

Task Scheduler: The utility that allows the user to schedule tasks such as backups, reports, file maintenance, or eligibility verification to be performed after hours.

View Backup Disks: The function that allows the user to view existing backups stored on various types of media, giving the file name, date, and size of each file contained within a particular backup.

Restore Data: The process of replacing the existing practice data with a backup copy.

Backup Root Data: The process of creating a duplicate copy of the Medisoft data inside the Medidata folder but outside of the practice folder. This includes the practice's shared files and registration files.

Restore Root Data: The process of replacing the existing root data with a backup copy of the root data.

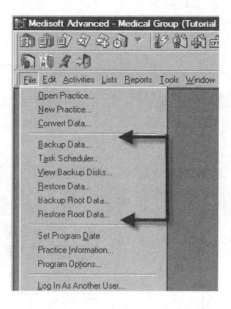

▶ Figure 7-1 **Backup and Restore Options**

PRACTICE EXERCISE 7-1   Becoming Familiar with the Backup and Restore Utilities

Medisoft contains six utilities that address backing up and restoring data, which were covered in the previous section. This exercise will familiarize you with these utilities.

1   Open up each utility one by one and click on the Help button.

2   Read the Help for each utility.

3   Write a brief paragraph for each utility outlining its function and importance.

Creating a Backup

The first step to backing up the Medisoft data is to go to File and then Backup Data. After clicking on Backup Data, a pop-up box appears, giving the user the following options (Figure 7-2):

Destination File Path and Name: This field allows the user to type in the designated location and name of the backup file, or it displays the backup location selected in the Find option.

Find: By clicking on this button, the user can view all available resources on the computer and select the backup location.

Password: The backup files may be password protected; this field allows the user to protect backups from being restored by another user.

Start Backup: Clicking this option creates the backup file.

Close: This button closes the Backup pop-up window.

Help: This option gives complete information and instructions to the user.

Once all the options are completed under Backup Data, the user will select Start Backup. Backup progress is indicated on the bottom toolbars (Figure 7-3).

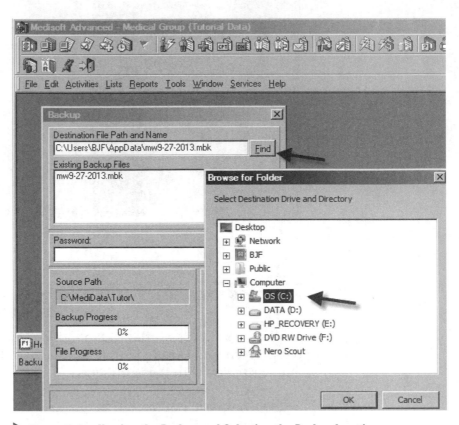

▶ Figure 7-2   Naming the Backup and Selecting the Backup Location

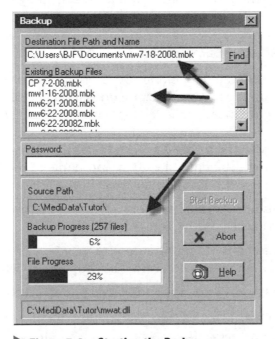

▶ Figure 7-3   Starting the Backup

Task Scheduler

Many of the tasks in Medisoft can take a considerable amount of time, especially for larger practices. Tasks such as File Maintenance, Backup, Eligibility, and Advanced Reporting Reports are best run when the office is closed. In addition to these tasks taking a long time to process, Medisoft or Office Hours cannot be used during these processes. Essentially, Task Scheduler enables the office to make the most of its system: Medisoft processes the needed tasks after hours, and the user is able to use Medisoft fully during working hours.

To access Task Scheduler, click on File on the menu bar, then Task Scheduler; the Medisoft Task Scheduler pop-up box (Figure 7-4) appears. In the Medisoft Task Scheduler, the options available are listed on the bottom toolbar. The following options are available:

Edit: Allows the user to change a previously scheduled task.

New: Allows the user to add a new task to the scheduler.

Delete: Allows the user to remove a previously scheduled task.

Cancel: Allows the user to exit the window without saving changes; the program will warn you that the tasks will not be performed.

OK: Allows the user to exit the window with saving changes and prepares Medisoft to perform the tasks.

Help: Opens to specific help on the Task Scheduler options.

Open on Startup: By checking this box, the Task Scheduler automatically starts when the computer is shut down and rebooted.

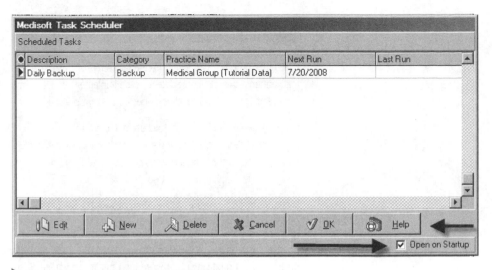

▶ Figure 7-4   **Medisoft Task Scheduler**

PRACTICE EXERCISE 7-2   Task Scheduler

In this practice exercise, the Task Scheduler is reviewed to show that offices can automate their critical and time saving processes to be performed when the office is closed.

1   First, go to File on the menu bar, then click on Task Scheduler. A pop-up box will appear, giving the Medisoft Task Scheduler options.

2   Next, click on New, and another pop-up box will appear, prompting you to Select Type of task to be scheduled (Figure 7-5). For the purpose of this exercise, you are going to add a Backup task. For now, select Backup, then OK.

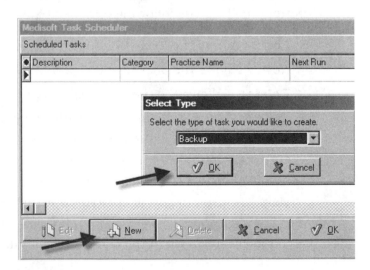

▶ Figure 7-5   **Select Type**

3   Another pop-up box appears, prompting you to Select Practice (Figure 7-6). Select the Medisoft Group (Tutorial Data), then OK.

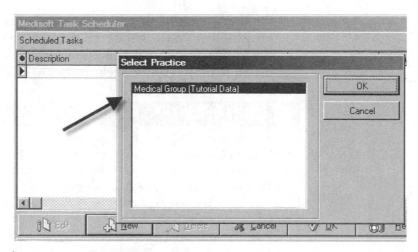

▶ Figure 7-6 Select Backup

4   Next, a pop-up box called the New Backup Task will appear (Figure 7-7). In this box, the description, frequency, time, start date, and destination need to be completed. The password line is optional. At this time, click the Help button to view complete details of each field. Then, name the backup Daily Backup, and set the program to create the backup every day at midnight starting tonight. Allow the Destination path to be the default. Click Save and view the scheduled task in the Medisoft Task Scheduler.

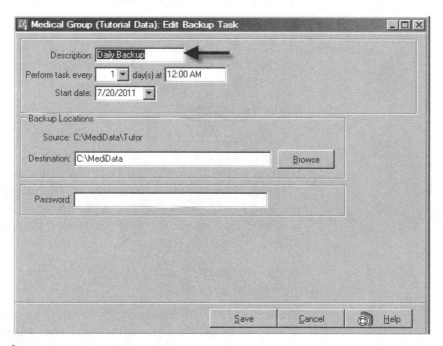

▶ Figure 7-7 New Backup Task

5   This step is critical in order for the function to work properly. Check Open on Startup, then use the OK button to exit the box. The Open on Startup means if the computer is rebooted, this task is reopened. The OK button means it is OK to process the tasks. Users frequently make the mistake of clicking the Cancel button; this cancels the task.

6 Finally, upon the discretion of your instructor, you can allow the backup to automatically create and view it tomorrow using the View Backup Disks, or you should delete the scheduled task to prevent multiple unnecessary backups being stored on the computer.

Medisoft Quick Tip Printing Backup Copies of the Registration

Three crucial items are important to running Medisoft: the Medisoft program, the Medisoft data, and the Medisoft registration. It is not important to backup the Medisoft program, because the program can be reinstalled from the disks or by downloading the latest copy from the Medisoft Knowledge Base. The Medisoft data is very important to backup daily, and one of the main topics in this chapter. However, the most overlooked component of Medisoft is the **registration**. The registration is created when the program is initially installed. The sequence of the clinic's name and serial number creates the registration code. Because the registration is a vital part of running Medisoft, it should be printed out with a copy kept onsite in the Medisoft case and a copy kept off-site with data backups.

PRACTICE EXERCISE 7-3 **Printing the Registration**

With Medisoft, if a computer crashes, there are two items of great importance: first is a backup copy of the software, and second is a printout of the registration. Complete this practice exercise by printing a copy of the registration for safe keeping.

1 After opening Medisoft, select Help from the menu bar.

2 Next, select Register Program from the drop-down menu.

3 Select Print from the pop-up box.

4 In a clinic setting, a copy of the registration should be kept in the Medisoft software box, and a second copy should be kept off-site with the backups.

View Backup Disks

View Backup Disks is a utility in Medisoft that allows the user to look at the details of the backups. It is particularly helpful if the user wants to restore a backup and needs to know the date and time the backup was created. To access this utility, go to File on the menu bar and View Backup Disks. A pop-up box will appear that states View Backup. Inside this pop-up box are the options to view available backups. A description of these options follows:

Source Path: Allows the user to enter the path where the backup is located.

Find: By clicking on this button, the user can view all available resources on the computer that may contain backup files.

Password: The backup files may be password protected; this field allows for a password to be entered.

View Backup: This button executes viewing the backup file.

Abort: This button stops the viewing.

Help: This option gives complete information and instructions to the user.

After the View Backup box is opened and the fields completed, the user will select the option to View Backup. This in turn brings up a second pop-up box, giving the desired information about the backup (Figure 7-8). The following information is given by the Backup View:

BU Date: The date the backup was created.

BU Time: The time the backup was created.

Data Path: The location of the backup file.

Total Files: The number of files contained within the backup.

Index: Numbering system used to identify Total Files.

File Name: The name of the file in the backup.

Time: The date of the file in the backup. (**Note**: File dates may vary depending upon when information in Medisoft was last saved to that file.)

Size: The size of the file in Kilobytes (**KB**).

Print: Prints the details of the backup files.

Close: Closes the Backup View pop-up window.

Help: Gives complete information and instructions to the user.

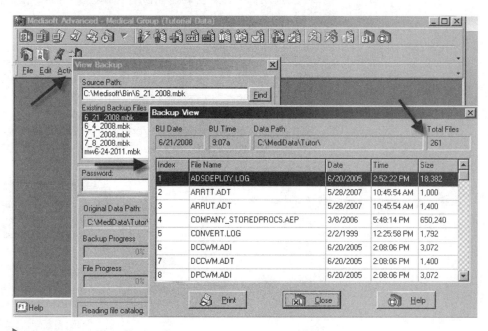

▶ Figure 7-8   **View Backup Data**

PRACTICE EXERCISE 7-4   Creating a Backup

This practice exercise will allow the user to review how to create a backup.

1   First, go to File on the menu bar and click on Backup Data. This will cause a pop-up box to appear.

2   After the pop-up appears, click on the Find button, and another pop-up will appear, showing the available drives to create a backup (Figure 7-9). Of course, the answer for which drive to select will vary by computer and the media type used. If unclear about the proper

location for the storage device, consult a computer technician. For the purposes of the example, click on the C drive, then click on the Medisoft folder, then OK.

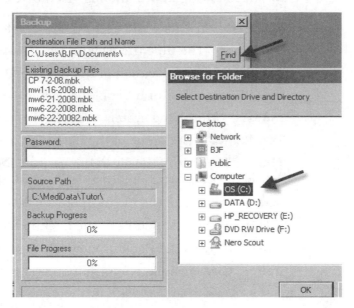

▶ Figure 7-9   Finding the Backup Location

3   Finally, click on Start Backup and Medisoft will automatically name the backup file using the convention mwDate.mbk (Figure 7-10) Remember, if there are multiple practices and multiple sets of data, manually name the backups to avoid overwriting an existing backup. After the process is complete, Medisoft will display a pop-up box stating that backup is complete; select OK.

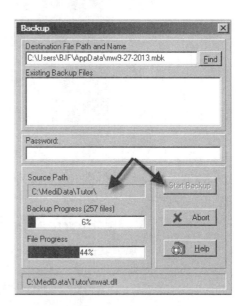

▶ Figure 7-10   Backup Progress

4   Option: If desired, the backup can be password protected. Practice creating a second backup with a password.

Reminder: If more than one set of data exists, this process must be run separately on each set of data, uniquely naming each backup.

Restoring a Backup

Restore gives the user the option to replace existing data files with selected backup files. Clinics use the Restore option for a few primary reasons, which include damaged or corrupted data, a damaged computer, or a transfer to a new computer system. In addition to these reasons, clinics sometimes want to test program features that make major changes in their data, such as purging or billing charges based on a practice data set different from their active data. Restore gives the clinic the option to create a duplicate set of data to practice on.

To access the Restore Data feature, click on File on the menu bar, then Restore Data (Figure 7-11). The following is a list of Restore options:

Backup File Path and Name: This field allows the user to type in the designated backup file, or it displays the backup file that has been selected through the Find option.

Find: By clicking on this button, the user can view all available resources on the computer that may contain backup files and select the appropriate one to restore.

Password: The backup files may be password protected; this field allows for a password to be entered in order to restore the file.

Start Restore: Clicking this option restores the selected backup file.

Close: This button closes the Restore pop-up window.

Help: This option gives complete information and instructions to the user.

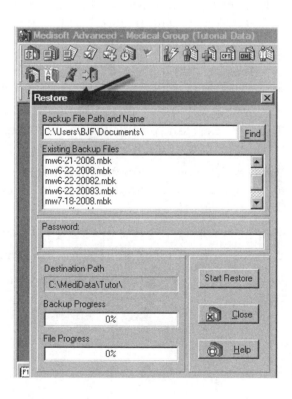

▶ Figure 7-11   Restore Data

Medisoft Quick Tip   Causes of Corrupt Data

With any software, damaged or corrupted data is one of the most common reasons to restore data. What causes corrupted data? Data corruption comes from Medisoft being shut down improperly either by the user, such as turning off the computer while Medisoft is running, a power outage, or a computer failure. Other possible causes include power surges or lags, networking card or cabling failures, improper networking, improper shutdown of the computer or network, hard drive, CPU, or other hardware failure.

If the data becomes corrupt, the only option is to restore it or have it repaired. Repairing the data can be very time consuming and costly, so it is imperative that the office have a good backup system.

Backup Root Data

Root data is data contained inside of the Medidata folder but outside the practice data folders. To fully understand this, it is important to understand how Medisoft is installed and set up. First, the Medisoft program itself is in a folder named Medisoft. However, the data for the practice is in a separate folder. If the clinic has more than one practice, each practice will have its own data folder. The practice data is all contained in one folder under the Medidata folder, which also contains the files shared by the practices. Examples of shared files are the registration files, the practice list, global login information, and EDI templates, to name a few. When the clinic performs a typical backup, it backs up the data files contained within the practice folder. It does not backup the entire Medidata folder. It is important to also backup the root data, which are the shared files in the Medidata folder.

For the user to Backup Root Data, click on File on the menu bar and then Backup Root Data (Figure 7-12). The following is a list of Backup Root Data options:

Destination File Path and Name: This field allows the user to type in the designated location and name, or it displays the backup file being created.

Find: By clicking on this button, the user can view all available resources on the computer and select the backup location.

Password: The backup files may be password protected; this field allows for a password to be entered in order to restrict other users from restoring it.

Start Backup: Clicking this option creates the backup file.

Close: This button closes the Backup Root Data pop-up window.

Help: This option gives complete information and instructions to the user.

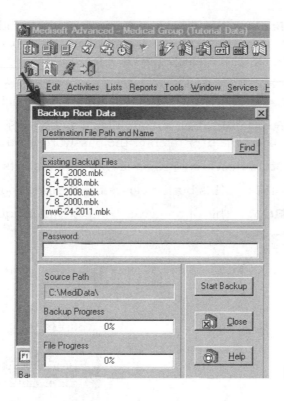

▶ Figure 7-12   Backup Root Data

Backing Up Multiple Practices

It is not uncommon to have Medisoft users billing for more than one practice. In these instances, each practice has its own database. Therefore, besides backing up the root data, the clinic needs to create a backup for each practice. Since Medisoft will default to automatically naming the backup for the user, this would create a problem for multipractice clinics because each practice would have a backup with the same name. This problem can be resolved by having the user enter the name and data of the backup rather than allowing Medisoft to automatically name it. An example of this is if there were two practices, one named Johnson Chiropractic and another named Jane Chiropractic, Medisoft would default to the name XX-XX-XXXX for both. Here is how the file name could be entered into the Backup Destination File Path and Name:

E:\johnson021110.mbk

E:\jane021110.mbk

The E represents the USB backup drive, the name represents the data being backed up, and the date represents the date of the backup. By creating backups in this manner, the office is assured to have a backup for each set of data that is easily identifiable by data set and date.

Restore Root Data

The reasons for restoring root data are similar to those of restoring the practice data. All of the items contained in the root data are important; however, the registration information is particularly valuable. To restore the root data, click on File on the menu bar, then Restore Root Data (Figure 7-13). The list of Restore Root Data options follows:

Backup File Path and Name: This field allows the user to type in the designated location and name of the backup, or it displays the backup file selected in the Find option.

Find: By clicking on this button, the user can view all available backup files and select the appropriate backup.

Password: The backup files may be password protected; this field allows the user to enter the password for the selected backup.

Start Restore: Clicking this option starts the restore process.

Close: This button closes the Restore Root Data pop-up window.

Help: This option gives complete information and instructions to the user.

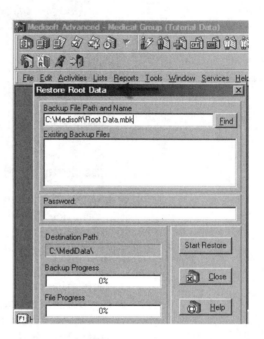

▶ **Figure 7-13   Restore Root Data**

Medisoft Quick Tip   Reminder for Getting Help with Medisoft

There is a great saying: "If I could only know what I have already learned." No one has all the answers all the time or can remember everything that has been taught. Therefore, it's important to remember the good resources for Medisoft. These resources have been listed previously in this text; however, it is especially important to list them again here because utilities such as Restore and File Maintenance are used infrequently, and it is a good idea to reread the details prior to performing these functions. So, once again, here are the three forms of assistance offered by Medisoft:

Medisoft Manual   included on the installation CD.
Knowledge Base   located at www.medisoft.com; click on support and Knowledge Base.
Help Key   located inside the program by clicking Help on the upper right menu bar or by hitting F1 any place within the program.

Because having the skills to find answers to questions is so important, this practice exercise will allow the user to review the methods of creating a backup by using the three forms of assistance offered by Medisoft.

1   Review how to create a backup on the manual contained on the Medisoft installation CD.

2   Review how to create a backup in Help within Medisoft.

3   Review how to create a backup on the Medisoft Knowledge Base.

4   Write a summary of how to make a backup, noting any differences found between the methods researched.

File Maintenance

File Maintenance is a utility inside of Medisoft used to optimize the performance of the program by purging data, removing deleted data, rebuilding the indexes, and recalculating the balances. This process should be run at least monthly prior to statements being printed. Some practices even run it weekly to optimize Medisoft's performance. It is very important to note that a backup should always be performed before processing File Maintenance. If File Maintenance is interrupted for any reason, a backup would be needed to restore the data.

The following steps outline how to access the File Maintenance utility: First, click on File on the menu bar, then click on File Maintenance. This causes the File Maintenance pop-up box to appear (Figure 7-14). Notice there are four tabs in the pop-up box, titled Purge Data, Rebuild Indexes, Pack Data, and Recalculate Balances. Review the following list of functions of each tab and their meanings:

Purge Data: Allows the user to purge various items in Medisoft including appointments, claims, statements, recalls, closed cases, and credit cards. This utility can be especially helpful in large databases to optimize the performance of different processes such as Claim Management; however, due to the large capacity of today's computers, this function is rarely used.

Rebuild Indexes: Recounts the record indexes of each table that exists in Medisoft; this process optimizes the system and can detect corrupt data.

Pack Data: This process permanently removes deleted records. Similar to emptying the Recycle Bin in Windows, this compresses the files and optimizes performance.

Recalculate Balances: Balances in Medisoft sometimes become miscalculated when charges and payments are deleted and reentered; this procedure adds the charges, payments, and adjustments again to calculate the proper balances.

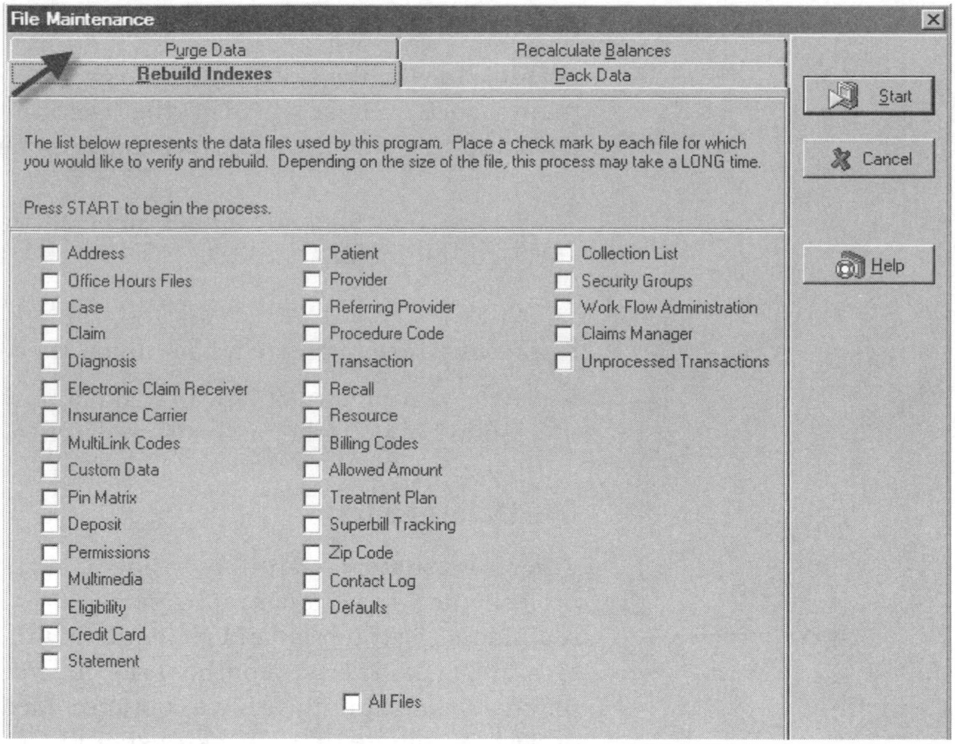

▶ Figure 7-14   File Maintenance

File Maintenance for Multiple Practices and Backups

File Maintenance is run on one dataset at a time, meaning that whichever data set is opened is processed. If a clinic has only one set of data, this is not an issue. On the other hand, if a clinic has more than one practice, the user must run File Maintenance within each dataset, being careful to also first make a backup of each practice.

PRACTICE EXERCISE 7-6   Running File Maintenance

In this practice exercise, you are going to run File Maintenance. Users have many different options when running this utility. This exercise covers the most common procedures used in processing File Maintenance.

1   Open File Maintenance by going to File on the menu bar and selecting File Maintenance in the drop-down list.

2   Notice there are four tabs at the top: Purge Data, Rebuild Indexes, Pack Data, and Recalculate Balances. Routinely, most clinics do not Purge Data. This is because with today's computers and memory it is not necessary. The most common procedure with File Maintenance is to run all the items on Rebuild Indexes, Pack Data, and Recalculate Balances.

3   On the Rebuild Indexes tab, click on All Files at the bottom of the screen (Figure 7-15).

4   On the Pack Data tab, click on All Files at the bottom of the screen (Figure 7-16).

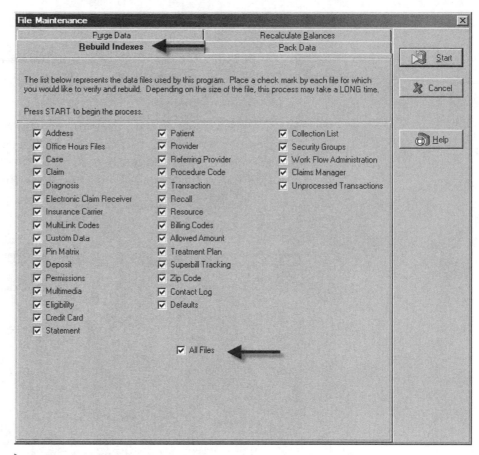

▶ Figure 7-15 **Select All Files in Rebuild Indexes**

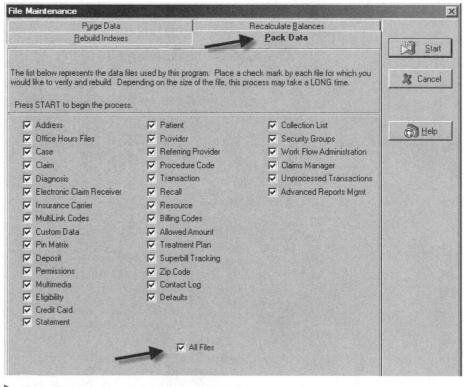

▶ Figure 7-16 **Select All Files in Pack Data**

5　On the Recalculate Balances tab, click all three boxes and then select Start (Figure 7-17).

6　This will complete the File Maintenance Process. After the process is complete, Medisoft will display a pop-up box stating it is complete; select OK.

Note: Always back up data prior to performing File Maintenance. File Maintenance should be run at least once per month prior to processing statements or more frequently to keep Medisoft performing optimally. If more than one set of data exists, this process must be run separately on each set of data.

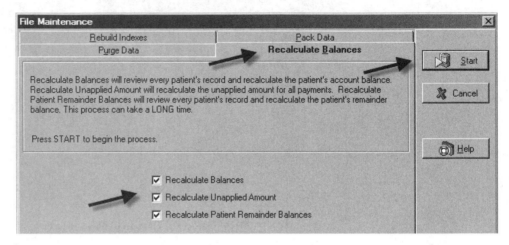

▶ **Figure 7-17**　**Select Recalculate Balances Boxes and Start**

▶ Test Your Knowledge 7-1

Imagine you start working at a new clinic and realize that it has not implemented a good backup or maintenance plan. Write a detailed plan for the clinic explaining how you will perform these functions and why you are going to do it in your defined manner.

CHAPTER REVIEW

Multiple Choice

1. What is the process used to create a duplicate set of the clinic data?
   a. Backup Data
   b. Backup Root Data
   c. View Backup Files
   d. Task Scheduler

2. Which process backs up the registration files?
   a. Backup Data
   b. Backup Root Data
   c. View Backup Files
   d. Task Scheduler

3. Which process should be run before statements are printed?
   a. Backup Data
   b. File Maintenance
   c. Both a and b
   d. Task Scheduler

4. What does View Backup Disks allow the user to see?
   a. Transaction data
   b. Patient data
   c. Modifiers
   d. File sizes

5. To restore the registration files, which process would be used?
   a. Restore Data
   b. Restore Root Data
   c. Backup Root Data
   d. Task Scheduler

6. Where should backup disks be stored?
   a. Desk drawer
   b. File cabinet
   c. Off-site
   d. Beside the computer

7. How often should you purge data?
   a. Daily
   b. Weekly
   c. Monthly
   d. Only if necessary

8. On average, how often should you run File Maintenance?
   a. Daily
   b. Weekly
   c. Monthly
   d. Only if necessary

9. When should Task Scheduler be set to run?
   a. After hours
   b. During business hours
   c. Only if needed
   d. Never

10. When selecting the backup location, the user should
    a. click Find and point to the location.
    b. click on My Computer and pick the location.
    c. type the backup and pathname into Destination File Path and Name.
    d. either a or c.

11. How many backup storage devices should the office have?
    a. Two
    b. One for each day of the week and one for the first of each month
    c. One for each month
    d. 30

12. After Task Scheduler is configured, what is clicked to exit the pop-up window?
    a. Cancel
    b. Open on Startup and OK
    c. Exit
    d. a, b, or c

13. When the computer is rebooted, which process will pop up for the user to approve?
    a. Backup
    b. File Maintenance
    c. Task Scheduler
    d. Backup Root Data

14. If an office has more than one set of data in Medisoft, how many backups need to be maintained?
    a. one for Medisoft
    b. one for each set of data
    c. one for the root data
    d. both b and c

15. What causes corrupt data?
    a. power or computer failure
    b. user error
    c. both a and b
    d. program failure

True/False

Identify each of the following statements as true or false.

1. File Maintenance should be run once a year.

2. Task Scheduler should run during business hours.

3. The office should have one backup for each business day of the week and rotate them.

4. The office should store backups in another location to protect them in case the office is destroyed.

5. After Task Scheduler is configured, click Cancel to exit the pop-up window.

6. Task Scheduler allows tasks to be run after hours.

7. File Maintenance should be run before a backup is done.

8. File Maintenance should be run before statements are printed.

9. The Medidata folder contains the registration files.

10. The practice folder contains the registration files.

Short Answer

1. Explain the three forms of support offered by Medisoft and where they are located.

2. Describe a good backup plan including rotating disks and storage of the disks types.

3. Explain the difference between Backup Data and Backup Root Data.

Resources

Medisoft: **www.medisoft.com**

This website provides additional information on the Backup and File Maintenance utilities. It can be found under the Knowledge Base, which is located under the Support button.

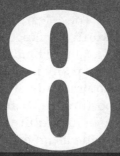

Chapter Eight

Billing Charges, Security Setup, and Other Little-Known Features

Learning Objectives

After completing this chapter, you should be able to:

♦ Define and spell the key terms in this chapter.
♦ Understand and define the special features outlined in this chapter, including Billing Charges, Small Balance Write-off, Security Setup, Group Setup, Permissions, and Audit Records.
♦ Explain and demonstrate the reasoning and mechanics of Billing Charges.
♦ Demonstrate Small Balance Write-off.
♦ Identify and describe how to set up security in Medisoft.
♦ Describe the reason behind setting up Groups.
♦ Create Permissions unique for a Medisoft dataset.
♦ Define the reports available in Audit Records.
♦ Explain how the Health Insurance Portability and Accountability Act (HIPAA) affects passwords.

Key Terms

Audit Records   a report feature that allows the user to audit patient records, track user logins, and view permission settings.

billing charge   interest or finance charge added to a patient's account.

Groups   the function in Work Administrator that allows tasks to be assigned to a pre-defined group of users.

Group Setup   an add-on to Security Setup that allows the practice to define groups of users.

Health Insurance Portability and Accountability Act (HIPAA)   a federal law passed in 1996 to develop standards among providers, health plans, clearinghouses, and employers regarding electronic transactions, security, and privacy.

Permissions   the utility inside of Medisoft that assigns tasks to user access levels.

Security Setup   the utility in Medisoft that sets up login rights for users, permission access levels, group assignments, and the ability to reset the user password.

Small Balance Write-off   a Medisoft feature allowing the user to mass write off small balances after setting the appropriate parameters.

Abbreviations

HIPAA   Health Insurance Portability and Accountability Act
PHI   Protected Health Information
TPO   Treatment, Payment, and Operations

■ ■ ■ ■

INTRODUCTION

Many of the items reviewed in this chapter will rarely be used in medical offices, even though some are absolutely required. These features can be considered the "cream of the crop" and are well worth learning. Why are they not always used? Many offices use Medisoft as limited billing software and do not explore all the extra features. Plus, many underutilize features pertaining to the security and privacy requirements of HIPAA and other employee management and billing opportunities. Learn and remember these features; if possible, implement them in a future job. These advanced skills will greatly increase your value as an employee, Medisoft user, and medical billing staff member.

OVERVIEW OF THE LITTLE-KNOWN FEATURES

Let us examine the little-known or seldom-used Medisoft features, including Billing Charges, Small Balance Write-off, Security Setup, Group Setup, Permissions, and Audit Records. Each of these features enables the user to be more productive.

Billing Charges

Billing charges are interest or finance charges that are assessed for delinquent payments. Medical offices should be viewed the same as grocery stores or gas stations: They supply a good or service, and the balance is due upon receipt. Billing charges encourage clients to pay in a timely manner. With the Billing Charge feature, if an outstanding balance is not paid after a specified amount of time, Medisoft can add billing charges to the patient statements. The rules covering if and when a clinic may add billing charges vary from state to state, and these rules must be strictly adhered to. However, consumers tend to pay off the bills first that have billing charges, and it is in the clinic's best interest to do the leg work to implement this policy into its practice. A good resource for this type of information is the state office or board of medical practices in the state in which the practice resides. **Note:** Billing charges are only assessed to patient balances, meaning the insurance responsibility is complete for the transaction.

Small Balance Write-off

Small Balance Write-off allows clinics to write off patient balances under a certain amount so statements are not printed unnecessarily. It would not make sense to print a statement with a 39-cent balance when the cost of a stamp is greater. In fact, with the printing, stuffing, stamping, and staff fee, many clinics do not send statements under $5.00. With this feature, Medisoft will mass write off minimum balances for the parameters set by the user.

Security Setup

Security Setup allows the practice to manage users that log into Medisoft. In addition to security, the practice is also able to set permission levels, monitor the activities the users are allowed to perform and to track or audit the users' activities.

Group Setup

Group Setup is an add-on feature of Security Setup. It allows the practice to develop groups of users to be assigned tasks such as scheduling, follow-up, or reporting in another utility named Work Administrator. Then, Work Administrator allows the work of the clinic to be collectively managed by both users and groups.

Permissions

Permissions works hand in hand with Security Setup. Once security is established in Medisoft, the user has five different levels of access that can be assigned to the user. The levels range from full permissions to very restricted permissions. In Permissions, specific tasks are assigned to each access level. In Security Setup, each user is assigned to a level. This gives the practice control over the functions the employees are allowed to perform. For example, the office may want only management staff printing financial reports.

Audit Records

Audit Records works hand in hand with Security Setup. Once security is established, the practice can monitor the activities and permissions of its users. Included in this section are three reports: The first report can show a variety of desired information such as how the user managed a particular patient's account or an overall view of items that were deleted or modified. The second report allows the clinic to view when staff members logged into Medisoft and logged out. The third report shows the current permission settings in Medisoft.

> ### Billing Insight   HIPAA
>
> In 1996, the federal government passed a law called the **Health Insurance Portability and Accountability Act** (**HIPAA**). This act created standards among entities including healthcare providers, health plans, employers, and clearinghouses with regard to how they conducted business relating to electronic transactions, privacy, and security. As with many laws, the complicating factor is the interpretation of the law. In addition, if state regulations are more restrictive than HIPAA, the state regulations take precedence. However, each practice should have a HIPAA policy manual, and it should contain within it how electronic transactions, privacy, and security are addressed. See Appendix D for information on HIPAA regulations.

DETAILING THE FEATURES

Now we will detail each of the features reviewed previously, remembering that there are three types of Medisoft: Basic, Advanced, and Network Professional. Not all types have all of these features; Basic has the fewest features, and Network Professional has all of the features.

Billing Charges: A Closer Look

Clinics can benefit greatly by adding billing charges, and the most important way is not by increased revenue, but by faster payments. Consumers do not like paying additional fees and prioritize paying their bills by paying off the highest fees first. Clinics that add billing charges tend to get paid first and have the ability to negotiate writing off the billing charges for faster payment.

Initially, a few important steps should be taken prior to billing charges being added to the patient statements. If an office suddenly decides to add billing charges without proper planning, it could create poor patient relationships and, at worst, break laws without knowing it. These steps include:

1. Research the laws of the state to be sure to comply with the regulations. There may be a limited billing rate, signatures required, and other various restrictions.

2. After the laws have been determined, the office should develop a clinic policy on how billing charges will be administered.

3. Next, a plan should be implemented to notify new and existing patients of the policy and retain signatures if needed.

4. Finally, a procedure code needs to be created in the Lists menu of Medisoft to track billing charges. This is an ad-hoc procedure code, not a CPT* procedure code. Patient billing charges should never be sent to an insurance company. Let's review how to create a new procedure code. First, on the menu bar select Lists, then Procedure/Payments/Adjustment Codes. Next, click on New at the bottom left of the screen. This will give a pop-up window allowing us to create a new procedure (Figure 8-1). Three items need to be entered in this box: Description, Code Type, and Patient Only Responsible.

*CPT is a registered trademark of the American Medical Association.

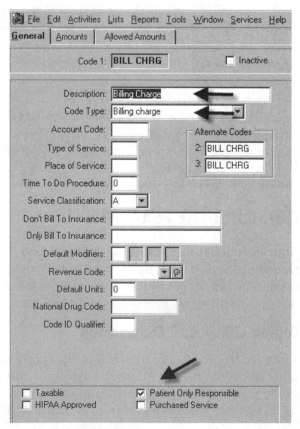

▶ Figure 8-1 Creating a Billing Charge Procedure Code

Once items 1 through 4 have been addressed, you are ready to create billing charges to fit the clinic's policy. Next, open the Billing Charges utility, select Activities on the menu bar, then Billing Charges. This brings up the Billing Charges pop-up window (Figure 8-2). The following options are available to the user:

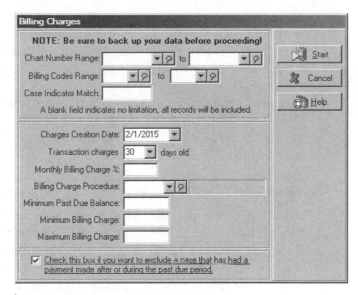

▶ Figure 8-2   Creating Billing Charges

Chart Number Range: To apply billing charges to a specific patient or range of patients, complete these fields.

Billing Codes Range: To apply billing charges to specific Billing Codes (from the Account tab of the Case), complete these fields.

Case Indicator: To apply billing charges to specific Case Indicators (from the Miscellaneous tab of the Case), complete these fields.

Charges Creation Date: Enter the day the billing charges will be posted to the patient accounts, generally the first day or last day of the month.

Transaction Charges: Enter the age a transaction must be before a billing charge would be added to the account.

Monthly Billing Charge: Enter the monthly percentage to be charged; i.e. if a clinic charges 18% annually, enter 1.5% (18 divided by 12 equals 1.5).

Billing Charge Procedure: Enter the procedure code the charges will be posted with; this is the code created in step 4 on page 186.

Minimum Past Due Balance: To apply billing charges for a minimum amount due and over, enter the amount here.

Minimum Billing Charge: To apply a minimum amount of billing charges per account, enter the amount here.

Maximum Billing Charge: To limit the amount of billing charges applied to a patient's account, enter the maximum amount here.

Check Box on Bottom: To exclude patients who are making current payments from receiving billing charges, keep this box checked.

Start: Initiates the procedure to add billing charges to the patient accounts.

Cancel: Exits the pop-up window.

Help: Gives complete explanation of the Billing Charges function.

Even though there are several options for creating billing charges, clinics most commonly complete these options: Charge Creation Date, Transaction Charges, Monthly Billing Charge, Billing Charge Procedure, and the Minimum Billing Charge.

It is also good practice to make a backup prior to performing this function. This function can change a vast number of accounts with the click of one button. Users want to have the option to restore a backup if a mistake is made.

PRACTICE EXERCISE 8-1   Billing Charges

Prior to processing Billing Charges, always remember to back up, run File Maintenance, and do the Small Balance Write-Offs. After these steps are done, you are ready to proceed with Billing Charges. For this practice exercise, assume that the clinic's policy is to charge billing charges on the first of each month for charges over 60 days old at the rate of 1.5% and a minimum charge of $3.00. Create billing charges for February 1, 2010. The clinic does not take into account if the patient has made a payment recently. Open the Billing Charges pop-up window by selecting Activities on the menu bar and Billing Charges from the drop-down menu (Figure 8-3). Then, follow these steps:

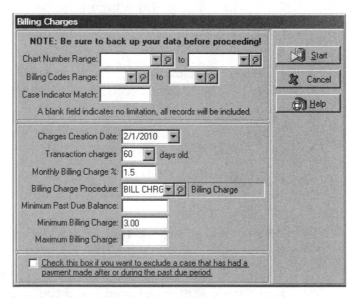

▶ Figure 8-3   **Creating Billing Charges**

1   Enter the appropriate criteria for Charge Creation Date, Transaction Charges, Monthly Billing Charge, Billing Charge Procedure, and Minimum Billing Charge.

2   Uncheck the box to exclude a case that has a payment.

3 Click Start to process the billing charges.

4 Finally, from skills learned in previous chapters, run a report showing the billing charges just created.

Small Balance Write-offs: A Closer Look

Processing patient balances, including printing and processing statements, answering phone calls, and posting payments, has a real cost to it. For smaller patient balances, it can cost more to bill the patient than it would to write-off the balance. Typically, clinics will write-off patient balances that are less than $3.00 to $5.00. Medisoft defaults the write-off amount to be anything less than $5.00; however, the user can change this and determine the amount to write-off.

As with Billing Charges, let's set some ground rules before we dive into the write-off procedure.

1. First the office should make sure that writing off a minimum balance does not conflict with any contracts it may have with insurance companies.

2. Next, the office should create a policy including the amounts, patient selection and dates the write-offs will be done.

3. Finally, just like in the Billing Charges example, a new ad-hoc procedure code for Small Balance Write-offs will need to be created by entering the Description, Code Type (Adjustment) and marking the option to Make Adjustment Negative (Figure 8-4).

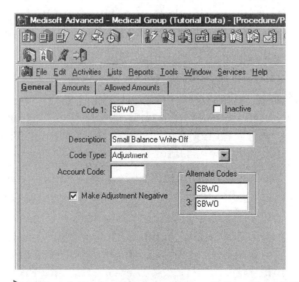

▶ Figure 8-4   **Small Balance Write-off Procedure Code**

After items 1 through 3 have been addressed, the user can proceed with the write-off procedure. To open the pop-up window allowing the Small Balance Write-off, Activities should be selected on the menu bar, then Small Balance Write-off in the drop-down list. This will open the window to perform the write-offs and reveal the options available to control the write-offs (Figure 8-5).

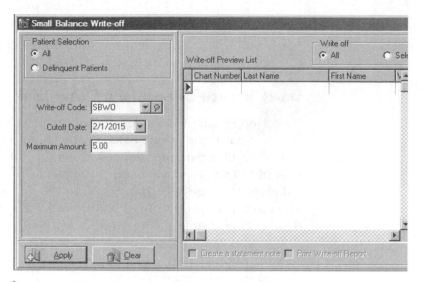

▶ Figure 8-5   Creating Small Balance Write-offs

Patient Selection: Gives the option to select all patients or just patients who have a delinquent payment plan.

Write-Off Code: Allows the user to enter the procedure code write-offs will be posted to.

Cutoff Date: Refers to the date of the last payment.

Maximum Amount: Allows the user to enter the maximum amount allowed to be written off.

Apply: Applies the criteria on the left hand column and displays matching patients in the right column.

Clear: Clears both the left and right columns.

Write-Off: Offers the user the option to select all patients or individually select patients.

Write-Off Preview List: Displays the information on the patients matching the small balance write-off criteria. The information includes Chart Number, Last Name, First Name, Write-off Amount and Last Patient Payment Date.

Create a statement note: Checking this box will cause Medisoft to add a note to each write-off adjustment that the statement is marked Done; if not checked, the statement will still be marked Done.

Print Write-Off Report: Checking this box will generate a report showing the write-offs done (if not checked, a report later can be pulled from Reports, Day Sheets, and Procedure Day Sheets and adding the desired procedure code).

Selected Count: Tells how many patients are selected and are ready to write-off.

Write-Off: Completes the write-offs.

Cancel: Exits the user out of the pop-up window.

Help: Gives the user complete details on the Small Balance Write-off.

Options: Gives the user additional options to only write off balances with applied payments and to use the cut-off date as an ending date range.

Since the tutorial data has a very limited amount of data, to view potential patients to write-off, increase the Maximum Amount to $50.00. Of course, a clinic would never write-off this amount; this is for viewing purposes only (Figure 8-6). Notice by changing the amount and viewing potential items to write-off, Medisoft displays the number of selected accounts. This provides a more realistic look at how write-offs are done in a clinic setting.

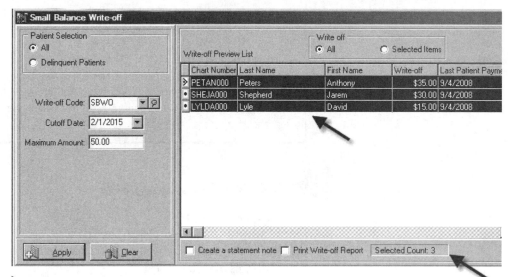

▶ Figure 8-6   **Viewing Potential Write-offs**

This is another area where clicking one button can make changes on several accounts. It is a good idea to make a backup prior to running this feature.

PRACTICE EXERCISE 8-2   Small Balance Write-Offs

In a typical clinic setting, there is a policy in place to write-off balances below a certain threshold such as $1.00, $3.00, or $5.00. Since the tutorial database does not contain balances this size, balances under $50.00 will be written off in this exercise.

1   Create a procedure code for Small Balance Write-off under the List menu.

2   Open Small Balance Write-off under the Activities menu.

3   Use the date of the first of the current month and the amount of $50.

4   Enter the criteria into the left side of the Small Balance Write-off menu and click Apply.

5 Review the items to be written-off, select Create a statement note, and if desired, select to print a report.

6 Click Write-off to finish the process.

▶ Test Your Knowledge 8-1

Now that accounts have had minimum write-offs, what reports could be printed to display the accounts affected? List two possible reports.

Medisoft Quick Tip HIPAA and Privacy

Many clinics feel they do not need to put user passwords on Medisoft because their computer is password protected. However, a quick look at the HIPAA privacy acknowledgment indicates otherwise. The privacy acknowledgment is a form the clinic is required to give each patient and request the patient to sign. The form tells patients their data can be seen and given to other parties in regard to Treatment, Payment, and Operations (**TPO**) without their written authorization. However, if the patient desires, a copy of the parties viewing their Protected Health Information (**PHI**) can be obtained. PHI is personal data defined in the HIPAA law. If Medisoft is not password protected, the clinic cannot give patients a copy of who has accessed their data. Password protecting Medisoft allows the user the ability to pull an audit report of the users involved with the patient data. This is also one reason that users should not share logins or passwords.

▶ Test Your Knowledge 8-2

Given what you have learned in Chapter 6 on Statement Management, Chapter 7 on Backup and File Maintenance, and this chapter on Small Balance Write-off, develop a clinic policy on how you would administer processing monthly patient statements with the practice of charging 1.5% interest on balances over 30 days old.

Security Setup: A Closer Look

Again, security allows the practice to manage who logs in to the program, specify what they are allowed to do, and generate reports about their activities while inside Medisoft. To start, open the pop-up window for Security Setup, select File on the menu bar, then click on Security Setup (Figure 8-7). Review the following options in Security Setup:

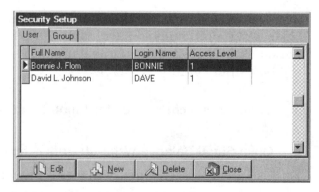

▶ **Figure 8-7 Security Setup**

User: Shows the user setup with security.

Group: Shows the groups in security (this tab will be covered more in the Group review).

Edit: Allows an existing user to edit.

New: Creates a new user.

Delete: Deletes an existing user.

Close: Closes the Security Setup pop-up window.

Next, within the User box are items that display the user currently set up. Here are the fields that can be viewed from this screen:

Full Name: Gives the full name of the user.

Login Name: Shows the security login of the user.

Access Level: Displays the permission level of the user (this will be reviewed in detail in the Permission Settings section).

Several notes should be mentioned. First, each data set needs to have at least one person who is an administrator and has full permission to make changes. If this is not done, a clinic could lock itself out of its own data. Second, each employee should have his or her own login. Some clinics like to think they can share logins—i.e., the front desk position would login as FRONTDESK. If more than one person uses the same login, this setup does not allow for the needed HIPAA privacy record of who has viewed or changed records.

PRACTICE EXERCISE 8-3   Security Setup

In this practice exercise, you are going to create security for two users. The first user will be Betty Newby with the password of "money@15" and an Access Level of 1. The second user will be Joe Again with the password of "billing@17" and an Access Level of 3. **Note:** You are encouraged to create passwords containing a combination of letters, numbers, and symbols, as this provides for greater security.

1 Open Security Setup under the File menu in Medisoft.

2 Select New to add a new user (Figure 8-8).

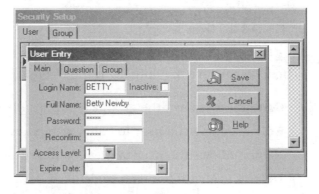

▶ **Figure 8-8   Creating a New User**

3 Fill in the appropriate information for the two new users under the Main tab.

Login Name: Generally the person's first name (i.e., Betty or Joe).

Full Name: The person's complete name (i.e., Betty Newby or Joe Again).

Password: The selected password (i.e., money@15 or billing@17).

Reconfirm: Repeat the password to eliminate the error potential.

Access Level: Corresponds with the Security Permissions Grid printed previously.

Expiration Date: Allows offices to terminate user accounts on a specific date; this is especially helpful for temporary employees.

4 Select the Question tab and pick a question to unlock your password in case it is forgotten.

5 Click Save and exit Medisoft.

6 Reenter into Medisoft that the password for one of the users was forgotten. Answer the question to unlock and reset the password.

Group Settings: A Closer Look

Groups are used within another utility called the Work Administrator. The Work Administrator is a tool that is used to manage the work within the practice and will be covered in detail in Chapter 11. Groups are created in the Security Setup window that was just reviewed under the Group tab. Let's open the group area by going to File on the menu bar, Security Setup in the drop-down list, followed by selecting the Group tab at the top of the pop-up box (Figure 8-9).

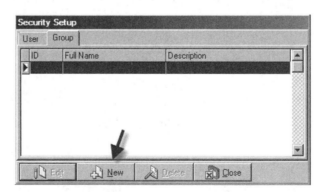

▶ Figure 8-9   **Group Setup**

The following are the options in the Group box:

Group: Displays the groups setup in this set of data.

Edit: Allows the user to edit a group already created.

New: Allows the user to create a new group.

Delete: Allows the user to delete a group.

Close: Closes the Security Setup pop-up box.

PRACTICE EXERCISE 8-4   Group Setup

In this practice exercise, we are going to create two Groups. The Groups will be named Front Desk and AR Management. The user Joe will be assigned to the AR Management group and Betty to the Front Desk group (Figure 8-10).

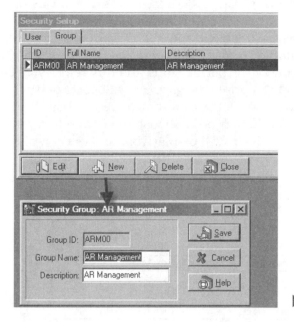

▶ **Figure 8-10   Group Entry**

1   Open Security Setup and select the Group tab.

2   Select New, fill in the Group Name and Description, and click Save. (**Note**: the Group ID automatically completes.)

3   Repeat step 1 to create the second group.

4   Next, click on the User tab and edit the user Joe Again (Figure 8-11).

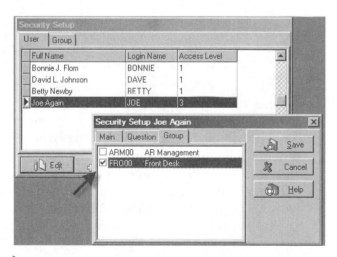

▶ **Figure 8-11   Adding a Group to a User**

5   In this pop-up window there are three tabs: Main, Question, and Group. On the Group tab assign the appropriate group to Joe Again.

6   Repeat the process with user Betty Newby.

Permissions: A Closer Look

Permissions are an essential part of Security Setup. In Security Setup, each user is assigned to a specific level from one to five. In Permissions, the specific tasks for each of the five levels are defined. Each user, particularly new users, should not have permission to do everything inside of Medisoft. Using Permissions is also a way of implementing checks and balances. The office manager should spend some time reviewing each task available in the audit report and deciding which staff members should be allowed to perform each function. Let's start by first printing a copy of the permissions and different levels currently allowed in Medisoft. To print this grid, go to Reports on the menu bar, then Custom Report List on the drop-down menu, then Security Permissions Grid in the Open Report box. Choose the option to preview the report, and an eight-page report will display that shows each of the permissions for each of the levels (Figure 8-12).

Happy Valley Medical Clinic
Security Permissions Grid
7/28/2008

Window	Process	Level 1	Level 2	Level 3	Level 4	Level 5
Activities	Billing Charges	X				
Activities	Quick Balance	X	X	X		
Activities	Quick Ledger	X	X	X		
Addresses	Delete Address Entry	X	X			
Addresses	Edit Address Entry	X	X	X		
Addresses	New Address Entry	X	X	X	X	
Addresses	View Address Entry	X	X	X	X	
Advanced Reporting						
Appointment Breaks	Delete	X	X			
Appointment Breaks	Edit	X	X	X		
Appointment Breaks	New	X	X	X	X	
Appointment Breaks	View	X	X	X	X	
Appointments	Delete	X	X			
Appointments	Edit	X	X	X		
Appointments	New	X	X	X	X	
Appointments	View	X	X	X	X	
Billing Codes	Delete Billing Code	X	X			

▶ **Figure 8-12   Security Permissions Grid**

After the office manager and/or owner has reviewed each of the Medisoft functions on the Security Permissions Grid and decided which level of staff member will have access to each function, it is time to modify the permission settings. To do this, the user should go to File on the menu bar and Permissions on the drop-down list. This will bring up the pop-up box for the Medisoft Security Permissions (Figure 8-13). Let's take a look at the components of the pop-up box:

Window: The left side of the pop-up box shows the window of activities in Medisoft.

Process: The right side of the pop-up box shows the processes attached to each activity in Medisoft and allows the user to check the permissions for each level.

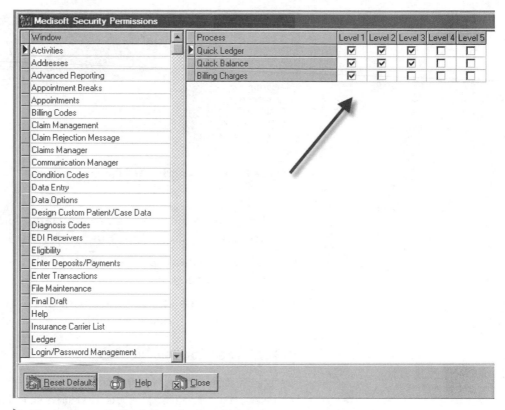

▶ Figure 8-13 **Medisoft Security Permissions**

Reset Defaults: Restores the Medisoft Security Permissions to its original settings.

Help: Gives a complete explanation of the options available in the Medisoft Security Permissions.

Close: Closes the pop-up window for Medisoft Security Permissions.

PRACTICE EXERCISE 8-5 **Changing Permissions**

Modifying the permission settings either gives or takes away the privileges of a user within a specific permission level. In this practice exercise, both types of modifications will be made. Remember from our previous discussion that there are five levels of permission assigned inside of Medisoft security, with levels ranging from one, where the user has the ability to do all tasks in Medisoft, to level five where the user has the fewest permissions. The following are the changes that will be made to the permissions settings:

Level Three: Remove the permissions to create a New Practice under Data Options.

Level Three: Add the ability to Backup Data.

Level Three: Add the ability to Index Files Only under File Maintenance.

1 Open Permissions under the File Menu.

2 Familiarize yourself with Process features listed under each Window item (Figure 8-14).

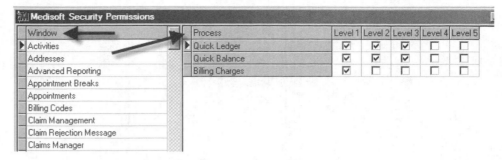

▶ Figure 8-14   **The Window and Process Features of Permissions**

3   Under the Window items, select Data Options and uncheck the permission to create a New Practice for the level three user.

4   Under the Data Options window, add the ability to Backup Data for the level three users.

5   Under the File Maintenance window, add the ability for the level three user to Index Files Only.

▶ Test Your Knowledge 8-3

Review each of the Processes under the Windows in the Permissions grid. Write three additional permissions you feel an entry-level user, level three, should be given and three that should be removed. State your reasoning for each.

Audit Records

Audit Records is the portion of Medisoft that complements Security Setup and Permissions. The options for Audit Records can be found by accessing Reports, then Audit Records in the drop-down menu (Figure 8-15). Each option gives a report for the user to print and pertinent information regarding security and permissions. Let's review the reports.

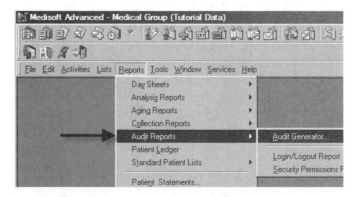

▶ Figure 8-15   **Audit Records Report Options**

Audit Generator: Allows the user to define the parameters for the Data Audit Report that will be created, showing the matching criteria for records that were deleted or updated.

Login/Logout Report: Shows the times users have logged into and out of Medisoft.

Security Permissions Report: Shows a detailed outline of features each user is allowed to access within Medisoft.

PRACTICE EXERCISE 8-6   Creating an Audit Report: Audit Generator

Of the three reports listed under the Audit Report section, the Audit Generator is the most frequently used. This is because users frequently want to know who made a change in a patient record or appointment or why a change was made. This area gives the complete details from the login name to the date and time the detailed change was made. For this example, you are going to create a detailed report of all the items entered or modified for patient Dwight Again for a time span from 01/01/2001 to 01/01/2011.

1   To generate a report, go to Reports on the menu bar, Audit Reports on the drop-down menu, and select the Audit Generator. This brings a pop-up box called the Audit Report Generator (Figure 8-16). The Audit Report Generator allows us to select from the following items:

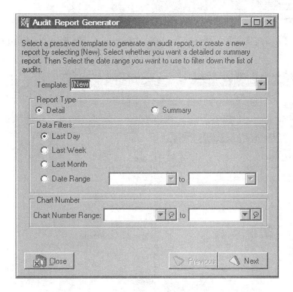

▶ **Figure 8-16   Audit Report Generator**

Template: Allows the user to select a previously created template or to create a new one; for the purpose of this exercise select (New).

Report Type: Allows the user to select if detailed information is desired or summary information; summary information only reports items changed by the user and not specifically which patients were affected.

Data Filters: Allows the user to designate the time frame for the report.

Chart Number: Allows the user to run reports for a specific patient or a span of patients.

2   After the items have been completed for the practice exercise, click Next. Now, select which users will be included in the report. This option is especially helpful for auditing a particular user. For the purpose of this exercise, select Add All, then click Next (Figure 8-17).

3   Our last option gives us the ability to select the tables to be included in the report (Figure 8-18). This is necessary to sort specific tasks

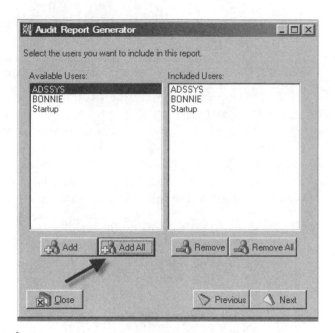

▶ Figure 8-17   Users Included in the Audit Report Generator

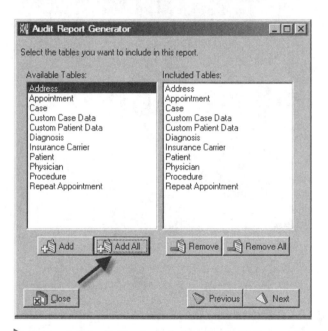

▶ Figure 8-18   Tables Included in the Audit Report Generator

done to specific areas of the program; i.e., deleted appointments or modified transactions. For this exercise, Add All and click Next.

4   In the final screen of the report generator, the user can save a new template created or simply press Print. Create a template called Dwight Again (Figure 8-19).

5   Press Print and view the report created.

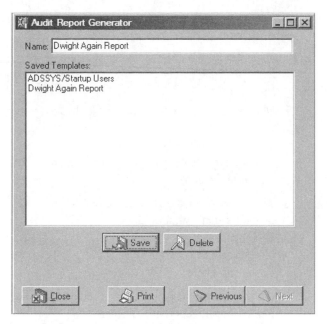

▶ Figure 8-19   Saving the Template

CHAPTER REVIEW

Multiple Choice

1. Which feature creates security for users in Medisoft?
   a. Permissions
   b. Security Setup
   c. Group Setup
   d. Billing Charges

2. Which feature creates a group in Medisoft?
   a. Security Setup
   b. Permissions
   c. Small Balance Write-off
   d. Audit Report

3. Which features gives a detailed list of the Permission settings?
   a. Audit Generator
   b. Permissions
   c. Security Permissions Grid
   d. Security Setup

4. To figure out when a user logged into and out of Medisoft, which would you use?
   a. Audit Generator
   b. Permissions Report
   c. Login/Logout Report
   d. Security Permissions Report

5. When writing off small balances, the clinic should
   a. determine policy for the amount to write off.
   b. make a new backup.
   c. run File Maintenance.
   d. all of the above.

6. How many levels of Permissions are provided by Medisoft?
   a. One
   b. Six
   c. Four
   d. Five

7. When adding Billing Charges, the clinic should
   a. make a backup.
   b. run File Maintenance.
   c. research local regulations surrounding billing charges.
   d. all of the above.

8. Where are groups used to track tasks?
   a. Work Administrator
   b. Security Setup
   c. Permissions
   d. Group Tracker

9. If a user wants to find out who changed a patient's account and when it was changed, which of the following reports should be run?
   a. Security Permissions Grid
   b. Login/Logout Report
   c. Audit Generator
   d. Transaction Report

10. Which of the following would be a good procedure to run before statements?
    a. Backup, Statements
    b. Backup, File Maintenance, Billing Charges, Small Balance Write-off, Statements
    c. Backup, File Maintenance, Small Balance Write-off, Billing Charges, Statements
    d. Security Setup, File Maintenance, Statements

11. When setting up security, the administrator should be level
    a. one.
    b. five.
    c. any level.
    d. six.

12. Greater security is provided by passwords that contain
    a. letters.
    b. numbers.
    c. symbols.
    d. all of the above.

13. If the clinic charges 12% annually, how much would be entered into the Monthly Billing Charge field under the Billing Charge pop-up window?
    a. 1.2%
    b. 12%
    c. 2%
    d. 1%

14. In Security Setup, which access level has the fewest privileges by default?
    a. One
    b. Three
    c. Five
    d. Six

15. In Small Balance Write-off, Medisoft defaults the write-off amount to be
    a. $5.00.
    b. $3.00.
    c. $10.00.
    d. $1.00.

True/False

Identify each of the following statements as true or false.

1. Clinics can assess their patients any amount of Billing Charges they decide.

2. Clinics can write-off any balance they decide without regard to their insurance contracts.

3. Billing charges are assessed to patients as well as insurance companies.

4. Billing Charges use the Code Type of Adjustment.

5. Small Balance Write-offs use the Code Type of Adjustment.

6. The Security Permissions Grid assigns the access level to each user.

7. Groups are used in the Work Administrator.

8. HIPAA addresses the access level for each user.

9. All users working the same position should use the same login and password.

10. The Audit Generator generates the security setting for each user.

Short Answer

1. Explain which tools are available to the medical office specialist to problem solve questions on the Medisoft utilities covered in this chapter.

2. If you, as the medical office specialist, accepted a position at a new clinic that had Medisoft and some of the features covered in this chapter were not available, explain why that may be and what you would look at to confirm your belief.

3. Describe the steps that should be taken prior to adding billing charges to patient statements.

Resources

HIPAA Information: **www.cms.hhs.gov/HIPAAGenInfo/**

Government website designed to disseminate HIPAA information to providers.

Chapter Nine

Reporting and Accounts Receivable Management

Learning Objectives

After completing this chapter, you should be able to:

♦ Define and spell the key terms in this chapter.

♦ Understand and describe how to manage accounts receivable.

♦ Explain the importance of a clinic follow-up policy.

♦ Demonstrate how to determine days in accounts receivable for a practice.

♦ Identify and describe reports and strategies for collecting accounts receivable.

♦ Describe the Simple Patient Aging report.

♦ Print Insurance Aging reports: Primary, secondary, and tertiary.

♦ Create a plan for follow-up on patient balances.

♦ Create a plan for follow-up on insurance balances.

♦ Explain reporting options for doctors and/or office managers.

Key Terms

accounts receivable (AR)   money owed to the clinic for services provided.

Collection List   a utility inside Medisoft that assists users in follow-up activities.

contract insurance category   the section of accounts receivable that has been billed to a contracted insurance company.

days in accounts receivable   the average number of days it takes for a clinic to receive its money, calculated as the total AR divided by the average daily revenue.

Fair Debt Collection Practices Act   a federal law controlling the collection of debt.

follow-up procedures   describes the steps of how unpaid accounts will be processed by the office in order to collect the outstanding balances.

non-contract insurance category   the section of accounts receivable that has been billed to a non-contract insurance company.

self-pay category   the section of accounts receivable that is entirely due from the patient guarantor.

ticklers   items within the Collection List.

Abbreviations

AR   accounts receivable

■ ■ ■ ■

INTRODUCTION

Many offices get swept away in doing the apparent "must do" tasks of Medisoft, such as adding new patients, entering charges and payments, and scheduling (refer to the Daily Medisoft Work Flow covered in Chapter 1). However, this is only half of the job; the other half entails following up on unpaid accounts, tracking receivables, and reporting. As with the familiar 80/20 principal, 80 percent of the accounts get paid the first time. But, the 20 percent not paid take 80 percent of the time. This chapter provides tools to track unpaid accounts, receive a faster turnaround on payments, and manage reporting to assist in these tasks.

AN OVERVIEW OF MANAGING ACCOUNTS RECEIVABLE

There are three parts to managing **accounts receivable.** First, clinic policies need to be established to outline the management of aging accounts; next **follow-up procedures** need to be implemented; and finally, the progress of the accounts receivable (**AR**) management needs to be followed by monthly reporting.

Creating Accounts Receivable Clinic Policies

Before the medical office specialist can manage accounts receivable, the office needs to have clearly defined policies regarding unpaid accounts. It is important for a clinic to have these policies in writing, so that all patients are treated consistently and fairly, and so that staff have a clear understanding of the steps to follow. All new staff should be trained as to what the follow up policies are, even if that is not their primary job, as patients may ask billing questions of clinical staff as well as office staff. It is a good idea to give patients a copy of the financial policy that applies to their category at the time the appointment is scheduled, so that clear expectations are established from the beginning. Any patient seen at a medical office falls into one of three accounts receivable categories: **self-pay category, non-contract insurance category,** or **contract insurance category.** Review the definitions of these three categories:

Self-Pay: Accounts due from the patient; hence, the patient either does not have insurance coverage or his or her insurance has finished processing charges.

Non-contract Insurance: Accounts outstanding from an insurance company with which the clinic does not have a contract.

Contract Insurance: Accounts outstanding from an insurance company with which the clinic does have a contract.

Why is it important to note if the clinic has a contract with the patient's insurance company? If the clinic has a contract with an insurance company, the insurance company is contractually obligated to process and settle the claim with the office. If the clinic does not have a contract with the insurance company, the clinic does not have to work with the insurance company to process and settle claims. In essence, with non-contract insurance companies, the contract is strictly between the patient and the insurance company, so the clinic is really doing "courtesy billing" on behalf of the patient and does not have the contractual obligation to follow-up on the claim. This should affect the way a clinic writes its accounts receivable management policies.

Although there are dozens of variations for follow-up policies, the following are basic examples with steps outlined.

Example 1: Self-Pay Follow-Up Policy

Step 1: Patients should pay their balance on the date of service. This expectation should be established at the time the appointment is made. If the patient fails to pay, proceed to Step 2.

Step 2: If the patient does not pay in full at the time of service, a statement will be sent on the first of each month. If the patient makes a payment, Step 2 will be repeated. If the patient does not make a payment within 30 days, proceed to Step 3.

Step 3: If the patient misses a payment at the Step 2 level, the patient will be sent a friendly reminder statement asking the patient to contact the office to help him or her set up a reasonable payment plan. The office can set up Medisoft to automatically print the friendly message on the statement as discussed in Chapter 6. After the friendly reminder statement is sent, if the patient makes a payment, statements will continue to be sent. If the patient does not pay within 30 days of the friendly reminder statement, proceed to Step 4.

Step 4: Once the patient has received two statements and failed to pay, the patient will be sent a collection statement giving the patient 10 days to pay or be turned over to a licensed collection agency. After the collection statement is sent, if the patient pays, continue to bill the patient. If the patient does not pay within 10 days, proceed to Step 5.

Step 5: Transfer the patient's outstanding balance to a collection agency and write off outstanding balance in Medisoft to a bad debt adjustment. Once the account is turned over to collection, the office can have no further follow-up with the patient. Any payments made must be channeled through the collection agency.

Billing Insight Rules and Regulations of Collection Accounts

Strict laws, both federal and state, surround the collection practices of medical offices. Prior to developing collection practices, a clinic should consult its local board of medical practice for direction in collection practices. In addition, the **Fair Debt Collection Practices Act** (see Resources at the end of the chapter) should be read and state laws consulted. If accounts are to be placed with a collection agency, again all collection laws must be strictly adhered to and in most states agencies must be licensed.

Example 2: Non-Contract Insurance

Step 1: Bill the non-contract insurance company within 24 hours of the patient's service; preferably electronically. If the insurance fails to pay within 30 days, proceed to Step 2.

Step 2: Post a denial in Medisoft showing the insurance failed to pay and the balance is due from the patient. This will mark the claim done and move the money due to a remainder statement.

Step 3: Send a remainder statement to the patient with a notice that his or her insurance has been billed and failed to pay, hence the patient is responsible to pay the balance.

Step 4: At this point, the account is considered self-pay, and self-pay policies should be followed starting with Step 2.

Billing Insight   Prompt Pay Laws

Most states have insurance commissioners or state laws that govern insurance companies and prompt payment. Often, prompt payment is defined as 30 or 60 days. It is a good idea for each office to have a copy of its state's rules in its policy manual and to know the recourse it has if the insurance companies do not follow the law. Also, for contract payers, each office should be aware of the terms and conditions of the contracts and make sure it receives payments in accordance with the contracts.

Example 3: Contract Insurance

Step 1: Bill the contract insurance company within 24 hours of the patient's service, preferably electronically. If the insurance fails to pay within 30 days, proceed to Step 2.

Step 2: Call the insurance company, documenting the phone number called, person spoken to, and the name of the insurance company in the Comment section of the Claim in Claim Management. Document the action that is needed to settle the claim and the action that will be taken, knowing there are only three possibilities: (a) the patient owes the claim, (b) the insurance owes the claim, or (c) the insurance needs more information to process the claim. Once these items are documented, proceed to Step 3.

Step 3: If the insurance states the balance is due from the patient, process a denial in Medisoft, marking the claim done, and moving the balance to the remainder statement. If the insurance states it is responsible for the balance, get a commitment to pay and document that with the other notes in the Comment tab. If the insurance states it needs additional information to process the claim, get the needed information as soon as possible and confirm the receipt of the information. If the claim is not paid within another 30 days, proceed to Step 4.

Step 4: The only balances that reach this step are those that the insurance has made a commitment to pay, or additional information has been sent to them. If the claim is not paid after 30 days, call the insurance again and thoroughly document the findings. Since this is a contract payer, review the contract terms and conditions and, if necessary, notify them if the contract has been broken. Step 4 is very seldom reached with contract payers.

Determining the Days in Accounts Receivable

After clinic policies are established, it is time to calculate the **days in accounts receivable** for the office and set standards for the office to maintain. There are several theories and ways to benchmark accounts receivable. For the purpose of this chapter we are going to divide the gross outstanding receivables by a 90-day average of daily revenue to get the average number of days to collect money.

First, start by printing a Practice Analysis and calculating the days in accounts receivable (Figure 9-1). To perform this function, select Reports on the menu bar, then Analysis Reports on the drop-down menu, followed by Practice Analysis. This brings the pop-up menu for the Date Selection Questions—Practice Analysis (Figure 9-2). Here you will find the data selection options for this report. However, for determining the days in AR, we will only modify two of the items to print the report, the Date From range and the check box for Show Accounts Receivable Total Page. The list below provides an overview of what is available.

Procedure Code Range: Allows the user to run a report for a single procedure code or range of codes.

Date Created Range: Gives the option to run a report based upon the dates transactions were entered into Medisoft (versus the date of the transaction).

Date From Range: Allows reports to be created based upon the date of the transaction (for the days in AR report, we will enter a range for the last three completed months of transactions).

Attending Provider Range: Runs the report for a single provider, range of providers, or all providers.

Place of Service Range: Allows the report to be compiled by a single place of service (POS) code or range of codes.

Transaction Facility Range: Allows reports to be filtered by the transaction facility.

Case Billing Code Range: Allows reports to be created by the Billing Codes inside of the patients' Case.

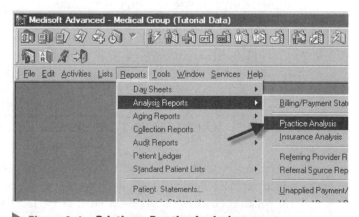

▶ Figure 9-1   **Printing a Practice Analysis**

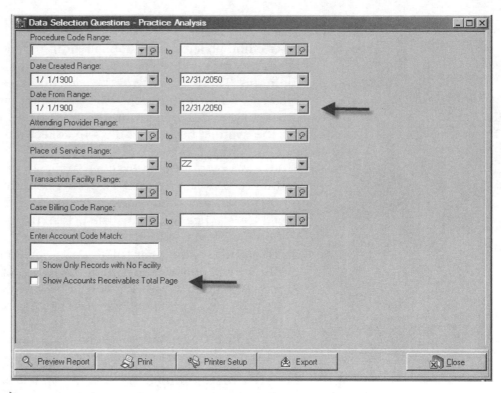

▶ Figure 9-2   Data Selection Questions—Practice Analysis

Enter Account Code Match: Directly related to the procedure code file; it allows the user to sort the practice analysis, the account code setup attached to the procedure code.

Show Only Records with No Facility: Creates a report for only those transactions that do not have a facility.

Show Accounts Receivables Total Page: Shows the current practice totals on the last page.

After printing the report, divide the Total Charge column by 90, which is the number of days in the report. (If a clinic were to run the report for one month, they would divide the Total Charges by 30 or 31.) This is the daily average revenue. Next, take the total accounts receivable shown at the bottom of the report and divide it by the daily average revenue. The result is the average number of days it takes for the clinic to collect its money. Days in AR will vary from one clinic to another depending on the contractual agreements a clinic has and whether the clinic transmits electronically. A general guideline to follow and a good starting point is for a clinic to have its days in accounts receivable below 60 days. Clinics should track their monthly AR and set a goal for employees to keep the days in AR below a certain point.

PRACTICE EXERCISE 9-1   Determining the Days in Accounts Receivable

Again, only two boxes need to be completed to compile the days in outstanding AR. Typically, a clinic would use the previous three months and the total accounts receivable. But, because the tutorial practice is limited in data, complete this practice exercise twice. First, use the entire date range, then use the month surrounding the data previously entered in Chapter 3: Transaction Entry.

1   First, the Date From Range should show the last three completed months. For example, if we are printing the report on February 5, 2010, the last three months completed would be November 1, 2009 through January 31, 2010. For the purpose of this exercise, leave the Date From Range as is for the first report and use 9/1/08 to 9/30/08 for the second report.

2   Next, we also need to know the total amount of accounts receivable on the books. That can be obtained by checking the Show Accounts Receivables Total Page in the data selection questions.

3   Select the Preview Report option.

4   After the report has been compiled, it is quite simple to calculate the days in AR. First, look at the last page of the report. The total charge column should be divided by 90. This gives the daily revenue average for the last 90 days. For the report created for September 2008, divide the charge total by 30.

5   Next, take the total accounts receivable shown at the bottom of the report and divide it by the average daily revenue. The result is the average number of days it takes for the clinic to collect its money.

▶ **Test Your Knowledge 9-1**

Imagine you work at a clinic that has three doctors. One of the doctors wants to know her days in accounts receivable versus the overall clinic's number. How would you arrive at the two numbers?

Medisoft Quick Tip   Fast AR Total
Once a clinic starts tracking its AR, the staff usually becomes enthused about watching the amount in accounts receivable drop. A quick way to see the total on the books without running reports is to go to Tools on the menu bar, then User Information. This gives a one-page summary of statistics for the practice, from patient count records to the total outstanding accounts receivable. Again, this report gives totals—for example, the total charges lists the total ever entered into the data set.

REPORTS AND STRATEGIES FOR COLLECTING ACCOUNTS RECEIVABLE

As explained in previous chapters, Medisoft offers three types of its program: Basic, Advanced, and Network Professional. This allows the program to be versatile and accommodate every type of practice from a single doctor cash practice to a large insurance practice with several doctors. With each type of practice, there are several suitable options to adequately perform follow-up on unpaid accounts. Although the Basic program could be used in all settings, Advanced or Network Professional would save offices considerable time and money by expediting cash flow and efficiency. Some clinics shortchange themselves by purchasing the least expensive program but end up spending more because of decreased productivity and cash flow. In this section, we will explore reports and methods used to perform follow-up.

The Patient Aging Report

Performing follow-up by using the Patient Aging report entails two steps. The first step is to set the Program Options to accommodate the clinic's policies. Program Options can be accessed and modified by selecting File on the menu bar, then Program Options from the drop-down menu. Once the pop-up menu for Program Options appears, select the Aging Reports tab (Figure 9-3).

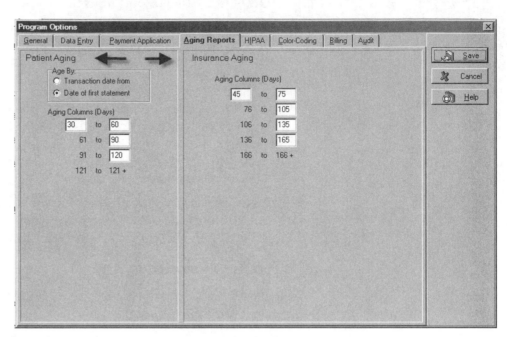

▶ **Figure 9-3   Setting Program Options—Aging Reports**

Notice that the Aging Reports tab is divided into two sections: Patient Aging and Insurance Aging. The Patient Aging tab gives the option to run a patient aging report by transaction date or date of first statement. If the date of first statement is chosen, only patients who have received statements will be listed on the report. For an insurance practice that runs remainder statements, this option would limit the number of outstanding balances placed on the report. Both the Patient Aging and the Insurance Aging tabs allow us to modify the data to be printed on the reports by setting the Aging Column Days. For example, if a clinic chooses to start the follow-up process at 45 days, the start day would be 45 rather than 30. In other words, it can be very beneficial to match the begin dates with the clinic's follow-up policies. This eliminates the accounts that do not need to be reviewed from printing on the reports.

PRACTICE EXERCISE 9-2   Setting the Aging Column in Program Options

In this practice exercise, the Aging Column Days will be set within Program Options. For the purpose of this exercise, you will work under the assumption that the office follows-up on patient balances over 30 days and insurance balances over 45 days.

1 Open Program Options by selecting it from the File menu.

2 Click on the Aging Reports tab.

3 Notice the two sections in the Aging Reports tab. Under the Patient Aging section, choose the option to run the report by Date of First Statement. (This will assist in filtering out patients who have not been billed yet.)

4 Under the Patient Aging section, enter the beginning Aging Column Days to be 30 and make the span every 30 days.

5 Under the Insurance Aging section, enter the beginning Aging Column Days to be 45 and make the span every 30 days.

6 Save the changes made in Program Options.

Now that Program Options are modified, the next step for a clinic would be to print an aging report to work the older accounts that fall within the set parameters.

PRACTICE EXERCISE 9-3   Printing the Patient Aging Report

In this practice exercise, a patient aging report will be printed. The Aging Column Days will be set within Program Options. For follow-up purposes, the clinic will want to print a report containing all balances over the minimum days designated in Program Options.

1 Reports are printed from the Reports heading on the menu bar. To print a Patient Aging report, select Reports from the menu bar, Aging Reports from the drop-down box, and Patient Aging from the side box (Figure 9-4).

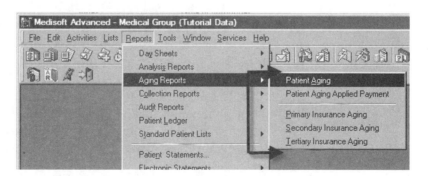

▶ **Figure 9-4   Printing the Patient Aging Report**

2 Once again, many filters can be entered to restrict the report's output. For follow-up purposes, the report needs to contain all balances over the minimum days designated in Program Options. So, the report can be previewed or printed without adding anything to the filters (Figure 9-5).

The following filters are available on the report:

Aging Columns: Correlates to the Aging Report setting in Program Options; it assists the clinic in processing the account through its policies.

Chart #:   Gives the Chart number for the outstanding account.

Happy Valley Medical Clinic
Patient Aging
August 02, 2008

Chart#	Name	Birthdate	Current 30 - 60	Past 61 - 90	Past 91 - 120	Past 121 +	Total Balance
AGADW000 Again, Dwight		3/30/1932	200.00	0.00	0.00	216.00	416.00
Last Pmt: -10.00 On: 4/10/2010		434-5777					
AU SAN000 Austin, Andrew		1/1/1950	48.00	0.00	0.00	0.00	48.00
Last Pmt: -10.00 On: 9/4/2008		767-2222			Unapplied Pmt/Adj: -35.00		
BORJO000 Bordon, John		1/20/1972	25.00	0.00	0.00	106.00	131.00
Last Pmt: 0.00 On:		(434)777-1234					
BRIEL000 Brimley, Elmo		9/29/1997	96.00	0.00	0.00	0.00	96.00
Last Pmt: -10.00 On: 9/4/2008		(222)342-3444					
BRISU000 Brimley, Susan			173.00	0.00	0.00	12.00	185.00
Last Pmt: -10.00 On: 9/4/2008		(222)342-3444					
CATSA000 Catera, Sammy		6/17/1964	40.00	0.00	0.00	71.00	111.00
Last Pmt: 0.00 On:		227-7722					

▶ Figure 9-5   The Details of the Patient Aging Report

Name: Gives the name of the patient for the outstanding account.

Birthdate: Gives the birthdate of the patient.

Amount Outstanding: Gives the amounts outstanding in each aging division along with the total due on the account.

Last Payment: Reports the last payment amount.

On: Reports the last payment date.

Phone: Gives the patient's phone number.

3   Preview the report noting the various columns and details on the report.

Once generated, this report can be used to work the follow-up policies designed by the clinic. Follow-up procedures will vary based upon program type, but it is important that each outstanding account is worked each month. It is equally important that the follow-up work is documented in the note section of Transaction Entry, Claim Management, or Statement Management. The Patient Aging report will give a complete list of accounts that need to be worked. The following sections of this chapter will include shortcuts available to clinics using Advanced and Network Professional Medisoft.

Medisoft Quick Tip   Modifying the Grid Columns

The best time-saving feature in Medisoft follow-up is the ability to modify the grid columns. The three most important places to modify grid columns are in Transaction Entry, Claim Management, and Statement Management. (Remember: The Basic Medisoft does not include Statement Management.) Let's review how to modify the grid columns.

The grid columns to modify can be easily selected from any of the aforementioned screens by clicking on the black dot located in the upper left corner of the grid (Figure 9-6). Once this dot is clicked, a pop-up box called Grid Column appears. This box gives the name of currently displayed fields along with the option to Add Fields or Remove Fields in addition to moving the field positions up or down. Also included in this pop-up box is the handy Help button to give additional information on this specific area. To speed the follow-up process, it is helpful to Add Fields. After the Add Fields button is clicked, another pop-up box will appear, allowing fields to be added. The following is a list of fields that can be helpful to add to the three pertinent utilities.

Transaction Entry: Claim Number, Statement Number, Remainder, Date of First Statement, Date of Second Statement.

Claims Management: Primary Submission Count, Amount, Date of First Service.

Statement Management: Submission Count, Days Old.

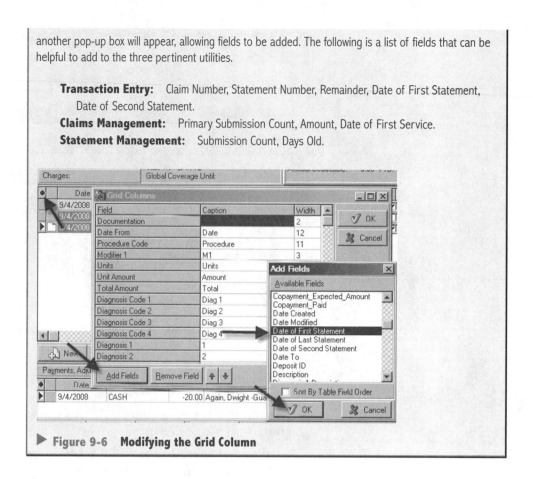

▶ **Figure 9-6   Modifying the Grid Column**

Printing the Insurance Aging Reports: Primary, Secondary, and Tertiary

After the Patient Aging report is printed, the next reports to compile are the insurance aging reports (Figure 9-7). There are three types of insurance aging reports: primary, secondary, and tertiary. Of course, the report name reflects the position of the payer within the patient case and claim. In addition, the aging columns have already been set from the early work done in Program Options. The Program Options, Aging Report tab was modified to reflect the clinic's policies on follow-up. To create an insurance aging, choose Reports on the menu bar, Aging Reports on the drop-down menu, and Primary Insurance Aging from the side menu. Again, filter options restrict the data output for the reports (Figure 9-8).

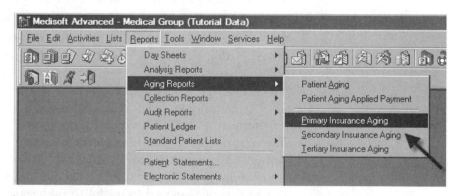

▶ **Figure 9-7   Insurance Aging Reports**

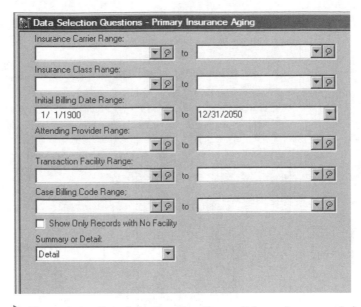

▶ Figure 9-8 Data Selection Questions—Primary Insurance Aging

The following filters are available:

Insurance Carrier Range: Allows the user to create a report for designated insurance carriers.

Insurance Class Range: This field is similar to a Billing Code for a patient; in List and Insurance Carriers, an Insurance Class can be assigned to group carriers into types, i.e., worker's comp, Medicare, commercial insurance, etc. This field allows the report to be filtered by Insurance Class Range.

Initial Billing Date Range Allows the report to be created for specific billing dates.

Attending Provider Range: Allows the report to be run for a single provider, range of providers, or all providers.

Transaction Facility Range: Allows reports to be filtered by the transaction facility.

Case Billing Code Range: Allows reports to be created by the Billing Codes inside the patient's Case.

Show Only Records with No Facility: Shows only records that do not have a facility associated with them.

Summary or Detail: Toggle field that gives the option of viewing the detail of each outstanding claim (Figure 9-9) or the summary of the outstanding claims (Figure 9-10); both options can be beneficial.

Let's compare the options provided by a detail versus summary aging report. The detail aging report provides all of the information needed for a staff member to call an insurance company on unpaid claims, including name of insurance, phone number and contact person, plus the policy number, date of birth, and outstanding transactions. This report would be very helpful if a medical office specialist did not have access to a computer and was assigned to assist in follow-up.

Primary Insurance Aging

August 02, 2008

Date of Service	Procedure	- Past - 45 to 75	- Past - 76 to 105	- Past - 106 to 135	- Past - 136 to 165	- Past - 166 +	Total Balance
Cigna (CIG00)						Bill S. Preston 234-5678	
BRIJA000 Jay Brimley			SS:				
Birthdate: 1/23/1964	Policy: 98547377				Group: 12d		
Claim: 3	Initial Billing Date: 3/25/2002			Last Billing Date: 3/25/2002			
3/25/2002	99214	$0.00	$0.00	$0.00	$0.00	$65.00	$65.00
3/25/2002	97260	$0.00	$0.00	$0.00	$0.00	$30.00	$30.00
		$0.00	$0.00	$0.00	$0.00	$95.00	$95.00
BRIJA000 Jay Brimley			SS:				
Birthdate: 1/23/1964	Policy: 98547377				Group: 12d		
Claim: 12	Initial Billing Date: 5/28/2007			Last Billing Date: 5/28/2007			
3/9/2007	99211	$0.00	$0.00	$0.00	$0.00	$25.00	$25.00
		$0.00	$0.00	$0.00	$0.00	$25.00	$25.00
	Insurance Totals:	$0.00	$0.00	$0.00	$0.00	$120.00	$120.00
Medicare (MED01)						Ted T. Logan (800)999-9999	
AGADW000 Dwight Again			SS:				
Birthdate: 3/30/1932	Policy: 780340761				Group: 23c		
Claim: 7	Initial Billing Date: 12/6/2002			Last Billing Date: 12/6/2002			
9/3/2002	73130	$0.00	$0.00	$0.00	$0.00	$45.00	$45.00
9/3/2002	99213	$0.00	$0.00	$0.00	$0.00	$60.00	$60.00
		$0.00	$0.00	$0.00	$0.00	$105.00	$105.00

▶ **Figure 9-9   Detailed Primary Insurance Aging**

Primary Insurance Aging Summary

August 02, 2008

Date of Service	Procedure	- Past - 45 to 75	- Past - 76 to 105	- Past - 106 to 135	- Past - 136 to 165	- Past - 166 +	Total Balance
Cigna (CIG00)						Bill S. Preston 234-5678	
Claim: 3	Initial Billing Date: 3/25/2002			Last Billing Date: 3/25/2002			
Claim: 12	Initial Billing Date: 5/28/2007			Last Billing Date: 5/28/2007			
	Insurance Totals:	$0.00	$0.00	$0.00	$0.00	$120.00	$120.00
Medicare (MED01)						Ted T. Logan (800)999-9999	
Claim: 7	Initial Billing Date: 12/6/2002			Last Billing Date: 12/6/2002			
Claim: 10	Initial Billing Date: 5/28/2007			Last Billing Date: 5/28/2007			
Claim: 18	Initial Billing Date: 7/7/2007			Last Billing Date: 9/1/2008			
	Insurance Totals:	$0.00	$0.00	$0.00	$0.00	$310.00	$310.00
U.S. Tricare (US000)							
Claim: 6	Initial Billing Date: 5/28/2007			Last Billing Date: 5/28/2007			
	Insurance Totals:	$0.00	$0.00	$0.00	$0.00	$85.00	$85.00
Report Aging Totals:		$0.00	$0.00	$0.00	$0.00	$515.00	$515.00
Percent of Aging Total:		0.00%	0.00%	0.00%	0.00%	100.00%	100.00%

▶ **Figure 9-10   Summary Primary Insurance Aging**

However, because of the detail, the report can be lengthy. The summary report also gives the name of the insurance, phone number and contact person, but only gives the claim numbers and claim billing dates. This report would be nice to work with if the computer was available. It groups the claims together by insurance company and shows the claim numbers to assist in documentation.

Once the primary insurance aging is printed and has been worked, the steps should be followed with the secondary and tertiary insurance aging. There are many ways to manage insurance follow-up, but a few basic principles should be followed: (1) Call each insurance monthly that fits the clinic's policy on contract follow-up, and (2) document the insurance called, phone number dialed, and person spoken with along with the response and any action taken on the clinic's behalf (e.g., billed patient, received commitment to pay, forwarded additional information to the insurance).

PRACTICE EXERCISE 9-4   Printing Insurance Aging Reports

Printing the insurance aging reports for primary, secondary, and tertiary payers completes the follow-up process. In this practice exercise, a detail and summary aging report will be previewed for each payer category.

1   Open the Primary Insurance Aging by going to Reports, Aging Reports, and Primary Insurance Aging.

2   Leave all the filters as is and select Preview Report. Note the last filter defaults to Detail.

3   Preview the Primary Insurance Aging again by changing the last filter to Summary.

4   Note the differences between the two reports.

5   Process the Secondary and Tertiary Insurance Aging in the same manner as the Primary.

6   Write a synopsis of how both the detail and summary reports could be useful.

▶ Test Your Knowledge 9-2

Imagine the clinic is having billing issues with its Medicare claims and needs to rebill all Medicare claims over 45 days. Write two different scenarios of how Medicare claims could be filtered in Medisoft to achieve this.

Insurance Follow-up Through Claim Management and Collection List

Although printing a report and having it available is beneficial, follow-up can also be done through Claim Management or the **Collection List** without printing a report. This is more earth-friendly and can be more efficient. Let's look at the two options to follow up without printing a report.

Claim Management

If payments are being posted properly, claims that are paid are marked Done. This affords us the opportunity to filter the Sent claims, sort them by the Bill Date, and implement the office policies. This can be accomplished by first going to Claim Management either under Activities or the Claim Management toolbar icon. Then, by selecting List Only on the Claim Management top toolbar, filters can be applied to sort claims that have been sent but not paid (Figure 9-11). After clicking on List Only, select Primary (or Secondary or Tertiary if that type of follow-up is being done) and select Sent. The Sent claims will be the claims that have not been paid by the insurance. Next, click on Bill Date 1 (Figure 9-12) (or Bill Date 2 for Secondary Claims or Bill Date 3 for Tertiary Claims) and the claims will be sorted oldest to newest or by clicking again it will sort newest to oldest. Using either option, now the insurance can be contacted on a list of claims according to the policies developed by the clinic. And, don't forget that it is imperative to add a note inside the claim stating the place called, phone number dialed, and person spoken with to document the follow-up call. In addition, the action that is needed to process the claim and action taken should be documented. Figure 9-13 shows an example of a follow-up note. Notice that you can see in Claim Management which claims have documentation.

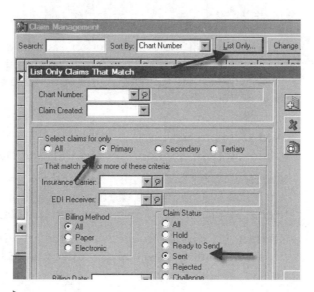

▶ Figure 9-11   Filtering Claims in Claim Management

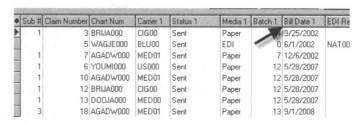

▶ Figure 9-12   Sorting Claims by Bill Date

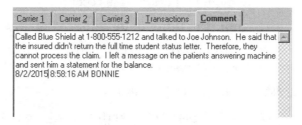

▶ Figure 9-13   Adding Documentation to Claims

Collection List

The next opportunity we have in Medisoft is to do paperless follow-up by utilizing the Collection List. There are two steps to utilizing the Collection List: First, we need to add items to the Collection List (by following the clinic policies, of course), and next, we need to work the items within the Collection List. The beauty of this process is that Collection List can contain all of the follow-up items for the clinic: self-pay accounts plus primary, secondary, and tertiary insurance accounts. And, if this isn't enough, Collection List functions can be assigned to the appropriate person in the office to do the task, and each person can filter his or her own accounts. As you can see, the Collection List is a great solution for follow-up, but as stated many times previously, not all Medisoft programs have Collection list, so both Collection List and Claim Management need to be learned.

To proceed with learning Collection List, select Activities on the menu bar, then Add Collection List Item from the drop-down menu. Next, a pop-up window will appear, giving options to complete. The following is a review of the options.

Add items based on ...:   Allows parameters to be set if items from Claim Management or Statement Management will be added.

Carriers: If Claim Management items are chosen in the first option, then this option allows the choice to add all matching claims or selected Primary, Secondary, and Tertiary claims.

Claim: If Claim Management items are chosen in the first option, this section allows all claim statuses to be selected or just the Rejected or Challenged statuses.

Range of:

Insurances: For Claim Management lists, a filter by insurance companies can be added here.

Initial Billing Date: Can apply to either Statement Management or Claim Management; it is useful for targeting accounts over a certain age.

Billing Date: Pertains to the last date billed.

Add item if submission count is greater than:

Enter Number: Applies to either Statement Management or Claim Management; this is particularly helpful in tracking the number of statements a patient has received.

Add item if patient remainder balance is greater than:

Enter Amount: Pertains only to remainder statements due by the patient; allows statements to be filtered by amount.

Add Delinquent Payments:

Missed Payments: Pertains only to patient balances that have a payment plan associated with them in the Chart; checking this box allows for filtering missed payments.

For Patient Payment Plan: Allows the selected Payment Plan to be monitored.

Assign to: Allows Collection List Items to be designated to a particular user.

Add Billing Comment to Office Notes: By checking this box, Medisoft will copy the Claim Management or Statement Management Notes into the Collection List.

Add items: Performs the Add Collection List Items task.

Cancel: Exits the pop-up window.

Help: Offers detailed help on Add Collection List Items.

Defaults: Resets the options inside the window.

PRACTICE EXERCISE 9-5   Adding Items to the Collection List

After reading the previous section, you will probably agree that Collection List offers the most streamlined approach for follow-up. In this practice exercise, we are going to add patient and primary insurance items to the list.

1 Open the pop-up window for Add Collection List Items by selecting Activities on the menu bar, then Add Collection List Items on the drop-down menu.

2 Next, add **ticklers** for patients who have received two or more statements. To do this: Select the Statements radio button and enter the number 1 in the Enter Number box. **Note:** This box states, "Add item if the submission count is greater than _____" (Figure 9-14).

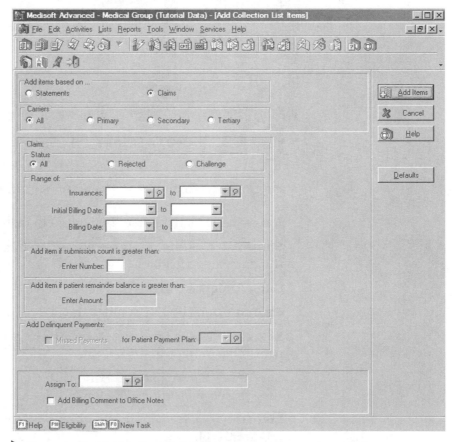

▶ **Figure 9-14   Add Collection List Items**

3 Now, click the select Add Items to complete the process.

4   Repeat the steps and add to the list insurance claims that have an initial billing date before 01/01/2000 and Add Billing Comment to Office Notes.

Once the items have been added to the Collection List, the next task is to work the items according to the clinic's follow-up policies. To access the Collection List, select Activites on the menu bar, then select Collection List from the drop-down menu. This gives the pop-up window for Collection List along with a wealth of information to assist in follow-up. The items that are contained in Collection List are known as ticklers. This is a term used historically by collection agencies and is a method used to track outstanding accounts (Figure 9-15).

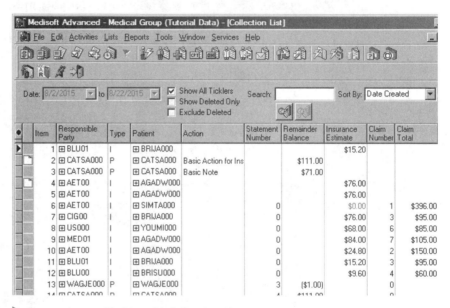

▶ **Figure 9-15   Working the Collection List**

The items available to view, filter, and sort in Collection List follow.

Date: Allows ticklers to be filtered by date.

Show All Ticklers: Shows all ticklers regardless of dates (shuts off the date range fields).

Show Deleted Only: Shows the deleted ticklers only.

Exclude Deleted: Excludes the deleted ticklers.

Search: Works hand in hand with the Sort By option; allows the user to search for items specified in the Sort By type.

Sort By: Works hand in hand with the Search option; allows the user to specify the type of item to be searched.

List Only: Gives another pop-up box that allows additional filters (Figure 9-16).

Change Status: Gives a pop-up box similar to the change status option in Claim Management allowing the status of the ticklers to be changed either one by one or in a group.

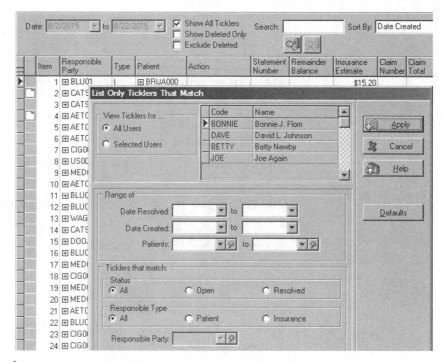

▶ **Figure 9-16   List Only Ticklers That Match**

Locate Field Value: The two search buttons directly below the Search box described above; allows another pop-up box to occur and specify more options to locate ticklers.

Item: gives each tickler a sequential item number in the Collection List.

Responsible Party: Lists either the guarantor or the insurance with whom the balance is pending; clicking the associated plus sign gives an additional pop-up window with additional information to assist in follow-up (Figure 9-17).

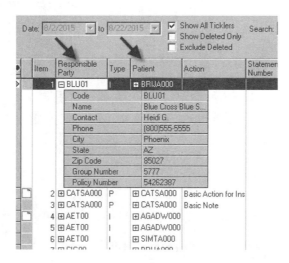

▶ **Figure 9-17   Plus Signs in the Collection Lists Give Additional Pop-Up Windows**

Type: Gives the type of tickler; I = pending insurance processing or P = pending patient payment.

Patient: Gives the Chart number for the patient and detailed information if the plus sign is selected.

Action: Displays the beginning of the note entered into the tickler.

Statement Number: For patient types; gives the associated statement number.

Remainder Balance: For patient types; gives the remainder due from the patient.

Insurance Estimate: For insurance types; gives the amount waiting to be processed by the insurance.

Claim Number: For insurance types; gives the associated claim number.

Claim Total: Shows the amount of the total claim billed to the insurance.

Status: Displays the current status of the tickler; options include open, deleted, or resolved.

Follow-Up Date: Gives the date the tickler was added to the Collection List.

Date Resolved: Gives the date the user documented that the actions needed on the tickler were complete.

User ID: Shows the user assigned to work the tickler.

Edit: Allows the user to open the ticker and process it; double-clicking any tickler allows it to be processed as well (Figure 9-18).

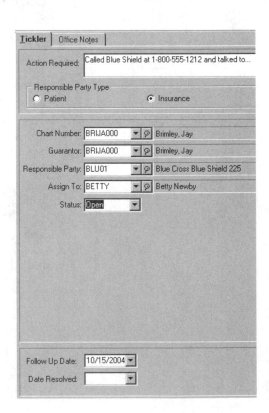

▶ Figure 9-18 **Editing the Ticklers**

New: Allows new ticklers to be added one by one.

Add Items: Allows groups of ticklers to be added.

Reassign: Changes the responsible user from one user to another.

Print Grid: Allows users to select fields to create a grid of the Collection List to print, preview, or export to a file

Print List: Allows users to print a Collection List Report; as with all reports, contains a list of filters available to sort contained data.

Delete: Deletes a tickler.

Close: Closes the Collection List pop-up window.

F1: This item is not displayed but it is available; F1 clicked within Collection List gives specific Help on this topic.

It is apparent that the Collection List utility in Medisoft has a full range of features to accomplish, document, and report on the follow-up policies of the clinic; it will work for both claim and statement follow-up.

Patient Follow-up Through Statement Management and Collection List

Again, once clinic policies are developed, a follow-up plan can be used as a guide. Patient balances can be tracked through two different utilities, Statement Management and Collection List. Remember, some of the types of Medisoft do not include these features.

Statement Management

If payments are being posted properly, those that are paid are marked Done. This provides the opportunity to filter the Sent statements, sort them by the submission count, and implement the office collection policies. To do this, first go to Statement Management either under Activities or the Statement Management toolbar icon. Once inside Statement Management, select List Only on the top toolbar; filters can be applied to sort statements that have been Sent but not paid (Figure 9-19). After clicking on List Only, select Sent, then Apply. Another option that can be performed at this time is to filter items that have a certain submission count, e.g., one or two statements. Again, this depends on clinic policy. Once the statements are filtered to match the desired criteria, any number of tasks could be implemented: Statements could be reprinted using a custom-created statement, giving the patient a friendly reminder notice

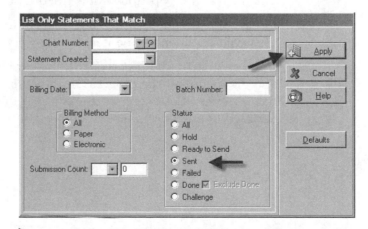

▶ Figure 9-19 **Filtering Statements in Statement Management**

or collection notice, or patients could be called regarding outstanding balances. At any rate, whatever the chosen method of follow-up, remember that documenting the actions taken is imperative. Use the Comment section of the statement to do this. To access Comment, simply double-click any statement, or highlight a statement and click Edit on the bottom toolbar (Figure 9-20).

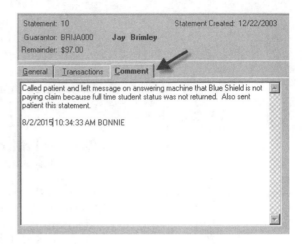

▶ Figure 9-20 Documenting Actions in Statement Management

Collection List

As reviewed in the previous section, Collection List is a great utility to manage both insurance and patient follow-up tasks. Again, to access Collection List, select Activities on the menu bar, then select Collection List from the drop-down menu, or click on the Collection List icon on the toolbar. Once inside this area, review the selection under the Claim Management follow-up section or select F1 to get comprehensive details of the Collection List.

PRACTICE EXERCISE 9-6   Resolving Collection List Items

Now that the items are added to the Collection List, it is time to resolve the ticklers.

1   First, we need to display only the open accounts. To do this, click on List Only on the top menu bar of the Collection List (Figure 9-21). This brings the pop-up window titled List Only Ticklers That Match.

2   In this box, select Open ticklers and All under Responsible Type. This will display only the items to be worked.

3   Open each item and proceed with the clinic's follow-up policy, making sure to document the progress in the Action Required and Office Notes boxes. Remember to change the Status to Resolved once the process outlined in the office policies has been accomplished (Figure 9-22).

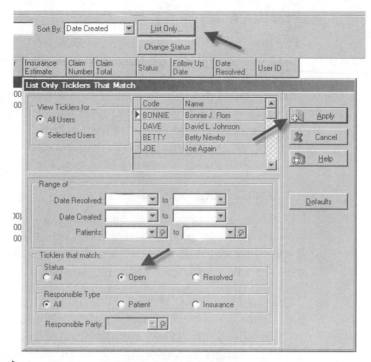

▶ **Figure 9-21** **List Only Ticklers That Match**

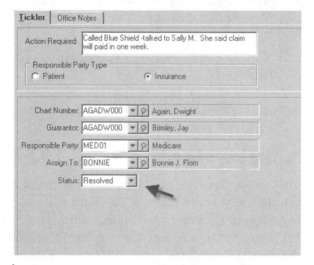

▶ **Figure 9-22** **Editing a Tickler**

REPORTS FOR THE DOCTOR AND/OR OFFICE MANAGER

Reporting is like accounting or banking: Each person has his or her own preference about what reports are desired and how frequently they are received. In addition, the purpose of the reports will dictate how often and which type of reports should be generated. In some specialties—i.e., mental health or chemical dependency—the practitioner often will collect balances from the patient. In these circumstances, more detailed and more frequent reports are useful. On the other hand, if the provider wants to just stay abreast of how much is outstanding in the accounts receivable, a simple report is warranted. The following sections describe the reports preferred by most offices.

Practice Analysis

The Practice Analysis can be found under Reports, Analysis, and Practice Analysis. A number of filters are displayed in the pop-up box. The most frequently selected are the Date From Range and the Show Accounts Receivables Totals Page. By completing these two areas, the doctor or manager is able to get a comprehensive view of the types of services performed, payments received, and adjustments written-off, along with a tally of these items and an outstanding accounts receivable amount. This report alone created at regular intervals will suffice for most reporting needs.

PRACTICE EXERCISE 9-7   Printing a Practice Analysis

Whether it is a report card or a report of the service work done on our car, reports provide us with an understanding of a situation. One of the best reports in Medisoft is the Practice Analysis, which was already covered in the reporting section of this chapter. However, because of its importance, you will print or display a practice analysis in this practice exercise.

1. Print a Practice Analysis for the clinic for the entire month of September 2008. (This will bring in the charge and payment information entered in previous chapters.) Begin by selecting Reports, Analysis Reports, and Practice Analysis.

2. After the pop-up window comes up, enter the appropriate Date Created Range and Date From Range.

3. Finally, check the box next to Show Accounts Receivable Total Page. This gives the total amount of charges, payments, adjustments, and the accounts receivable.

Again, this report fills most reporting needs for a doctor or manager. It gives a quick snapshot of the status of the practice.

Patient Day Sheet

This report has been reviewed previously to perform audits of our daily charges and transactions. The data selection questions can be accessed by going to Reports, Day Sheets, and Patient Day Sheets. The most useful filters for this report are the Date Created Range, Date From Range, Attending Provider Range, and Show Accounts Receivable Totals. Completion of each field depends upon the purpose for which the provider is using the report. This report is frequently used by providers to collect on the date of service because it gives details of charges, payments, and the patients' balance.

User Information Report

If a user only wants to see a snapshot of the details of the Medisoft data, this report is perfect. It can be viewed by selecting Tools from the menu bar and User Information from the drop-down menu. A variety of information can be viewed on just one page: practice information, data information, storage information, and practice totals.

CHAPTER REVIEW

Multiple Choice

1. Who creates the clinic follow-up policies?
   a. The federal government
   b. The insurance companies
   c. The clinic owners and managers
   d. All of the above

2. What is one way to determine days in AR?
   a. Divide the total practice AR by 90
   b. Divide the total charges by 90
   c. Divide the total AR by the charges and 90
   d. Divide the total charges for three months by 90, and divide the total AR by that number

3. A clinic should try to get their AR days below
   a. 30.
   b. 50.
   c. 60.
   d. 90.

4. How often should the days in AR be calculated?
   a. Daily
   b. Weekly
   c. Monthly
   d. Semi-annually

5. AR stands for
   a. Account Rite.
   b. All Right.
   c. Accounts Receivable.
   d. All Ready to collect.

6. Where are the columns set that print on the patient and insurance aging?
   a. Filters on the Report
   b. Aging Reports tab
   c. Dates in Collection List
   d. All of the above

7. How many types of insurance aging reports under the Reports menu can be printed in Medisoft?
   a. 2
   b. 3
   c. 4
   d. 5

8. Which claim status means it is processed?
   a. Done
   b. Sent
   c. Ready to Send
   d. Hold

9. Which statement status means it is sent but not paid?
   a. Sent
   b. Unpaid
   c. Due
   d. Ready to Send

10. Which of the following filters the date the claim or statement was last billed in Add Collection List Items?
    a. Initial Billing Date
    b. Billing Date
    c. Follow Up Date
    d. Date Resolved

11. Items in the Collection List are referred to as
    a. claims.
    b. statements.
    c. ticklers.
    d. collection items.

12. By clicking on the plus signs in Collection List, the program does which of the following?
    a. Adds all the claims for a patient
    b. Adds all the items together into one list
    c. Adds all the statements for a patient
    d. Expands information for the area selected

13. Which item shows in the Action displayed in the Collection List?
    a. The beginning of the Action Required note in the tickler
    b. The action taken with the tickler
    c. Both a and b
    d. The action needed with the tickler

14. The button to click to change an item on the Collection List to another user is called
    a. Change User.
    b. Change Item.
    c. Reassign.
    d. Redo.

15. Which report alone can suffice for most reporting needs?
    a. Patient Aging
    b. Practice Aging
    c. Insurance Analysis
    d. Practice Analysis

True/False

Identify each of the following statements as true or false.

1. The collection policies in all states are the same.

2. Two categories should be addressed in clinic follow-up policies: patient and insurance.

3. It is not important to track the days in AR.

4. The Aging Reports tab located in Program Options contains three tabs: Patient, Contract Insurance, and Non-Contract Insurance.

5. Doctors and managers want the same reports each month.

6. The Collection List is available to all Medisoft users.

7. The User Information Report is a handy, one-page report that gives a snapshot of the clinic's data and practice totals.

8. A properly compiled Practice Analysis report can suffice for most reporting needs by owners and managers.

9. CPT codes tell an insurance company what service was provided to the patient.

10. Only two items should be documented when calling an insurance company: the name of the insurance and the phone number.

Short Answer

1. If you had three medical office specialists in the office, each handling a different segment of the insurance follow-up (primary, secondary, and tertiary), explain the most efficient process to assign and track these duties.

2. If a user needs additional help within a Medisoft utility, what is the best way to get detailed help?

3. Explain in detail how to modify the grid column of Statement Management to include the submission count.

Resources

Fair Debt Collections Practices Act

www.ftc.gov/bcp/edu/pubs/consumer/credit/cre27.pdf

This is the website for the government Fair Debt Collection Practices Act.

10

Report Designer

Learning Objectives

After completing this chapter, you should be able to:

♦ Define and spell the key terms in this chapter.

♦ Understand and define how reports are created and modified.

♦ Explain how to access Design Custom Reports and Bills and the available features.

♦ Demonstrate how to open an existing report and make minor and major changes.

♦ Identify and describe reasons clinics may modify or create new reports and bills.

♦ Describe how to add a field, such as a company logo, to a report.

♦ Create a new report.

♦ Copy a report from one data set to another data set.

♦ List the various report styles available in Design Custom Report and Bills.

Key Terms

Bands   a tab inside Report Properties that allows the user to define the height of the header, detail, and footer sections of the report or bill.

claim footer   the bottom portion of the Format Grid in an insurance form.

claim header   the top portion of the Format Grid in an insurance form.

Custom Report List   a feature in Medisoft that allows the user to open and print existing reports.

data field   the information contained within the Medisoft tables and items that are selected on the Format Grid.

Data Field Properties   the pop-up window associated with each data field that allows the user to define and modify the field.

Data Filters   a tab inside Report Properties that allows the user to establish criteria used to generate the report.

data path   location in the computer to find desired data.

Design Custom Reports and Bills (DCRB)   a utility in Medisoft that allows the user to customize new or existing reports.

detail   the middle section of a report.

Detail File   companion or sub-file to the Master File.

footer   the bottom section of a report.

Format Grid   the section of DCRB where the user adds the fields.

General a tab inside Report Properties that allows the user to make major changes in the appearance of the report or bill; some of the options include changes in margins, paper size, or page orientation.

header the top section of a report.

Master File identifies the Medisoft table from which data fields for the Format Grid may be selected.

Report Properties a utility within DCRB that allows definitions and changes to be performed on the report being modified or created.

Report Style the default settings for the Format Grid assigned in the Report Properties of the report created; each report (e.g., labels or lists) has its own characteristics.

transaction detail the line in the insurance form that contains the charges on the claim.

transaction header a buffer before the transaction detail allowing for increasing and decreasing the margin.

Abbreviations

DCRB Design Custom Reports and Bills

■ ■ ■ ■

INTRODUCTION

So far, this text has covered the tasks needed to track patient appointments and information along with the financials. In other words, you have studied the must-know information in patient billing. This chapter covers a utility that affords offices a way to manipulate the data for other reasons, including marketing, sending newsletters or birthday cards, or making statements attractive by adding a company logo. In addition, it explains how to customize the printing of the claim form and statement. This Medisoft utility is called **Design Custom Reports and Bills (DCRB)** and is found under the Reports option on the top menu bar.

OVERVIEW OF DESIGN CUSTOM REPORTS AND BILLS

First, it is important to note that the existing reports available for modification are those found in the **Custom Report List** under the Reports menu. The reports found under other sections, such as Day Sheets and Analysis Reports, are not available to customize. Many report styles can be customized, such as Label, Statement, Ledger, and Superbill. Now we are going to explore one of the most thrilling features of Medisoft where the users express their creativity and computer savvy all in one utility!

Accessing Design Custom Reports and Bills

To access Design Custom Reports and Bills, go to Reports on the top menu bar and select Design Custom Reports and Bills (Figure 10-1). For this utility, there is no icon on the toolbar. However, if the toolbar is customized, an icon may be added.

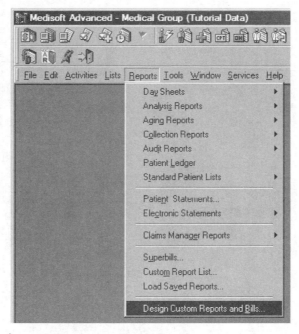

▶ **Figure 10-1** **Accessing Design Custom Reports and Bills**

PRACTICE EXERCISE 10-1   **Customizing the Toolbar**

1   A great feature of Medisoft allows users to customize the icons that appear on the toolbar. This feature is very flexible, and programs outside of Medisoft may even be added. In this exercise, Design Custom Reports and Bills will be added to the toolbar. Right-click on an empty space on the toolbar and select Customize (Figure 10-2).

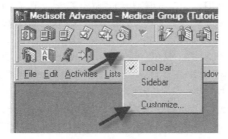

▶ **Figure 10-2**   **Customizing the Toolbar**

2   Select the Commands tab (Figure 10-3).

3   In the left box, review the available categories that can be added, noting the numerous options in the companion Commands window. Select the Report field in the list.

4   Under the Commands window, select Design Custom Reports and Bills and drag it to the toolbar.

5   Go back to the categories and review all the Commands options once again under each category.

6   Finally, add the calculator to the toolbar.

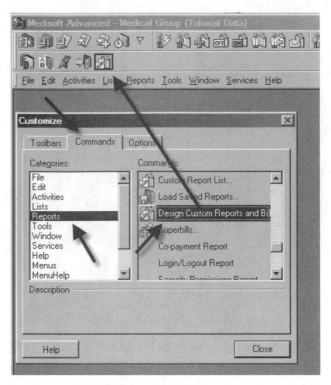

▶ Figure 10-3   Adding Design Custom Reports and Bills to the Toolbar

An Overview of Design Custom Reports and Bills

Once inside the Design Custom Reports and Bills (DCRB), it is very important to note that the rest of the Medisoft program cannot be used, even though the Medisoft icon can be viewed on the bottom toolbar of Windows. If a user tries to access Medisoft while DCRB is open, Medisoft will appear as if it is frozen. Many users at this point will reboot their computer with Medisoft open; the resulting damage could be data corruption. A key point to remember is to always exit DCRB when finished.

Another important feature that sets DCRB apart from other Medisoft features is it appears to be an entirely separate program operating with its own menu bar and toolbar. Let's review the look and feel of DCRB (Figure 10-4). On the menu bar, you can see the File, Edit, Insert, Window and Help Options. A complete description of all the items contained within these options can be found in Help. In addition, we will review the most pertinent items.

The toolbar, located directly below the menu bar, contains shortcuts for some of the items found within the menu bar. It starts with creating a new report and opening a report, and ends with the various items that may be inserted into a report. Open DCRB and take a moment now to review the icons on the toolbar by placing your mouse directly over them one by one. As this is done, each shortcut name will be displayed.

Directly under the toolbar is the **Format Grid,** which is where the report will be developed. The top section is the **header** to the report and usually contains the report name and details such as date and time. The middle section of the report is called the **detail** and is known as the "meat" of

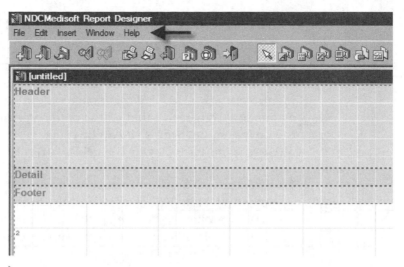

▶ Figure 10-4 **Overview of Design Custom Reports and Bills**

the report. It displays the data for which the report was created—i.e., transaction list, label, letter. The bottom section of the report is the **footer** and contains any data the creator would like to see, such as file name or date. In addition to these three general fields, some reports, such as the insurance form and statement forms, contain additional headers to a section: i.e., the insurance form has a **transaction header.** The transaction header is a buffer right before the **transaction detail,** allowing the user to increase or decrease the margin.

PRACTICE EXERCISE 10-2   Becoming Familiar with DCRB

An important aspect to learning any new software is to become familiar with the tools and options of the program. In this practice exercise, you will explore DCRB and become familiar with its features.

1   Open DCRB from the Reports menu.

2   Click on each of the menu bar items (File, Edit, etc.) and acquaint yourself with the drop-down menus.

3   Point your mouse to each of the toolbar items and decipher each one's purpose.

4   Click on the Help option and review the help files available for DCRB.

5   Click on File and Open Report.

6   Select any report and click OK.

7   Familiarize yourself with the properties of the various items on the report you choose by right-clicking and selecting Properties from the drop-down menu.

8   Close DCRB, remembering that Medisoft is locked while DCRB is open.

Opening an Existing Report and Making Minor Adjustments

Now that we have discussed how to open DCRB and what it contains, let us take a look at an existing report and how small modifications can be made. Minor adjustments are made on the Format Grid by moving, adding, deleting, or modifying a field within the various bands (header, detail, or footer) allotted by the report type.

PRACTICE EXERCISE 10-3   Opening and Viewing a Report

In this practice exercise, you are going to open and review the most commonly changed form in DCRB, the CMS-1500 form. The reason this form is so often modified is because there are dozens of printers made by several manufacturers, and all of them have unique alignment. If sending paper claims, it is imperative that all the data be printed within the boundaries of the boxes on the form, so it can be properly read by an OCR scanner. Consequently, clinics are moving the fields within DCRB to align to the claim form.

1   To start, let's open an existing report. There are two ways to open an existing form: Either click on the Open icon on the toolbar (Figure 10-5) or click on the Open Report item under the File menu (Figure 10-6). This will cause a Open Report pop-up window appear, and the form can be selected.

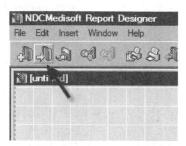

▶ **Figure 10-5   Open Icon on Toolbar**

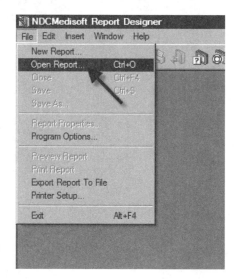

▶ **Figure 10-6   Open Report under the File Menu**

2   The user could arrow down the long list of options containing all the report styles. The better option is to click on the radio button below Show Report Style that says Insurance Form, and limit our choice only to that form style. (Figure 10-7). Select the most commonly used insurance form in Medisoft, the CMS-1500 (Primary) form. As we learned from Chapter 4, the CMS-1500 is the new form implemented in the billing industry in spring of 2007. Although we have the option to use the CMS-1500 (Primary) Medicare Century, most offices take one form and modify it to fit all the primary circumstances.

3   Once this form is open, review the Format Grids (Figure 10-8). The top portion of the grid is known has the header, or, in this case, the **claim header.** It holds the information found in boxes 1 through 23.

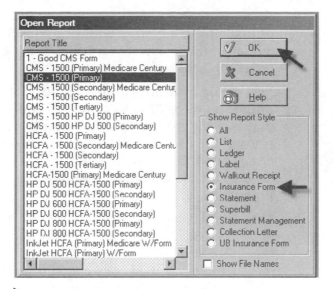

▶ **Figure 10-7   Selecting the Form**

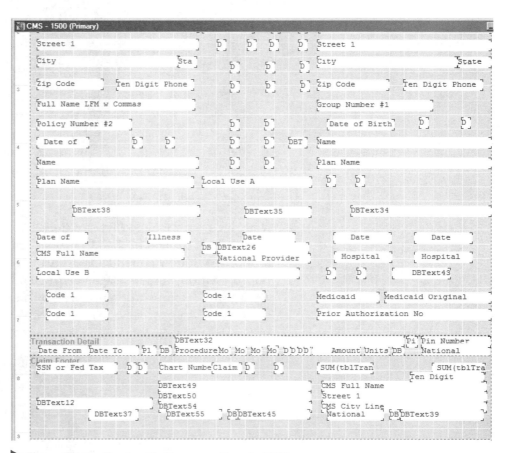

▶ **Figure 10-8   Viewing the Insurance Form in DCRB**

The next section is called the transaction header and does not appear on the paper claim form. Data is typically not put into this area; it is used strictly to increase or decrease the space between the claim header and the transaction detail. The transaction detail located directly below the transaction header holds all the charges on the claim, and this line repeats itself six times. The transaction detail prints in box 24, lines 1-6. Finally, the **claim footer** is located at the bottom of the insurance form and holds the items that are located in boxes 25 to 33 on the claim form.

An existing insurance form in DCRB looks exactly like what is printed on the CMS–1500 form. The only difference is that, rather than specific patient data, field names are listed. Once the report is opened, the user can make minor adjustments by adding, deleting, or moving items within the form view. Or, major changes can be done by changing margins, bandwidths, and data filters in **Report Properties.**

4   Now, let us delete a field. There are two ways to delete a field: One option is to click on the desired field so it is highlighted and press the delete key; another option is to highlight a field, choose the Edit menu, and select the Delete option from the drop-down menu (Figure 10-9). Select any field and delete it.

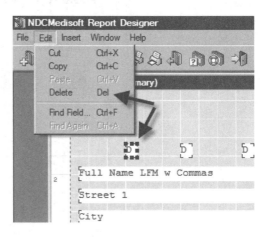

▶ Figure 10-9   **Deleting a Field**

5   Now, let's practice modifying a field. To modify a field, just right-click on the desired field and go to properties (Figure 10-10). This initiates a pop-up window called **Data Field Properties** (Figure 10-11). This pop-up window offers a wide arrange of options to use to modify the **data field,** from printing options to the selection of the Medisoft field or creating an expression. To view the complete array of options, press Help in this window. Pick any field and practice modifying it.

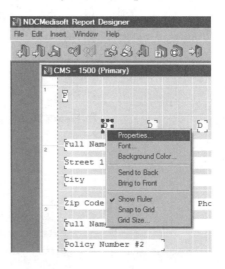

▶ Figure 10-10   **Modifying a Field**

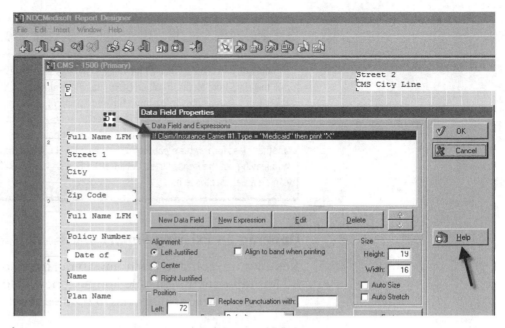

▶ **Figure 10-11   Modifying Data Field Properties**

6   Now, practice moving a field. Moving a field is simple; just click on the field to be moved and make sure it is highlighted, then either drag and drop the field to the preferred position or use the arrow keys on the keyboard to move the field (Figure 10-12). Practice moving fields by both dragging and dropping them and by selecting them and using your arrow keys.

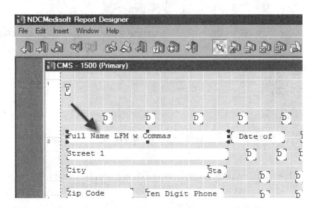

▶ **Figure 10-12   Moving a Data Field**

▶ **Test Your Knowledge 10-1**

What are three common reasons that clinics modify reports or bills in DCRB? Why are the modifications beneficial?

Opening an Existing Report and Making Major Adjustments

Next, we are going to learn how to make major adjustments to a report. Major adjustments include adding a new field; changing the bandwidths, filters, page size, or margins, to name a few.

Adding a Field

Adding a new field would be simple if there weren't so many options, but these options add creativity and flexibility. To add a new field, either click on Insert on the menu bar and select the field type or click on the toolbar and select the field type (Figure 10-13).

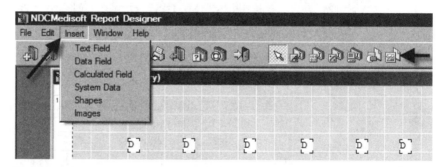

▶ Figure 10-13   **Adding a New Field**

The following available Field Types can be inserted or added:

Text Field: Allows the user to add free text to the report or bill.

Data Field: Allows the user to add Medisoft Data Fields to the report or bill.

Calculated Field: Enables the user to add, average, or count a field, plus calculate maximums and minimums.

System Data: Displays the data contained in the system such as date, report title, and page number, to name a few.

Shapes: Allows the user to add shapes—circles, rectangles, and lines, to name a few

Images: Inserts images (JPG, TIF, or GIF, to name a few) available from the computer's resources—hard drive, external hard drives, flash drives, etc.

Using Report Properties

Three tabs inside Report Properties allow the user to make major changes in reports or bills. They are **General**, **Bands**, and **Data Filters** (Figure 10-14).

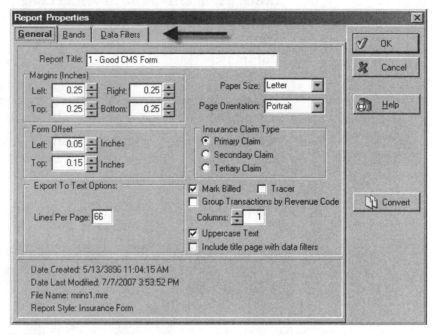

▶ Figure 10-14   Options Inside Report Properties and the General Tab

The following items are covered under the General tab:

Report Title: Gives the user the option of renaming the report.

Margins: Allows the user to define margins for the report including top, bottom, right or left margins of the reports or bills; new feature added in Version 14.

Form Offset: Similar to the Margins options, but only allows the print area to be offset from the left or top.

Export to Text Options: This option was created to have statements and claims in particular sent to a print image file in a predictable form (i.e., 66 lines per page); assists outside developers in creating import programs.

Paper Size: Allows the user to select the paper size of the report.

Page Orientation: Allows the user to select the report to print in either portrait or landscape orientation.

Insurance Claim Type: Permits the user to select the claim type of the bill; this correlates to whether Claim Management will print the primary, secondary, or tertiary claim based on the radio button chosen (option shown for insurance form bills only).

Statement Type: Permits the user to choose the statement type to be a standard or a remainder statement; this correlates to whether the statements were created as standard or remainder (option shown for statement bills only).

Marked Billed: Allows the user to check this box if Medisoft should process the bills and mark them as complete.

Tracer: Filters the use of the report to reprint only claims that have been printed at least once (option only in the insurance form).

Group Transactions by Revenue Code: If using the UB-04 claim form to bill facility charges, check this option to group transactions that have the same revenue code together.

Columns: Permits the user to create multiple horizontal columns; particularly helpful with labels.

Uppercase Text: Checking this box makes all characters on the report uppercase; this is required with insurance forms.

Include title page with data filters: Allows user to print a cover page on the report showing the report details, title page, practice name, date of report, and data filters selected on the reports.

The following items are covered under the Bands tab (Figure 10-15):

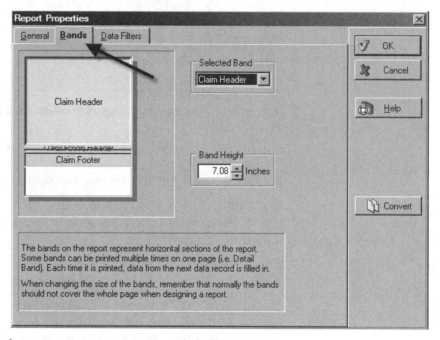

▶ Figure 10-15   **Options of the Bands Tab**

Selected Band: Gives the user the option to select the band on the Format Grid that will be modified (i.e., header, detail, or footer).

Band Height: Allows the user to define the height of the selected band on the Format Grid

The following items are covered under the Data Filters tab (Figure 10-16):

Data Filter Questions: Lists the current questions assigned to the report.

New Question: Allows the user to create a new filter for the report.

Delete Question: Deletes the above highlighted questions.

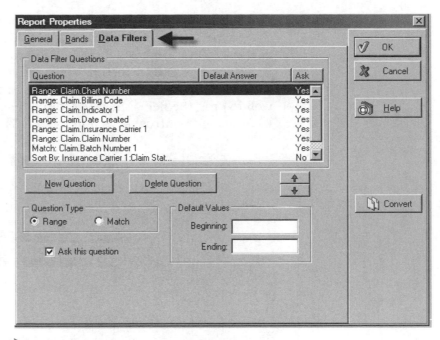

► **Figure 10-16 Options of the Data Filters Tab**

Question Type: Allows the user to define the filter by a range or a matched response.

Default Values: These questions correlate with the Question Type field, allows the user to enter default values so they do not have to be completed.

Ask this question: If this box is checked, the question will be listed in the range of filters when the report is created and the user may complete; if the box is not checked, the filter will still be applied but the user may not be aware of it. This also allows the report to be created with default values working in the background.

To clarify the difference between making minor changes on the Format Grid or major changes within Report Properties, an analogy can be drawn that Report Properties can be likened to building the features of a theatrical stage (width, height, layout, etc.), and Format Grid is the stage itself that is being modified.

PRACTICE EXERCISE 10-4   Modifying the Insurance Form

Insurance claim forms are more difficult to print than most forms because there is a smaller margin to print the information in—namely, small boxes. In addition, each printer aligns a little bit differently. It is not uncommon for a clinic to get a claim form aligned and then need to replace the printer and have to realign the claim form. It is often a process of trial and error to get the alignment correct. In this practice exercise, we are going to move the patient's name to the right three clicks, and we are going to move all of the charges down by .09 inches.

1   As reviewed in Practice Exercise 10-1, open DCRB and open the Insurance Form titled "CMS-1500 (Primary)."

2   First, click on the patient's name and hit the right arrow button three times. There are several ways to identify what is contained in each field: first, right-click and go to properties, or second, compare the Medisoft DCRB screen to the claim form. In this example, the patient name says "Full Name LFM w Commas." It also works perfectly well to drag the fields; however, dragging a field allows less control than using the arrow keys (Figure 10-17).

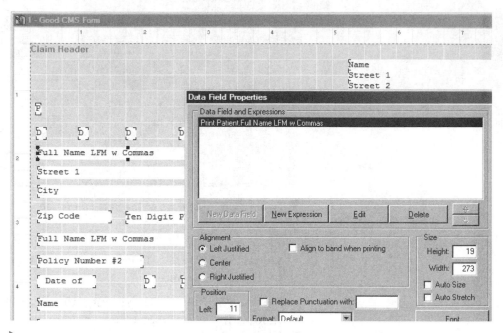

▶ **Figure 10-17**   **Previewing Data Field Properties**

3   Next, we want to move all of the transactions down in box 24, lines 1–6. If a mass change should be made, use Report Properties. To access Report Properties, select File from the menu bar and Report Properties from the drop-down menu.

4   Each section of the claim form is defined by a different Band. So, select the Bands tab.

5   In the Bands area, there are four possible areas to adjust. Review them now with the idea that the transactions need to be moved. The height of the Transaction Detail should never be changed. This is clearly stated in the Help section of Report Properties. So, the only area we can adjust for the transactions is the Transaction Header.

6   Select the Transaction Header in the Select Band drop-down, then adjust the band height from .01 to .10.

7   Upon exiting DCRB, there will be a prompt to name to new report. Do this, and then print or preview the original and modified report to see the changes.

Most Common Labels

Although DCRB can be used to print on any size of label, the most commonly used labels are three labels across and ten labels down on 8.5 × 11-inch paper. Therefore, the labels already created with DCRB are designed for this size. It is easiest to remain with this type of label and customize data to print in those formats. However, if different sizing is desired, Medisoft can be set to accommodate the new labels by changing Report Properties under the File menu.

Creating a New Report

Usually it is easier to take an existing report and make modifications to it rather than create a new report. However, there are times when the desired report does not exist or the user wants to make many modifications. In this case, it only makes sense to start with a blank Format Grid. To create a new report, Medisoft offers two options: the menu bar option or the icon option. To create a new report from the menu bar, select File from the menu bar, then select New Report (Figure 10-18). Or, click on the New Report Icon on the toolbar. It has a plus sign next to it (Figure 10-19). Clicking on either of the two options will give users a pop-up window titled Create New Report.

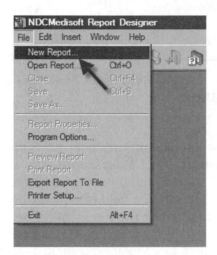

▶ **Figure 10-18   Creating a New Report from the Menu Bar**

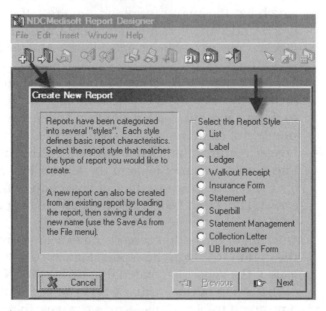

▶ Figure 10-19   **Creating a New Report from the Toolbar and the Create New Report Box**

In this window, select the **Report Style** (Figure 10-20). This really means the default settings for the Format Grid, which is located in Report Properties. For example, the Report Style for a label will set up the report to have three labels across and ten labels down, whereas the Report Style for a list contains a header, footer, and a detail area in the middle for the list to print. To illustrate this example, Label will be selected.

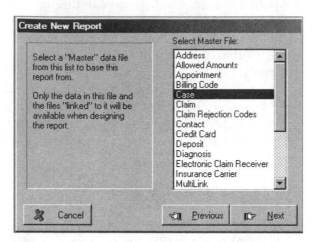

▶ Figure 10-20 **Available Fields for the Master Files Comes from the Selected Medisoft Table (Medisoft Lists)**

This in turn will make another pop-up window appear. This window requests the user to Select **Master File.** The Master File points to the Medisoft table from which data fields will be chosen for the Format Grid. A good way to identify the fields that may be selected from the Master File is to consider where the items might be found under the Lists menu in Medisoft. Each item under Lists is contained in a table. So, if we wanted to create a label to send postcards to people that bring revenue to the clinic—namely, the guarantors—we must first consider under which list the guarantor data is entered. If you recall, guarantors are listed under the Personal tab of the Case. Therefore, to create guarantor labels, Case would be selected as the Master File.

For all of the reports except Label and Ledger, the report could now be created by selecting a Create button. However, with the Label and Ledger, each has another pop-up window. Label requires the user to define the number of columns in the label and the label height (Figure 10-21). The Ledger requires the user to select a **Detail File** (Figure 10-22). The Detail File is an associated table to the Master File and offers the Data Fields for the user to place in the Detail section of the Format Grid. As stated above, Label and Ledger are the only reports that entail an extra screen.

Once all of the option screens have been completed, the final screen gives the option to create the report (Figure 10-23). When this option is selected, the report is created (Figure 10-24). Notice on this blank report each section of the Format Grid is designated by a varying color from lime green to blue. This assists the user to differentiate various segments of the report (i.e., Header, Detail, and Footer).

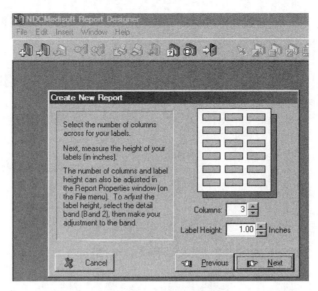

▶ Figure 10-21   **Additional Pop-up Window for Labels**

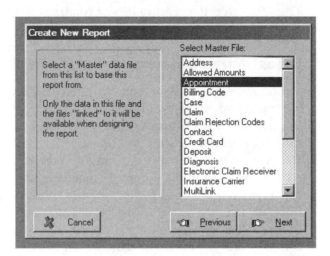

▶ Figure 10-22   **Additional Pop-up Window for Ledgers**

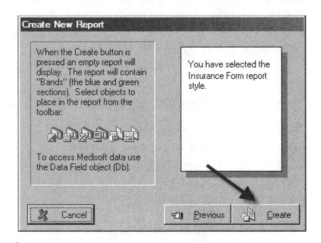

▶ Figure 10-23   **Create a New Report**

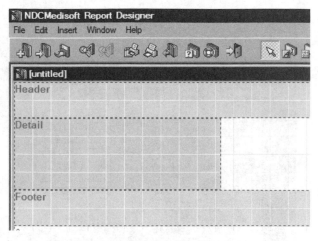

▶ Figure 10-24   **The Newly Created Report**

The final step to creating a new report is inserting the Data Fields onto the Format Grid. This will be demonstrated in Practice Exercise 10-6.

Logos, Warning Statements, and Other Options to Customize

There are numerous reasons to use DCRB to customize an office's report. Here are two examples. First, many businesses are conscious of branding the documents produced by their offices. Branding is a process of making sure all information disseminated contains a similar look and feel, which provides recognition and comfort to the reader. So, if a clinic's letterhead contains a company logo, the statement should as well. With Medisoft, adding the logo to the statement can easily be accomplished. Second, rather than printing or purchasing warning labels and statements, clinics can create a "Friendly Reminder Statement" and a "Collection Statement" inside of DCRB with the desired wording printed in bold on the statement. In addition to the time saved by not having to stick on the label, this option also affords the clinic the option to print the statements on different-colored paper that makes the notice stand out from a normal statement. With the combination of adding the logo and warning notices to the statement, the office will make a statement to its consumers that it is a professional organization.

PRACTICE EXERCISE 10-5   Adding a Company Logo to Statements

Businesses that invest time and resources into creating a logo for their company image want to use that logo wherever possible. Each month, offices send out dozens of statements, and so logically the statement is an ideal place to add the company logo. In this practice exercise, you will add a logo to a remainder statement.

1   Open DCRB from the Reports menu.

2   Select Open Report from the File menu or the Open Report icon and then select the Remainder Statements (0, 30, 60, 90), making sure that the radio button for Statement Management is selected right under Show Report Style.

3 After the statement is opened, take a look at the layout of the statement. You want to put the logo to the left of the clinic's name and address. There isn't enough room for both of them as they currently appear. In this step, we are going to move the clinic name to the right. First, drag the Practice Name to the right to a location that appears to give enough space for a logo. (You are going to use Medisoft's logo for the practice logo.)

4 Next, while holding the shift key down, click first on the Practice Name and then the address information. This will cause all of the items to have a gray shadow (Figure 10-25).

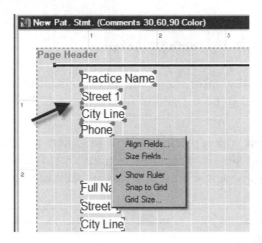

▶ **Figure 10-25** **Moving the Clinic's Name and Address**

5 Right-click while all of the items are shadowed, select Align Fields, then select Left sides. This will move the address fields into alignment with the Practice Name.

6 Now, we are going to insert the logo. There are two ways to do that. First, Insert can be selected from the menu bar and the images; second, the icon for images can be chosen on the toolbar (Figure 10-26).

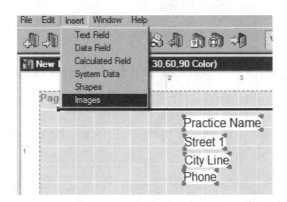

▶ **Figure 10-26** **Inserting the Image**

7 Once this button is clicked, it appears to do nothing. The user must then click on the Format Grid to indicate where the object should appear, then it is planted there. Medisoft will display it as empty box. Next, right-click and go to Properties. This box allows you to select the image. For this purpose, select the Medisoft image in the Bin folder under Medisoft (the program should default to that location) (Figure 10-27).

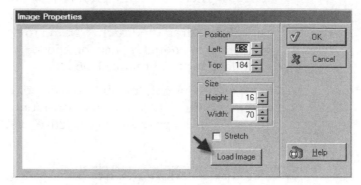

► Figure 10-27   **Loading the Image**

8   Finally, after the image is loaded and OK is selected, the box may need to be resized to fit the picture. To do this, stretch the corners as needed.

9   Now, upon exiting DCRB, Medisoft will ask you to rename the report and save it. After this is done, go to Statement Management and try to preview a statement using the one just created (Figure 10-28).

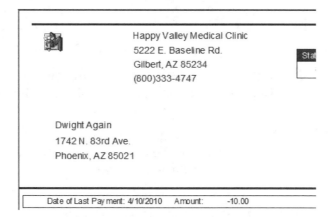

► Figure 10-28   **Previewing the Statement**

Copying a Report or Bill from One Practice Set to Another

If an office uses more than one Practice or dataset in Medisoft, it often creates a report in one practice and wants to copy it to another practice. This saves hours of time and keeps the format and layout for the report consistent.

To copy a user report, select Tools on the user menu inside Medisoft, then Add/Copy User Reports under the drop-down menu (Figure 10-29). The enables a pop-up window titled Medisoft User Reports (Figure 10-30). Inside this pop-up window, the user is given the following options.

Report Title: Lists the reports available in the open data set to be copied to another data set (only shows the user-created reports; each data set already contains the Medisoft-created reports).

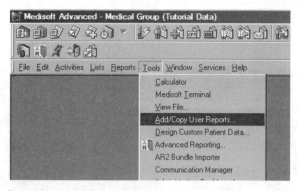

▶ Figure 10-29　Add/Copy User Reports

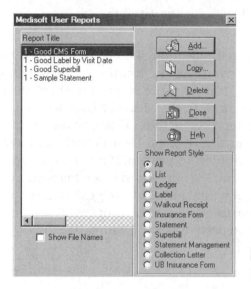

▶ Figure 10-30　Medisoft User Report Pop-up Window

Show File Names:　Broadens the report window to display the file name associated with the report.

Add:　Allows the user to add a report from another dataset to the opened dataset.

Copy:　Permits the user to copy a report from the open dataset to another dataset.

Delete:　Allows the user to delete a report from the open dataset.

Close:　Closes the Medisoft User Reports window.

Help:　Gives detailed information on the Medisoft User Reports options.

Prior to adding or copying a report, it is important to understand where the report exists. The report is always located in the Practice folder under another folder titled UReport. The difficult part is determining where the Practice folder exists. This depends on where the Medidata folder exists and, more importantly, if Medisoft is on a single workstation or a network. But, thankfully, Medisoft affords a shortcut. To find the Practice data folder, click on File on the menu bar and Open Practice on the drop-down menu (Figure 10-31). Then hold the left mouse button down while pointing to a practice. This make the program display the **data path** in two places, just below the practice name and at the bottom of the Medisoft window.

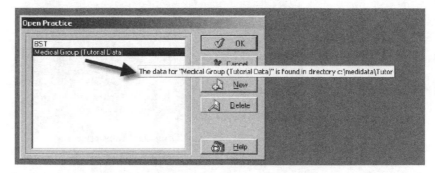

▶ Figure 10-31 Practice Data Path

The data path location should be identified before beginnning the add/copy process. Once the location is identified, users begin the process by selecting Tools from the menu bar, then Add/Copy User Reports. This brings us back to the Medisoft User Reports window reviewed earlier in the chapter. It is helpful to click Show File Names here. Then, click on Add under the Medisoft User Reports window; this will cause the Add Reports window to pop-up. If no custom reports have been designed on your system, the screens you see here will not look exactly like yours. Your screen may not show any existing reports, but they are shown here to familiarize you with the process. The following options are available in the Add Reports window (Figure 10-32).

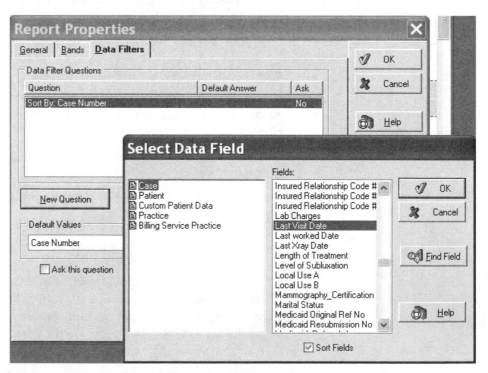

▶ Figure 10-32 Add Reports Window

Browse: Allows the user to select the data path for the desired report.

All: Selects all the reports to add.

None: Selects none of the reports.

Report Title: Permits the user to select the report to add.

File Name/Type/Last Modified: Displays additional information on the reports found under Report Title.

To review, in order to add or copy a report, begin by selecting Add/Copy User reports from the Tools menu. This brings up the Medisoft User Reports window. Check the box to Show File Names and select the report style desired under Show Report Style. If copying, select the name of the report(s) desired. You can press and hold the Control key to select non-sequential file names, or press the Shift key to select all reports between two selected file names. Then click Copy, which opens the Copy Reports To window where the destination directory can be selected. If adding a new report you will not select any files from the current window, you will simply click Add, which opens the Add Reports window. Click the Browse button to find the data path for the report, select the report title desired, then click Add.

▶ Test Your Knowledge 10-2

Imagine you are the office manager for a clinic that just had a new logo designed, and you are assigned to add it to all the applicable Reports Styles to create a new image. In addition, you want to make sure the logo is present in all areas of the clinic's collection policies to lend recognition to the office. Write a list of reports or bills you would add the logo to and which Report Style each would be found under.

PRACTICE EXERCISE 10-6 **Printing Labels for Fliers and Newsletters**

Clinics often want to send fliers and newsletters to their patients, and therefore would use labels from Medisoft's database. However, the difficulty comes when they try to filter the labels by only the adults. The labels that come pre-loaded with the Medisoft program are patient labels only. Of course, clinics aren't going to want to send open house invitations to 15-month-old babies. If patients are sorted by age, the user may inadvertently omit parents if only the children, not the parents, are patients. Therefore, a label needs to be created to print to the responsible adults only. This would be the guarantors, of course. Also, clinics often want to print labels for patients seen within a certain timeframe. If they sent fliers to someone seen six years ago, there is a good chance he or she may have moved.

In this practice exercise, create a new label for guarantors that have had clinic visits within the last twelve months.

1   Open DCRB as indicated in Practice Exercise 10-1 and click on New Report by selecting the appropriate item on either the menu bar or toolbar.

2 Once a new report is selected, a pop-up window will appear and ask which Report Style will be created; select Label and press Next.

3 Now, we need to tell the program which Master File to pull the Label information from. Since the guarantor information is found in the Case, select Case under the Master File options and click Next.

4 The next option asks the label to be defined. Leave the label definition as it is, select Next, and Create.

5 Notice there are three colored areas on this report. The top and bottom blue areas are the header and footer. The middle area is for the detail that contains the guarantor information. To add the guarantor information, insert three separate Data Fields similar to the way an image was inserted in Practice Exercise 10-5.

6 Next, align the left columns of the three areas similar to the instructions used to align fields in Practice Exercise 10-5.

7 Once the data fields are aligned, right-click on the first item and go to Properties. The top data field will be the Guarantor's Full Name, the second data field will be the Guarantor's Street 1 line, and the third data field will be the Guarantor's City line. After Properties is clicked, a pop-up window titled Data Field Properties will appear. Click on New Data Field and another pop-up window will appear titled Select Data Field. This is where the items for each box will be selected (Figure 10-33).

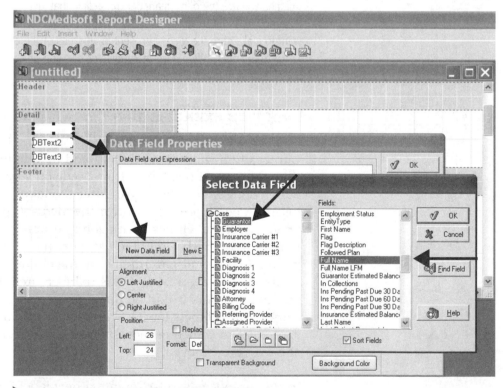

▶ Figure 10-33   **Adding Data Fields to the Report**

8 Repeat step 7 until all three data fields have been assigned. Then, go to Reports Properties as discussed in Practice Exercise 10-2 and select the Data Filters box. Since the label itself prints only guarantor information, we do not need to filter by guarantor. However, we need

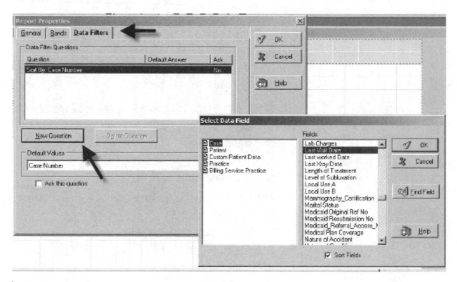

▶ Figure 10-34   **Adding Data Filters to a Report**

to add a filter of the Last Visit Date. This is done by adding a new question, selecting the appropriate items, and then clicking OK to exit Report Properties (Figure 10-34).

9   DCRB can now be exited; enter a report name when prompted. Now, go to Custom Reports and display the label just created with a Last Visit Date of the last twelve months.

CHAPTER REVIEW

Multiple Choice

1. Which is an example of a DCRB?
   a.   Patient Day Sheet
   b.   Procedure Day Sheet
   c.   Practice Analysis
   d.   Patient Label

2. To access DCRB, click on
   a.   File on the menu bar and DCRB.
   b.   Reports on the menu bar and DCRB.
   c.   icon for DCRB on the toolbar.
   d.   both b and c.

3. Which of the following is a minor adjustment?
   a.   Change the Bandwidth
   b.   Move Name to Right
   c.   Delete a Data Field
   d.   Both b and c

4. To open an existing report within DCRB, click on
   a.   File on menu bar and Open Report.
   b.   Open icon on toolbar.
   c.   Report on menu bar and Open Report.
   d.   Both a and b.

5. To insert a line across a report, click on Insert on the menu bar, then
   a. Lines.
   b. Text.
   c. Shapes.
   d. Objects.

6. Which of the tabs in Report Properties allows report questions to be added or removed?
   a. General
   b. Bands
   c. Data Filters
   d. Data Questions

7. Which two Report Styles have an extra window when created?
   a. List and Label
   b. Ledger and Label
   c. Statement and Label
   d. Superbill and Label

8. Where are custom reports located in the computer?
   a. UReport under Medisoft
   b. UReport under Medidata
   c. UReport under Practice Data
   d. UReport on the C drive

9. Which tab in Report Properties allows the user to set the margins for the report?
   a. General
   b. Margins
   c. Bands
   d. Data Filters

10. Which master file does the guarantor information come from?
    a. Patient
    b. Transaction
    c. Statement
    d. Case

11. Where can a clinic add its logos?
    a. Claim
    b. Statement
    c. Both a and b
    d. Neither a nor b

12. The most common labels have how many labels across?
    a. 2
    b. 3
    c. 4
    d. 5

13. To add the page number to the report, select Insert on the menu bar, then
    a. System Data.
    b. Page Numbers.
    c. Report Page.
    d. Data Field.

14. Which of the following does not exist on the Insert list of the menu bar in DCRB?
    a. Shapes
    b. Logos
    c. Text Field
    d. System Data

15. To align data fields, the user should
    a. highlight the items and select Align from the menu bar.
    b. highlight the items, go to Report Properties, then Align.
    c. either a or b.
    d. highlight the items and right-click, then select Align Fields.

True/False

Identify each of the following statements as true or false.

1. The Practice Analysis is one of the favorite reports to be modified in DCRB.

2. Without customization, Medisoft does not have an icon for DCRB.

3. Medisoft can be used simultaneously with DCRB.

4. DCRB comes out of the box with labels clinics use for marketing fliers.

5. To add a logo to a statement, the user must go to Report Properties.

6. To add a new field to a report, the user must go to Report Properties.

7. To add a logo, the user opens the report to be modified, selects Insert on the menu bar and Images.

8. Sometimes the height of the Transaction Detail needs to be changed.

9. After an item is selected from the Insert menu, the user must click on the Format Grid to place the item.

10. The Patient Day Sheet is modified in DCRB by going to Open Report on the File menu and selecting the report.

Short Answer

1. Explain why the patient labels that come with Medisoft do not suffice for sending a clinic flyer.

2. Briefly describe the steps to take to create a new report.

3. Briefly describe how to make minor changes to a report.

Resources

Medisoft Knowledge Base **www.medisoft.com**

This is a great resource for questions involving DCRB.

Medisoft Manual: Comes with each Medisoft installation CD and has an entire chapter devoted to DCRB.

Help within Medisoft: Located inside Medisoft on the menu bar and within utility. By clicking on Help or pressing F1 from inside Medisoft, assistance is given for any Medisoft function including DCRB.

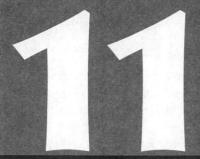

Chapter Eleven

Work Administrator, HIPAA, and Electronic Transactions

Learning Objectives

After completing this chapter, you should be able to:

◆ Define and spell the key terms in this chapter.
◆ Understand and define Work Administrator.
◆ Explain how to add assignments manually and automatically to Work Administrator.
◆ Create a new assignment.
◆ Create filters and process assignments in Work Administrator.
◆ Demonstrate how to create a rule.
◆ Identify and describe HIPAA.
◆ Describe the EDI transactions affecting medical billing.
◆ Explain the EDI enrollment process.

Key Terms

Assignment List   the pop-up window that displays after the Work Administrator utility is launched.

assignments   tasks performed by users in Work Administrator.

audit/edit report   feedback from the clearinghouse to the provider documenting the progress of individual claims that have been submitted. This report documents changes to be made or additional information to be submitted on a claim.

clean claim   a claim that has no data errors when submitted to an insurance carrier.

clearinghouse   a company that receives claims from multiple providers, evaluates them, and batches them for electronic submission to multiple insurance carriers.

code set   defined by HIPAA as an approved collection of codes used in the healthcare industry to communicate information, e.g., diagnosis, procedure, or place of service.

covered entity   an organization subject to the HIPAA law—e.g., insurance companies, clearinghouses, hospitals, and clinics.

dirty claim   a claim that is incorrect or is missing information when submitted to an insurance carrier.

Edit Rule   pop-up window under Task Rules List that allows the assignments to be created based on the criteria specified.

Edit Task   allows the user to process the work by marking the work done and documenting the details.

EDI transactions   data transmitted electronically in a specific format that is used by providers, insurance companies, and clearinghouses to communicate healthcare information including eligibility, claims, claims status, and remittance.

Filter Selections   allows the user to specify tasks that will be displayed in the Assignment List.

Groups   the function in Work Administrator that allows tasks to be assigned to a pre-defined group of users.

health plan   an organization that provides insurance coverage including employer plans, insurance plans, or government plans.

List Rules   button to execute the Task Rules List within Work Administrator.

New Task   utility in Work Administrator that allows the user to create a new assignment.

protected health information (PHI)   under HIPAA, individually identifiable health information transmitted or maintained in any form or medium, which is held by a covered entity or its business associate.

Repeat Setup   pop-up window under New Task that allows assignments to be set up to repeat automatically.

Rules   items created under the Task Rules List that have circumstances associated to them that will trigger an assignment if met.

Task Rules List   allows the user to view, delete, edit, or create Rules in Work Administrator.

Users   individuals' setup in the Medisoft security utility that allows the program to manage and track activities performed.

Work Administrator   utility in Medisoft used to assign, track, and manage clinic work.

Abbreviations

EDI   Electronic Data Interchange
ERA   electronic remittance advice
HIPAA   Health Insurance Portability and Accountability Act
PHI   protected health information
TPO   Treatment, Payment, and Operations

■ ■ ■ ■

INTRODUCTION

This chapter reviews two completely different but very necessary topics. One topic creates faster workflow; the other, faster office transactions.

First, **Work Administrator** will be reviewed. Work Administrator manages **assignments** given to the users or groups within Medisoft. This utility works completely separately from Medisoft, akin to Office Hours, and syncs to the data tables contained in Medisoft to share the data files. Assignments are tracked and managed inside of Work Administrator. Work Administrator is a big time saver because much can be communicated and accomplished without the staff members' needing to take the time to discuss each item. In other words, Work Administrator promotes working instead of talking. In addition, users can be held accountable for assigned work.

The last section of this chapter discusses the Health Insurance Portability and Accountability Act (**HIPAA**), and the Electronic Data Interchange (**EDI**) **transactions** portion of the law will be reviewed in more detail. Many payers and states are now requiring EDI transactions. Whether the transaction involves eligibility, claim transmission, claim status, or electronic remittance, clinics will soon be required to invest the time and resources to become EDI compliant. The origin of EDI transactions, the definitions of each transaction, and an implementation plan to assist offices through the process will be reviewed in this section.

OVERVIEW OF WORK ADMINISTRATOR

Work Administrator looks like a spreadsheet and displays the assignments given to users and groups of users (Figure 11-1). It can show all the assignments or may be filtered to show only selected assignments. Both options are needed because managers will want to view all of the assigned work for the clinic and monitor the progress. Workers can look only at the work assigned to them and develop a plan for the work day. Work Administrator is very accommodating and flexible. Items may be added manually or automatically. Learning proper setup of Work Administrator makes it much more effective.

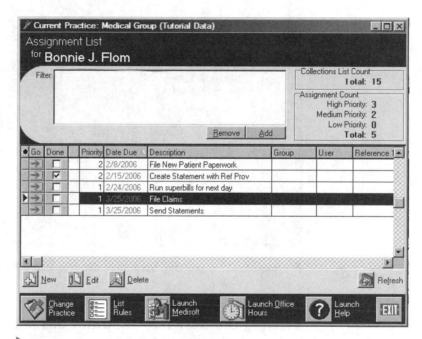

▶ Figure 11-1   A Look at Work Administrator

Creating Users and Groups

Prior to using Work Administrator, **Users** and **Groups** need to be created in Medisoft as discussed in Chapter 8. Work Administrator assigns tasks to specific Users and/or Groups.

Accessing Work Administrator

Work Administrator can be accessed in three ways. The first is to click on the Work Administrator icon on the Desktop (Figure 11-2). The second and third options come from within Medisoft either by selecting Work Administrator from the Activities menu or by selecting the Work Administrator icon (Figure 11-3).

▶ Figure 11-2　**Accessing Work Administrator from the Desktop**

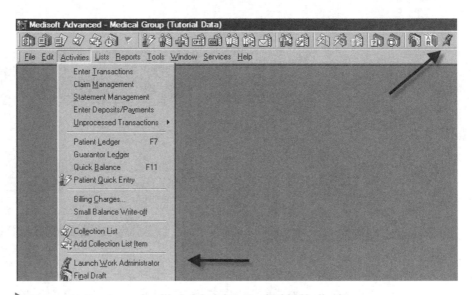

▶ Figure 11-3　**Accessing Work Administrator Inside Medisoft**

Viewing the Work Administrator Dashboard

Once Work Administrator is opened, an immediate assessment can be taken of the assigned work. Here are definitions for each area.

Assignment List for:　Displays the user logged into Work Administrator.

Filter:　Allows criteria to be specified for the user to only view selected items such as only show items not done or items with a high priority.

Collections Lists Count:　Displays the number of items assigned to the User in the Collection List.

Assignment Count:　Shows the number of assignments for the user for each of the three levels of priority, high, medium, and low, and a total count for all.

High Priority:　Tasks assigned a level one and should be done first.

Medium Priority:　Tasks assigned a level two and should done second.

Low Priority: Tasks assigned a level three and can be done last.

Total: Shows the total assignments in Work Administrator.

Work Grid: Displays the items that match the assigned filters; several fields are available including Go, Done, and Description; further clarification of these fields will be given when a new task is added. **Note:** Clicking on the Go arrow of the Work Grid will open the associated table in Medisoft.

New: Allows a new task to be created for the assignment list.

Edit: Permits an existing task to be modified.

Delete: Deletes a task in the assignment list.

Refresh: Updates the view in the assignment list; the view is stored in memory and needs to be refreshed occasionally to reflect changes.

Change Practice: Allows users to move between practices.

List Rules: Automatically creates items that add tasks to the assignment list.

Launch Medisoft: Opens Medisoft.

Launch Office Hours: Opens Office Hours.

Launch Help: Opens Help specifically for Work Administrator.

Exit: Closes Work Administrator.

PRACTICE EXERCISE 11-1   **Becoming Familiar with Work Administrator**

Work Administrator is very much like Office Hours in that it can be used as standalone software without having Medisoft open. As with any new software, it is best to start by familiarizing yourself with the features. In this practice exercise, we will become familiar with the features of Work Administrator.

1   Launch Work Administrator.

2   Click on Launch Help (Figure 11-4) and double-click on the topics under the Work Administrator book.

3   Review each of these topics.

4   Within Work Administrator, click on each area (Filters, New, Edit, etc.) and review the available options.

Billing Insight   Patient Flow

In considering the items to be added to the Work Administrator, the patient flow for the office needs to be reviewed. For example: Patients are first scheduled, then appointments are confirmed, the patient is seen, and finally a recall appointment needs to be set for each patient every two months. How might Work Administrator assist in this flow? A rule could be created to confirm the patient appointments and another rule could be created to set two-month follow-up appointments. An important part of utilizing Work Administrator is identifying situations such as these that can be streamlined by creating rules and then implementing them.

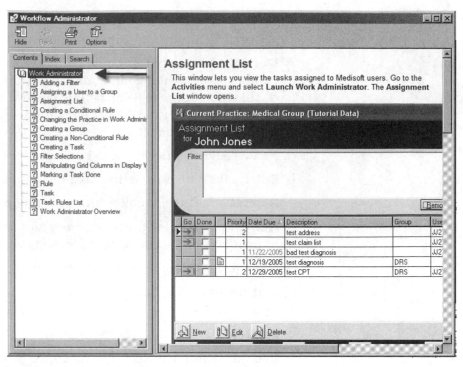

▶ Figure 11-4   Launch Help for Work Administrator

▶ Test Your Knowledge 11-1

Imagine yourself working at a clinic. Draw a work flow of the daily activities at a clinic and write three areas you can visualize the need to manage.

Adding Assignments Manually to Work Administrator

Assignments that are added manually can be broken into one of two categories: unplanned work or items that are planned but are not linked to the Medisoft tables and do not require special conditions. Examples of unplanned items are patients or insurance companies calling and needing special assistance with phone calls, records, or payment plans. Planned assignments include predicable work such as taking out the trash, entering charges and payments, or printing statements. Basically, the entire work flow for the office may be tracked and managed.

To add an assignment manually, click on the New button located at the bottom left of the assignment window. This will cause a pop-up window titled **New Task** to appear. Once the pop-up window appears, another pop-up window comes up called **Repeat Setup** (Figure 11-5). The following is a list of options you need to understand and complete:

New Task:

Done: Allows user to mark a completed assignment done.

Remind: Signals program to prompt user the number of days desired before the assignment is due.

User: Person assigned to the task.

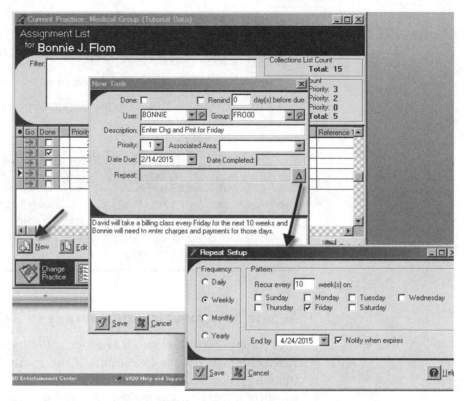

▶ Figure 11-5   Adding Assignments Manually to Work Administrator

Group: Group of users assigned to the tasks (users are assigned to groups in Security Setup).

Priority: Categorizes assignment by three levels of priority: low (3), medium (2), or high (1).

Associated Area: Associates a Medisoft function to the assignment.

Due Date: Date the assignment needs to be completed.

Date Completed: Date the assignment is actually completed.

Repeat: Allows the assignment to be re-created based upon the settings.

Free Text: Allows users to communicate directions or additional information regarding the assignment

Save: Saves the assignment.

Cancel: Cancels the assignment and closes the window.

Help: Gives complete details of how to set up a New Task.

Repeat Setup:

Frequency: Defines how often the assignment will be repeated.

Pattern: Further defines the frequency such as if weekly is chosen, this area will request the user to select which day of the week and for how many weeks.

End by: Allows the user to set a day the assignment will stop.

Notify when expires: Allows the user to request being prompted when the assignment is done.

Save: Saves the Repeat Setup screen.

Cancel: Closes the Repeat Setup screen without saving.

Help: Displays the Help for Repeat Setup.

Medisoft Quick Tip Defining the Work Administrator Rules by Office Policies

Work Administrator really shines when it comes to managing the office follow-up policies. To manage this, the user needs to first review the policies and identify how many rules need to be written to accommodate follow-up. Here are some ideas for follow-up rules: sending Friendly Reminder Statements, processing Collection Letters, marking non-contract payers Done and calling on contract payers.

Adding Assignments Automatically to Work Administrator

Assignments will be issued automatically by creating a **Rule** in the **Tasks Rules List**. In the medical billing field, many times claims get denied, are missing information, are missing referrals from outside doctors, or are missing authorization codes, to name a few. Some of these items will be caught in the electronic edits, but many of the items, such as needing a referring physician or authorization, are conditional to the situation, and the edits will not catch the errors. Plus, in some situations time is of the essence and the information needs to be obtained prior to the visit. In the example given, an assignment will be created if the patient doesn't have a referral within five days of the service. This allows time for the staff to get this task done.

To create a rule, the user first clicks on the **List Rules** button at the bottom of the Work Administrator. This will cause a pop-up window to appear (Figure 11-6). The following are the options in the Tasks Rules List.

Tasks Rules List:

Search For: Filters the rules by allowing the user to enter fields to locate.

Rules Grid: Displays the items that match the assigned filters; several fields are available including Code, Description, and Priority, to name a few; further clarification of these fields will be given when a new rule is added.

New: Creates a new rule.

Edit: Edits a rule.

Delete: Deletes a rule.

Help: Provides assistance on Task Rules List.

Close: Closes the Task Rules List.

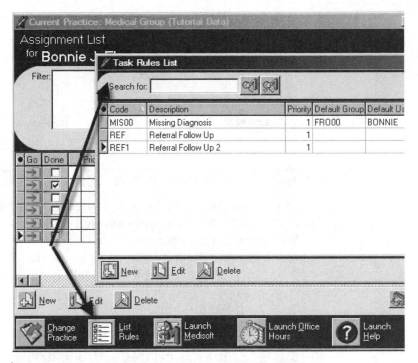

▶ Figure 11-6 **Adding Assignments to Work Administrator**

Edit Rule:

Task Code: Unique identifier used to track rules; may be assigned by the user or auto assigned.

Priority: Sets the urgency to the rule at either high (1), medium (2), or low (3).

Description: Defines the rule.

Notify when expires: Allows the user to request being prompted when the assignment is done.

Default Group: Selects a Group for the assignment.

Default User: Selects a User for the assignment.

Due in: Allows the user to select when the assignment will be created; allows user to define negative to positive days and define from which date.

Note: Free text box allows for comments regarding the rule.

Condition: Allows the rule to be defined by associated area, type, field, operand, and value.

Associated Area: Defines the Medisoft table associated to the rule.

Type: Allows the user to select whether the rule is conditional or nonconditional.

Field: If the rule is conditional, selects a field to place the condition upon.

Operand: Allows a variety of options from less than, equal to, and greater than conditions to be applied.

Value: Defines the filter to be placed on the Field.

Display Condition: Allows the user to view the Condition created.

Event: Defines if the Rule will be implemented based on a new event, deleted event, or edited event (i.e., when an appointment is created, deleted, or edited).

Save: Saves the rule.

Cancel: Closes the New Rule window without saving.

Help: Allows Help on New Rule to be viewed.

PRACTICE EXERCISE 11-2 Creating a New Assignment

In this practice exercise, you are going to create an assignment. It has come to the doctor's attention that Dwight Again's blood counts are too low to receive chemo. He wants Dwight to be contacted and his treatment rescheduled. The lab tech needs to create an assignment for the schedule group to call him. Complete the following steps (Figure 11-7):

1 Open Work Administrator.

2 Click the New button at the bottom of the assignment window.

3 Select Betty as the User and/or FR000 as the Group to assign the task.

4 Enter the Priority (1) and Associated Area (Appointment Edit).

5 Select the Appointment Date to be rescheduled, which for this exercise is 08/03/2015.

6 Select the Chart Number for Dwight Again. The chart number is AGADW000. (Important: The Chart number will not appear if the Associated Area is not selected correctly.)

7 Select the Due Date to reschedule the appointment. The due date is 08/01/2015.

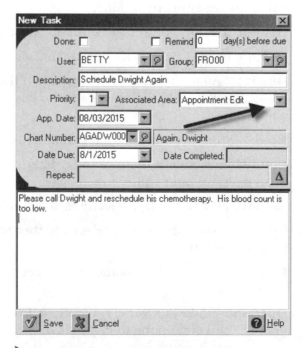

▶ **Figure 11-7   Creating an Assignment**

8 Repeat does not apply to this scenario.

9 Enter the following pertinent notes in the free text area: "Please call Dwight and reschedule his chemotherapy. His blood count is too low."

10 Save the Task.

Filtering Assignments

Filtering assignments can be an enormous time saver. Users typically want to see only tasks that are not done and tasks that are assigned to them. In addition, it is helpful to be able to filter by priority status, date due, or group association. In this section, we will learn how to filter assignments.

To start with filtering assignments, make sure Work Administrator is open, then click on Add to create a new filter. This will bring up a pop-up box titled **Filter Selections** (Figure 11-8). The following options are available.

Filter Selections

Select the field you want to filter on: Allows the user to select one of six areas to filter assignments.

> *Assigned User:*   User assigned to the task.
>
> *Assigned Group:*   Group assigned to the task.
>
> *Associated Area:*   Medisoft table associated to the task.
>
> *Date:*   Due date associated to the task.
>
> *Priority:*   Priority status assigned to the task.
>
> *Status:*   Done, not done, or all.

Select the values for the condition: The condition depends on the selected field; the appropriate options may be selected.

Click "Add" to add the filter below: Just as the description implies, click the Add button to execute the options selected in items one and two.

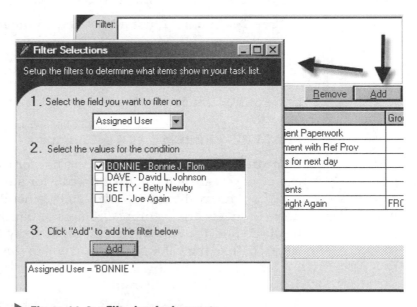

▶ **Figure 11-8   Filtering Assignments**

Display box: Shows the options added in item three.

Remove: Removes selected items.

Save: Saves the filter.

Cancel: Closes the Filter Selections window without saving.

Help: Displays Help for Filter Selections.

PRACTICE EXERCISE 11-3   Filtering Assignments

Work Administrator is a place where managers and other staff members can make it clear to each other what is expected of them. In this practice exercise, filters will be applied to view the tasks assigned to each staff member.

1   Open Work Administrator.

2   Edit each existing task and assign it to a user. Make sure each user has at least one task.

3   Select Add under the Filter column, check first user in the list and add it to the filters, then choose Save.

4   Review the tasks given for the user noting that only the current user's name is displayed in the user column.

5   Repeat the exercise for the other users.

Processing Assignments

Finally, after the assignments have been given out and the user filters the assignments that need to be done, the assigned work should be processed, marked done, and documented. **Edit Task** allows the work to be processed. To access Edit Task, highlight the desired assignment and click Edit on the bottom of the Assignment List (Figure 11-9). The following items should be completed in the Edit Task window to document that an assignment is complete.

Done: Put a check in the Done box.

Date Completed: Enter the date completed.

Free Text Box: Enter a brief note in the free text area documenting the work completed.

▶ **Test Your Knowledge 11-2**

List five potential rules that could be created at a clinic and how the rules would benefit the office.

PRACTICE EXERCISE 11-4   Creating a Rule

Some insurance companies may not pay for routine care. In this practice exercise, you are going to create a rule for any claim that is created that has the primary diagnosis code V70.0, general medical exam. This diagnosis code tells the insurance company that the patient received routine medical care. The rule will ask users to verify the accuracy of the diagnosis. Complete the following steps to create this Rule (Figure 11-10).

1   Open Work Administrator.

2   Complete the Description by entering "Missing Diagnosis."

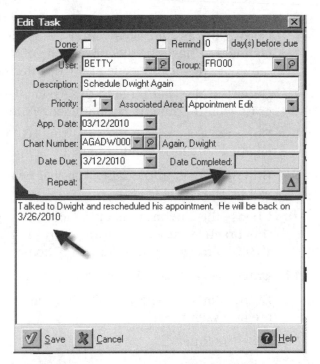

▶ Figure 11-9   **Processing the Assignments**

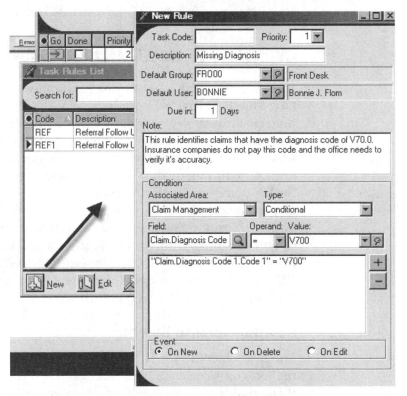

▶ Figure 11-10   **Creating a Rule**

3   Select the Default Group FR000.

4   Select the Default User.

5   Select the Due In Days (1).

6 Enter the reason the rule is created and the expectations for processing the assignments. Enter the following: "This rule identifies claims that have the diagnosis code of V70.0. Insurance companies may not pay for this code and the office needs to verify its accuracy."

7 Enter the Medisoft table in the Associated Area to instruct the program what is going to be managed. Enter "Claim Management."

8 Enter the Type of management that will be done on this table. In this example it will be conditional.

9 Enter the Field in the table that will be managed. In this example, it will be Diagnosis Code 1.

10 Choose the Operand, meaning less than, greater than, or equal to. In this practice exercise you want any claims with a diagnosis equal to V70.0 to trigger an assignment. Choose equal to.

11 Enter the value for the operand to match. Enter V70.0.

12 Event should be specified On New, meaning on any new claims, create an assignment.

13 Save the Rule.

▶ Test Your Knowledge 11-3

Review the required fields on a CMS-1500 form and list three rules that would ensure claim accuracy.

OVERVIEW OF HIPAA AND EDI TRANSACTIONS

HIPAA is the Health Insurance Portability and Accountability Act (Public Law 104-191) that was published in August 21, 1996, and has been phased-in in stages ever since. There are still some provisions of HIPAA that have not been fully implemented. The original purpose of the law was to protect workers when they changed or lost their jobs. HIPAA guarantees health insurance access, renewal, and portability by prohibiting health plans from denying coverage or charging extra based on present or poor health. This original purpose of HIPAA is expressed in the law's name. Then, the law was expanded to other areas of the healthcare industry to simplify the exchange of information and to ensure privacy of healthcare records and confidential information. Each specific area of HIPAA will be further defined in the sections that follow, and Appendix D explains more on HIPAA regulations.

Health Insurance Reform

The first objective for HIPAA was to protect health insurance coverage for millions of Americans by ensuring that if they change or lose their jobs, their insurance access will be portable and renewable by:

- Limiting the use of pre-existing conditions and/or exclusions

- Prohibiting group health plans from denying coverage or charging extra for coverage based on past or poor health

- Guaranteeing certain small employers and certain individuals who lose job-related coverage the right to purchase health insurance

- Guaranteeing that employers or individuals who purchase health insurance can renew their coverage regardless of health conditions.

Administrative Simplification

Next, HIPAA wanted to simplify the way organizations within the healthcare industry communicated with each other regarding transactions and **code sets**. Code sets are collections of codes used to communicate healthcare information such as diagnosis, procedure, place of service, or modifiers. The term *transactions* refers to electronic transactions and are the form of communication transmitted between **covered entities**. Examples of communications are verifying eligibility, checking on claim status, and electronic claims. Prior to HIPAA's defining electronic claims, insurance companies had over 450 formats in place to accept electronic claims. It is easy to understand why a single standard was needed to simplify electronic transactions and reduce the cost of maintaining multiple formats.

Privacy and Security

The Administrative Simplification section of HIPAA also deals with the privacy and security of medical records and personal health information. HIPAA defines **protected health information (PHI)** as the patient's individually identifiable health information transmitted or maintained in any form or medium, which is held by a covered entity or its business associate. PHI can be shared for purposes of treatment, payment, and operations (**TPO**) of the health care provider, but cannot be disclosed for other purposes without the patient's explicit written authorization. In addition, the government wanted to create the opportunity for access to all patient records with regard to government operations. This opened up the arena for the government to track diseases and outcomes, morbidity, and mortality. HIPAA gives the government rights to the patient records. However, it also gives rights back to patients. If the patient wants to know which entities have viewed his or her records, an accounting of the records may be requested. This portion of the law also:

- Gives patients the right to access their medical records, to request a modification of their medical records, and to request an accounting of the use of their medical records.

- Limits the use and release of PHI to unauthorized parties.

- Restricts most PHI disclosures to the minimum needed for the intended purpose.

EDI Transactions

Standardizing EDI transactions was an important part of the HIPAA Administrative Simplification and has reduced the expense for medical offices to transmit healthcare information electronically. HIPAA currently does not require that all covered entities transmit electronically; however, it does mandate if the covered entity chooses to communicate electronically it does so in the HIPAA-approved format. HIPAA has defined ten standard transactions for EDI transmission of healthcare data.

In the defined EDI transactions, some are used by healthcare providers, and some are used by **health plans**. Eligibility, claims, payment and remittance advice, and claim status transactions are the EDI transactions used by healthcare providers. *Eligibility* is the transaction used to verify insurance coverage; *Claims* is the transaction used to transmit claims; *Payment and Remittance Advice* is the transaction used to process insurance payments and denials; and *Claim Status* is the transaction used to verify the processing point of a claim.

EDI Transactions in Medisoft

Medisoft has its own **clearinghouse** that synchronizes directly with Medisoft to handle all the EDI transactions: claims, electronic remittance advice (**ERA**), eligibility, and claims status. Currently, there are two ways in which Medisoft accepts electronic transactions. First, a separate utility called Claims Manager has a unique Internet-based dashboard that works outside Medisoft. Note that the Claims Manager utility is a different function than the Claim Management feature within the Medisoft program. Claims Manager comprises all of the EDI transactions, and enrollment is done all at once. In addition to all the EDI transactions being covered, Claims Manager also has a claims scrubbing feature to edit claims for correct coding (Figure 11-11).

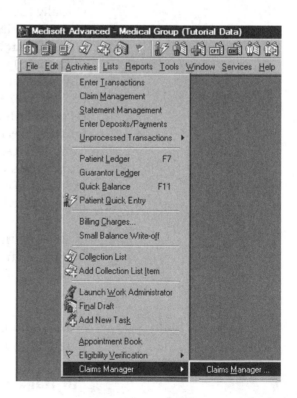

▶ **Figure 11-11   A Look at Claims Manager**

The other option for EDI transactions in Medisoft is more of a piecemeal system. Clinics enroll one service at a time and utilize them in separate places within Medisoft. Electronic claims and ERA can be found in Claim Management, and eligibility verification is found on the Activities menu. Claim Status is not available yet, and may not be developed as a separate product. In addition to these items, electronic statements are available.

Electronic statements do not have a defined ANSI format and are not a required electronic transaction.

The EDI Enrollment Process

Many small offices are still sending paper claims, and the notion of verifying eligibility or checking claim status has not occurred to them. How can the small office that doesn't have the resources to hire an IT department start sending claims?

If the offices have Medisoft, there are numerous benefits to utilizing Medisoft's clearinghouse: EDI interfaces directly with Medisoft, allowing reject notes to be entered into Claim Management and allowing data to be corrected in one place, just to name a few. Many providers also use other third-party clearinghouses.

A clearinghouse is a company that receives claims from providers, puts them through a series of audits to check for errors, and then forwards them to the appropriate insurance carrier in the carrier's required data format. Clearinghouses may charge a flat fee per claim or charge a percentage of the claim's dollar value. It is very important for the physicians' practices to negotiate the best possible fee for using a clearinghouse's services.

The clearinghouse conducts an audit to determine if any data on the claim is incorrect or missing; such a claim is referred to as a **dirty claim**. The results of the audit are sent back to the provider from the clearinghouse in the form of an **audit/edit report**. The audit/edit report shows which claims need corrections and which claims have been forwarded on to the appropriate carrier. The medical office specialist will need to correct any claims with incorrect data, as indicated on the audit/edit report, and resubmit them to the clearinghouse.

Dirty claims will not be transmitted to the carriers. When the claims are corrected and resubmitted to the clearinghouse, they are considered **clean claims**, which are then formatted and forwarded to the carrier. Each time the claim is returned there is an additional charge, so the medical office specialist should ensure that clean claims are transmitted initially.[*]

The following are the basic steps to begin the process of working with a clearinghouse:

1. The provider contacts the desired clearinghouse, signs a contract with it, and begins the enrollment process. Sometimes, a third-party vendor may represent the clearinghouse.

2. The provider identifies each of its contract payers to the clearinghouse and completes and signs any EDI agreements required by their contract payers.

*Source: Vines, Deborah; Braceland, Ann; Rollins, Elizabeth; and Miller, Susan. *Comprehensive Health Insurance: Billing, Coding, and Reimbursement*, 1st edition. © 2008 Pearson Education, Upper Saddle River, NJ. Reprinted with permission.

3. The provider submits a batch of sample claims for multiple payers, claims that will not be fully processed or paid, to the clearinghouse to test data integrity.

4. The clearinghouse activates live submission for non-contracted payers.

5. Contracted payers may require an additional testing period during which providers submit more sample claims for that specific payer to demonstrate data integrity with the particular payer.

6. The provider is approved by the contract payers to transmit electronically.

7. The clearinghouse activates live submission for contract payers.

Billing Insight   Garbage In/Garbage Out

A common complaint of new EDI submitters is that it doesn't work. Why? Usually there are numerous errors in the database, including invalid procedure codes, invalid diagnosis codes, missing dates of birth, missing entity types, etc. These errors printed just fine on paper claim forms (of course, they didn't get processed just fine). Brand new EDI submitters must painstakingly clean up the errors first, then they can enjoy much faster claims processing and payment time.

▶ **Test Your Knowledge 11-4**

It is not uncommon for the front desk person at a clinic to be in charge of setting the clinic up to transmit electronically. Write a detailed plan on how you would accomplish this task.

CHAPTER REVIEW

Multiple Choice

1. To setup Work Administrator to add items automatically, choose
    a.   New and then Repeat.
    b.   List Rule.
    c.   Automatic.
    d.   both a and b.

2. Which option in Work Administrator allows the User to view only his or her assignments?
    a.   Filter (Add/Remove)
    b.   New
    c.   View
    d.   List Only

3. Which would be created to tell a co-worker to return a patient phone call?
    a.   Rule
    b.   New Task
    c.   Reminder
    d.   All of the above

4. Which of the following would be created to watch for missing birthdates on claim forms?
   a. Rule
   b. New Task
   c. Reminder
   d. All of the above

5. Which utilities can be opened from Work Administrator?
   a. Claim Management
   b. Medisoft
   c. Office Hours
   d. All of the above

6. Which box is checked when an assignment is completed?
   a. Finished
   b. Completed
   c. Done
   d. Close

7. HIPAA was published as Public Law 104-191 on
   a. August 21, 1997.
   b. August 21, 1986.
   c. August 21, 2002.
   d. August 21, 1996.

8. Which portion of HIPAA defines the CPT?[*]
   a. Privacy
   b. Security
   c. Transactions and Code Sets
   d. Identifier

9. Which of the following is an example of a transaction?
   a. Scheduling Appointment
   b. Medical Record
   c. Payment
   d. Eligibility

10. Which is an example of a code set?
    a. Grid Colors
    b. Diagnosis
    c. Payment Code
    d. Both b and c

11. Which of the following was the initial reason HIPAA was created?
    a. To make health insurance portable
    b. To simplify transactions
    c. To provide privacy
    d. To provide security

12. Which portion of HIPAA addresses PHI?
    a. Code sets
    b. Transactions
    c. Security
    d. Privacy

[*]CPT is a registered trademark of the American Medical Association.

13. Which portion of HIPAA addresses claim status?
   a. Code sets
   b. Transactions
   c. Security
   d. Privacy

14. Which portion of HIPAA addresses electronic payment and remittance advice?
   a. Code sets
   b. Transactions
   c. Security
   d. Privacy

15. Which portion of HIPAA allows the government to access medical records?
   a. Code sets
   b. Transactions
   c. Security
   d. Privacy

True/False

Identify each of the following statements as true or false.

1. For a user to view his assignments, he can filter the assignments or print a copy with his user name.

2. State and federal governments can request copies of patient records without the patients' authorization.

3. Patients can refuse to allow their medical records be given to the government.

4. There are many different formats to transmit claims electronically.

5. Clinics must transmit claims electronically.

6. To create a rule, click on List Rules on the Work Administrator.

7. To create a rule, click on New in the Work Administrator.

8. Medisoft has its own clearinghouse.

9. HIPAA helps to ensure health insurance coverage if someone loses his or her job.

10. To send electronic claims, a doctor needs to complete special forms for his or her non-contract payers.

Short Answer

1. When is it more appropriate to create a Rule versus a New assignment?

2. Explain how Work Administrator and Collection List complement each other.

3. Briefly define HIPAA, outlining each of the provisions that directly affects medical billing.

Resources

Electronic Transactions: **www.cms.hhs.gov/ElectronicBillingEDITrans**

Government website that provides detailed information about electronic billing.

Transaction Code Set Standards: **www.cms.hhs.gov/
TransactionCodeSetsStands**

Government website that provides detailed information about the transaction code sets.

HIPAA: **www.hhs.gov/ocr/hipaa/**

Government website that provides HIPAA documentation.

Public Law 104-191: **http://aspe.hhs.gov/admnsimp/pl104191.htm**

Provides the text of the written law published on August 21, 1996, defining HIPAA; includes a table of contents and summary.

12

Office Work Flow Using Medisoft

Learning Objectives

After completing this chapter, you should be able to:

- ◆ Define and spell the key terms in this chapter.
- ◆ Understand and define the typical daily routine in a medical office regarding utilizing Medisoft.
- ◆ Demonstrate all of the key tasks done by a medical office specialist.
- ◆ Describe the use of the Collection List.
- ◆ Describe the Practice Analysis report.
- ◆ Describe and run the task of File Maintenance.
- ◆ Describe how to implement Work Administrator to enhance office work flow.
- ◆ Explain when to use the Small Balance Write-off function.
- ◆ Discuss when to use Security Setup.
- ◆ Explain when Design Custom Reports and Bills might be used in the clinic.
- ◆ Demonstrate how to create a new practice.
- ◆ Demonstrate how to switch between practices.
- ◆ Set the Program Date in Medisoft.
- ◆ Explain how to customize the Menu and Toolbar.
- ◆ Edit Program Options to enhance the efficiency of the clinic.
- ◆ Describe Final Draft word processing software available within Medisoft.

Key Terms

clinic follow-up policies   procedures defined by the office to collect self-pay, non-contract, and contract accounts.

Customize   feature that allows user to customize the menu, toolbars, and sidebars.

Final Draft   word processing software that interfaces with Medisoft.

New Case   the function that adds the insurance information, facility, referring doctor, and other details to the patient.

New Patient   the feature that allows users to add patient information such as name, address, and phone number.

New Practice   the utility that allows another set of data to be created.

Open Practice   the utility that allows users to switch from one practice to another.

Practice Analysis   the most commonly used Medisoft report to analyze information.

Program Options   a comprehensive utility that lets users define settings for Medisoft.

Set Program Date   function that allows the Medisoft date to be changed.

statements   invoices sent to patients/guarantors.

trending the days in AR   keeping a running log of the outstanding days in AR.

■ ■ ■ ■

INTRODUCTION

Anyone who has been employed for any length of time has experienced the fellow employee who seems to know all the tips and tricks of the trade. Of course, these employees are more valuable to the company and their paychecks probably show it!

There are several ways to become a seasoned medical office specialist and Medisoft user. Plan A would be to work at a clinic for a number of years, billing and using the program and hopefully picking up a number of secrets. Plan B would be to study the program by reading, watching videos, or attending classes. Either Plan A or Plan B could help the user to become a seasoned medical office specialist and Medisoft user who has expertise and efficiency in managing the clinic's patient tasks and account receivables (AR). Comparatively, Plan B would be much faster. By studying this textbook, you can start out being a knowledgeable employee and add value to the office place. And get there years faster!

This chapter is designed to serve as a review and checklist of "must-know" information by tying together the information presented in the previous chapters and providing a realistic look at office work flow by placing the user in a mock scenario about Sunny Life Clinic where the user is a new employee at the clinic. First, this chapter provides a brief overview of the daily tasks the user will do on his or her first day on the job. Second, it presents practice exercises that serve as a review of knowledge acquired in earlier chapters. And finally, this chapter will review features in Medisoft that are incredibly useful, but underused. Miscellaneous tips and tricks are presented. Armed with the information in this book and chapter, even a new medical office specialist and Medisoft user could appear to be a skilled employee.

YOUR FIRST DAY ON THE JOB

Imagine it is your first day on a new job and you work for Sunny Life Clinic. Sunny Life Clinic is a family practice and has medical doctors on staff who see patients for typical family doctor visits such as physicals, broken arms, or colds and flu. There are two doctors at the clinic, Marijane S. Anderson, M.D., and Charles W. Pearce, M.D. The doctors have hired you to work at their front desk and to do the billing. You arrive at your first day on the job and complete all of the necessary new employee forms. They welcome you to Sunny Life Clinic and show you where you will "live" for 40 hours of your life each week, and then they are off to their busy day at the clinic.

Help! Where do you start? Well, after you breathe deeply a few times, you can relax and focus. Everything you do with Medisoft for a medical office has already been reviewed in prior chapters. You just need to break it down into small, manageable tasks.

You will be responsible for scheduling, adding patients, entering charges and payments, submitting claims and statements, and reporting all of these items to inquiring minds. The inquiring minds may be your superiors (which are the doctors at Sunny Life Clinic), insurance companies, patients, or other state or federal agencies. In addition, you may be required to be the Information Technology person for your office and will need to back up Medisoft and run File Maintenance. With the working knowledge you now have, you will be a vital participant in the daily functions of the clinic. Review each of the sections below which provide an overview of the specific daily tasks, then complete the practice exercises to demonstrate your understanding of key concepts presented throughout the text.

Scheduling Appointments

Let's get started! The phone rings and you cheerfully answer providing your name and stating "How may I help you?" On the other end, a patient wants to see the doctor. It is your job to schedule and keep track of the patients. You begin by getting pertinent information such as the patient's name and type of appointment needed. Next, you look into the schedule for available times and schedule the patient, Dwight Again, into Office Hours (Figure 12-1).

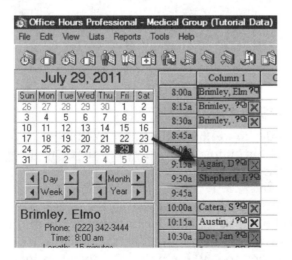

▶ Figure 12-1 **Scheduling Appointments**

Entering Patient Information

Dwight Again shows up at the front desk, and you have him sign in and complete his new patient forms. You pull his chart for Dr. Pearce. His chart is the folder of information that contains all his medical information. It contains the patient forms completed by Dwight on his first visit, lab reports, all the documentation by the doctors at Sunny Life Clinic, as well as any other documentation that other clinics or labs may have sent to Sunny Life Clinic to review. Dr. Pearce does his exam, documents his medical notes, and sends the patient back to you. Next, Dr. Pearce hands you the chart and tells you to handle it (Figure 12-2). You proceed with adding a **New Patient** and **New Case** in Transaction Entry.

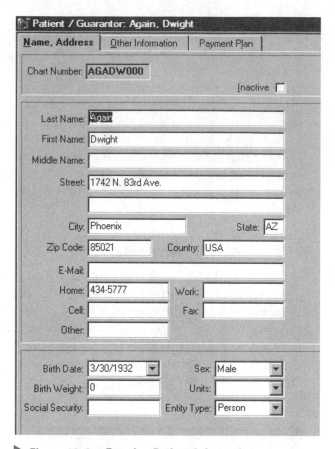

▶ Figure 12-2   **Entering Patient Information**

Charges and Payments

In addition to filing the chart in the appropriate drawer, you are responsible for billing for the services that Dwight Again received. So, you look at the superbill (Figure 12-3).

You think of your last visit at the doctor's office and remember the doctor had a clipboard that he or she checked and made notes on while speaking with you. Undoubtedly, the doctor checked off the services that were provided to you, including the doctor exam, X-rays, lab tests, and so forth. Dr. Pearce has done the same thing for Dwight. You enter the charges at the front desk and ask Dwight to pay his $20.00 co-pay. Then you enter the payment Dwight made into Medisoft. After Dwight leaves, you will open the mail and post any payments received.

PRACTICE EXERCISE 12-1   Adding Patients, Scheduling, and Printing Superbills

In this practice exercise, you will prepare for the next day by printing superbills. Pretend that the clinic started seeing patients on Saturday. This exercise will have you schedule three new patients and print their superbills.

1047	Happy Valley Medical Clinic 5222 E. Baseline Rd. Gilbert, AZ 85234 (800)333-4747	

AGADW000	Again, Dwight	7/29/2011	9:15:00 AM

EXAM	FEE	PROCEDURES	FEE	LABORATORY	FEE
New Patient		Anoscopy	46600	Aerobic Culture	87070	
Problem Focused	99201	Arthrocentesis/Aspiration/Injection		Amylase	82150	
Expanded Problem, Focused	99202	Small Joint	*20600	B12	82607	
Detailed	99203	Interm Joint	*20605	CBC & Diff	85025	
Comprehensive	99204	Major Joint	*20610	CHEM 20	80019	
Comprehensive/High Complex	99204	Audiometry	92552	Chlamydia Screen	86317	
Initial Visit/Procedure	99025	Cast Application		Cholesterol	82465	
Well Exam Infant (up to 12 mos.)	99318	Location Long Short		Digoxin	80162	
Well Exam 1 – 4 yrs.	99382	Catherization		Electrolytes	80005	
Well Exam 5 – 11 yrs.	99383	Circumcision	*53670	Ferritin	82728	
Well Exam 12 – 17 yrs.	99384	Colposcopy	54150	Folate	82746	
Well Exam 18 – 39 yrs.	99385	Colposcopy w /Biopsy	*57452	GC Screen	87070	
Well Exam 40 – 64 yrs.	99386	Cryosurgery Premalignant Lesion	*57454	Glucose	82947	
		Location(s):		Glucose 1 HR	82950	
Established Patient		Cryosurgery Warts		Glycosylated HGB (A1C)	83036	
Minimum	99211	Location(s):		HCT	85014	
Problem Focused	99212	Curettement Lesion w /Biopsy	CTF	HDL	83718	
Expanded Problem Focused	99213	Curettement Lesion w o/ Biopsy		Hep BSAG	86278	
Detailed	99214	Single	*11050	Hepatitis Profile	80059	
Comprehensive/High Complex	99215	2 – 4	*11051	HGB & HCT	85014	
Well Exam Infant (up to 12 mos.)	99391	> 4	*11052	HIV	86311	
Well Exam 1 – 4 yrs.	99392	Diaphram Fitting	*57170	Iron & TBC	83540	83550
Well Exam 5 – 11 yrs.	99393	Ear Irrigation	69210	Kidney Profile	80007	
Well Exam 12 – 17 yrs.	99394	ECG	93000	Lead	83655	
Well Exam 18 – 39 yrs.	99395	Endometrial Biopsy	*58100	Liver Profile	82977	
Well Exam 40 – 64 yrs.	99396	Exc. Lesion w /Biopsy	CTF	Mono Test	86308	
		w /o Biopsy		Pap Smear	88155	
Obstetrics		Location Size		Pregnancy Test	84703	

▶ Figure 12-3 **Superbill**

1 Pick the Saturday closest to the current day in the schedule.

2 Schedule three appointments for new patients, adding their Chart information from appointment entry. Be creative and use fictitious information.

3 Print the Superbills for the Saturday appointments in preparation for pulling the patient charts.

Checks and Balances—Daily Reports

The day is coming to an end, and Happy Valley Medical Clinic has been incredibly busy. The phones rang dozens of time, new and old patients have come and gone, and you've entered dozens of appointments and charges and payments into Medisoft. Hopefully, it's all correct. And, hope is exactly what many clinics do. But, at Sunny Life Clinic, you do things better! At the end of each day, you run a checks and balances of your system to make sure that you have everything you need done and it is correct. The checks and balance will be done by printing reports of your schedule (Appointment List), deposits (Deposit Report) and transactions (Patient Day Sheet) (Figure 12-4). Reports in Medisoft show you the details of the information entered into the system.

First, you make sure there are charges on the Patient Day Sheet for everyone on the Appointment List. The charges on the Patient Day Sheet

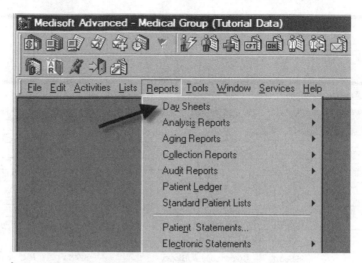

▶ Figure 12-4   **Printing Reports to Balance the Day**

match the superbills, and the Deposit Report totals equals the payment amount applied to the patients on the Patient Day Sheet.

Claims and Statements

You have done a great job on his first day and everything is in Medisoft. What's next? Well, you need to send out the bills. You will send insurance claims and if Sunny Life Clinic does cycle billing, send **statements** to patients (Figure 12-5). So, Claim Management and possibly Statement Management will be used to create claims and statements. If Sunny Life Clinic does not send cycle bills, statements will be created on the first of the month.

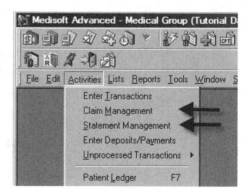

▶ Figure 12-5   **Sending Claims and Statements**

Back Up Medisoft

Your next task is very simple but incredibly critical. You must back up Medisoft every day (Figure 12-6). In addition, Sunny Life Clinic will have someone who takes the backups off-site so that if the building or computer is destroyed, the very vital data can be restored. Plus, you will want to rotate backups in a manner that will ensure that if there is a bad backup, you will still be able to retrieve the majority of your data. This is one of those areas that will show your employers that you are a professional.

At this point, we have come full circle with the typical daily job of a medical office specialist and Medisoft user at a clinic.

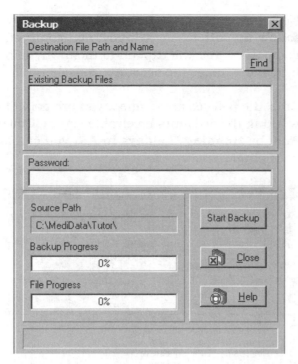

Backup

Destination File Path and Name

[   ] [Find]

Existing Backup Files

[   ]

Password:

[   ]

Source Path
C:\MediData\Tutor\

Backup Progress
[0%   ]

File Progress
[0%   ]

[Start Backup]

[☒] Close

[☉] Help

▶ **Figure 12-6 Backing Up Medisoft**

PRACTICE EXERCISE 12-2   Creating a Backup

This practice exercise will demonstrate a task that is vital to the operation of every clinic, backing up data. If available, back up the data to a flash drive or a CD. If those resources are not available, obtain permission to back up to the local hard drive. For the purpose of this exercise, "media" will refer to your resource choice to back up. Check with your instructor to find out what media you should use on the school's computers.

1   Open Backup Data under the File menu.

2   Review the Help information on Backup.

3   Select Find in Backup Data and choose the appropriate media source to back up to.

4   Click Start Backup and write the name of the backup created.

5   When finished, open My Computer and find the backup.

6   Write a rotation plan for making, storing, and rotating the backups.

Defining Clinic Policies and Collection List

It's just your first day at Sunny Life Clinic but, prior to your arrival, the person before you was diligently billing insurance companies and patients. Many payments have come in to reimburse Sunny Life Clinic for its hard work. However, many payments have not come back. Why? The person before you only did the daily Medisoft work flow and didn't follow-up on unpaid balances.

You are going to first start by figuring out the number of Days in AR. Then, you will start a grid to calculate the AR days on the same day each month to trend your progress.

Next, you will need to work with your employers on creating **clinic follow-up policies** for self-pay, non-contract, and contract insurance companies. You will explain to them why it is important to follow-up policies and manage the accounts consistently.

After the policies are defined, you are going to set off painstakingly working the accounts receivable via the Collection List (Figure 12-7). And, by **trending the days in AR,** you can prove your value (literally) to your employers.

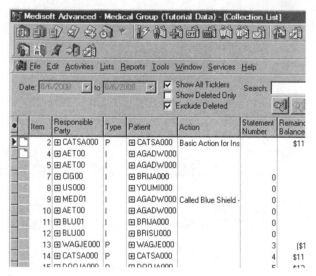

▶ **Figure 12-7   The Collection List**

Billing Insights   Days in AR and Trending

A clinic's financial health can be determined by its Days in AR. AR is the amount of money on the books, or the Accounts Receivable. The Days in AR is defined as the average number of days it takes for the clinic to receive its money. It is very helpful to track this number and trend it throughout the year. A typical practice that has a mix of insurance and patient payments wants to have less than 60 days in AR. How are the days in AR calculated? There are a number of formulas. One formula was presented in Chapter 9. Another formula is to take the last three months of charges and divide it by three. This gives you the average billing for 30 days. Next, take the total amount on the clinic's books and divide it by the 30-day average. This will give you a monthly AR ratio such as 1.3 or 3.2. Then, take the AR ratio and multiply it by 30 days. This will give you your Days in AR. If this is done diligently, it will help the practice monitor its financial health as well as help trend seasonal changes, such as when deductibles are due the first of the year, when patient health status changes, and when payer contracts change.

Reports

Next, Dr. Anderson and Dr. Pearce are at your desk. They want to know how much they billed out last month and how much money was collected. Plus, they want to know which insurance companies owe the most and how far behind they are paying. All these answers can come from any number of reports in Medisoft. The most comprehensive and commonly liked report is the **Practice Analysis** (Figure 12-8). However, each clinic has different preferences, and those will be learned on the job site.

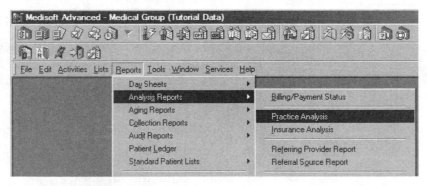

▶ Figure 12-8 The Practice Analysis

File Maintenance

Many things in our life need maintenance; some examples of these are our teeth, our car, and our home. With Medisoft, maintenance tasks also need to be performed. A critical task to keep your program running smoothly is File Maintenance (Figure 12-9). File Maintenance is a tool that rebuilds indexes, packs data, and recalculates balances. Most database software on the market contains tools that run similar processes. However, just like many of us are guilty of putting off getting oil changes for our cars, many clinics are guilty of either not knowing about this utility or not utilizing it. Here's another place you can shine as a skilled professional.

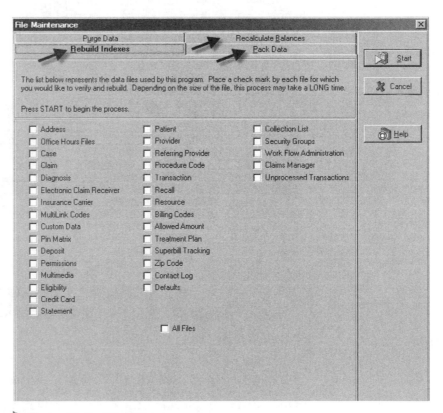

▶ Figure 12-9 File Maintenance

PRACTICE EXERCISE 12-3   Running the Task of File Maintenance

File Maintenance is a task similar to the system tools of Windows. Running the task will keep your system running faster and smoother. File Maintenance should be run at least once a month. Some clinics run it weekly to optimize their systems.

1   Select File Maintenance from the drop-down menu under File.

2   Select Rebuild Indexes and All Files.

3   Select Pack Data and All Files.

4   Select Recalculate Balances and all three options under the tab.

5   Select Purge Data and read the Help for it. Due to the size and efficiency of today's computers, most clinics do not use this function. However, it is nice to be acquainted with it.

6   Click Start.

Work Administrator

When you arrive at your new job, you notice notes and "stickies" all over the computer and desk area. You immediately implement the Work Administrator (Figure 12-10). Not only does it clean up all those notes and stickies, but you set it up to catch appointments that didn't have referrals and to show claims missing authorization numbers. Once again, you prove your worth to your employers.

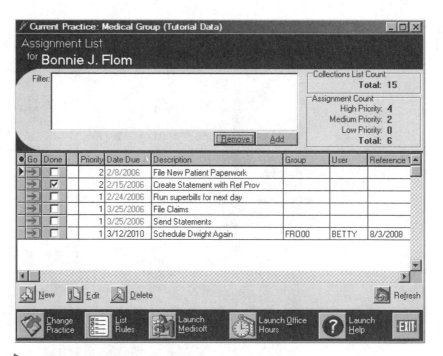

▶ Figure 12-10   Work Administrator

Billing Charges and Small Balance Write-off

Once you start working the Collection List, you realize that many patients aren't paying on a timely basis, so you decide to implement billing charges. But, first, of course, you check with the state office to find out the rules surrounding billing charges and write a clinic policy on billing charges. (Figure 12-11).

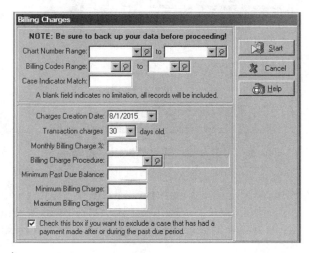

▶ Figure 12-11   Billing Charges

Next, you realize that the clinic was wasting money on printing, sending, and getting calls on statements that were under $2.00. You check with your boss and get approval to write off small balances. You utilize the Small Balance Write-Off (Figure 12-12) function to do this automatically for several accounts at once. Once again, you save money for the clinic.

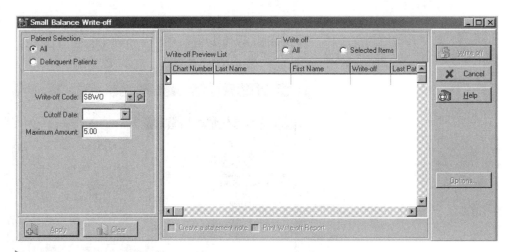

▶ Figure 12-12   Small Balance Write-off

Security, Groups, and Permission Settings

Sunny Life Clinic had a security setting when you started the job. However, the security code was set up by the previous biller, and everyone in the clinic used the same login. You know this is not HIPAA compliant and also know that Medisoft entries could not be tracked or work assigned given the current arrangements. So, you sit down with everyone in the clinic and set up unique security codes and match appropriate permission settings to each user. Then, you modify Security Setup. Plus, you identify areas where groups would be beneficial in the Work Administrator and created those too (Figure 12-13).

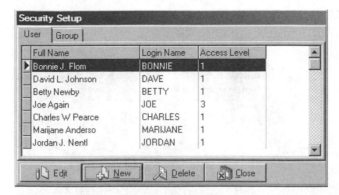

▶ **Figure 12-13   Security and Group Setup**

Sunny Life Clinic can now create an audit report of changes made to a patient's data, be assured that the proper employees were performing the correct functions, and assign work to users and groups. You are a hero!

Design Custom Reports and Bills

Finally, you have all of the AR in good order and the clinic's policies and procedures are all running smoothly with the aid of Medisoft. So, you think you will tackle a marketing campaign for Sunny Life Clinic. The holiday season is approaching and you want to hold an open house for the all the patients seen in the last two years. Sunny Life Clinic has added some new services and now would be a great time to bring them to light.

You decide you will make labels to send postcard invitations. Design Custom Reports and Bills is the perfect place to design some labels (Figure 12-14).

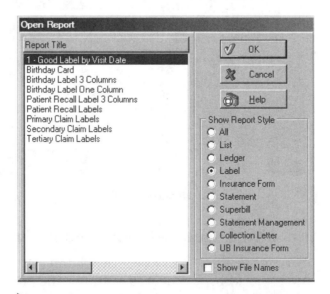

▶ **Figure 12-14   Design Custom Reports and Bills**

This last item does it for you—it puts you over the top in your employers' eyes, and they decide to give you a raise. The moral of this story, as is often true in life, the more you give, the more you get. Or, better said, the more you learn, the more you are able to give and get.

▶ Test Your Knowledge 12-1

Soon, you will be getting your first job at a medical office. Visualize yourself working at a clinic utilizing Medisoft. Write your own short story of your first week at work, demonstrating the knowledge you have learned with every feature of Medisoft and tying each one into the daily work flow.

TIPS AND TRICKS

Medisoft has several features that do not fit into any of the typical daily processes. That's because most of them are done infrequently. However, these tips and tricks can be very useful and save users hours of time.

Setting Up a New Practice

There are three possibilities for setting up a new practice: Medisoft is first being installed in an office, the office is adding another business entity, or the data currently used by the office is damaged and a new set needs to be restored from a backup.

PRACTICE EXERCISE 12-4   Creating a New Practice

Creating a new practice is simple, and it is recommended to have a test practice to restore a backup every week or two to make sure your backup system is working properly. Complete the following steps to set up a new practice (Figure 12-15).

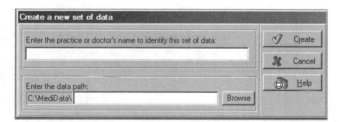

▶ Figure 12-15   Setting Up a New Practice

1   On the menu bar, choose File and **New Practice.**

2   In the top line of Create a New Set of Data enter the practice name, i.e., Sunny Life Clinic.

3   In the bottom line, enter the first name of the practice, i.e., Sunny.

4   Click Create.

5   Medisoft will give you a message stating this data does not exist. Do you want to create a new set of data? Click yes.

6   Medisoft will create the set of data and the Practice Information screen will appear. Enter the practice information.

7   Go to Help on the menu bar and Getting Started in the drop-down menu. Medisoft gives step-by-step instructions on how to set up a practice (Figure 12-16).

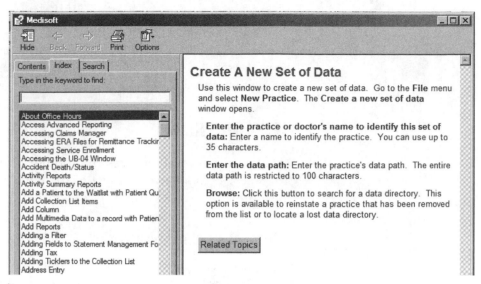

▶ Figure 12-16　**Step-by-Step Procedures to Set Up a Practice**

Switching Between Practices

Once Medisoft contains more than one dataset, it is imperative to understand how to switch between data sets. Switching between data sets is
similar to switching between documents or spreadsheets: Go to File on
menu bar and select **Open Practice.** A pop-up box will appear (Figure
12-17). This window displays all of the available practices. Simply select
the desired practice and click OK.

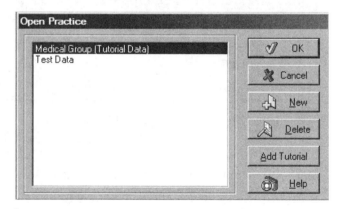

▶ Figure 12-17　**Switching Between Practices**

PRACTICE EXERCISE 12-5　Switching Between Practices

It is also common to have multiple practices in Medisoft. With billing services becoming ever more popular and more small businesses forming,
many offices share resources. Medisoft is among those resources. If two
doctors who have separate practices share the same office, receptionist,
and Medisoft program, there will be two sets of data to switch between.
Perform the following steps to complete this exercise.

1   Click on File on the menu bar.

2   Click on Open Practice in the drop-down menu.

3   Select the practice to open and click OK.

Setting the Program Date

Offices are often a day or two behind in posting mail payments. Setting the Program Date is a great little utility Medisoft offers to change the date inside Medisoft, but not on the computer itself. If the user wants to post payments from two days ago, all he or she has to do is change the program date, and the deposits and transactions will be posted to the proper day.

Set Program Date can be accessed by clicking on File on the menu bar and then Set Program Date from the drop-down menu. Next, select the date in the calendar that pops up in the bottom right window of Medisoft (Figure 12-18). Remember, the beauty of this feature is the computer date remains unchanged so emails or correspondence outside Medisoft will not be affected.

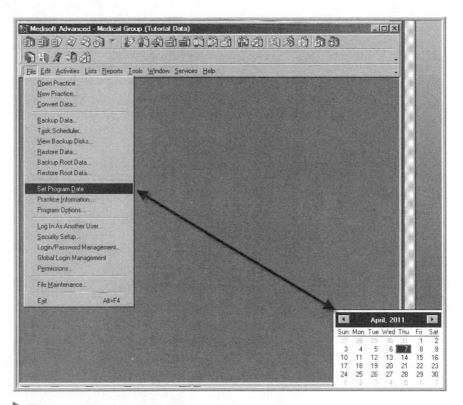

▶ Figure 12-18   **Setting the Program Date**

PRACTICE EXERCISE 12-6   Setting the Program Date

Setting the Program Date is one of the most common features that offices use. Most clinics are usually a day behind in entering charges and payments for several reasons: doctors not turning in superbills, employees out sick, and the list goes on and on. Complete the following steps to set the date in Medisoft.

1   Click on File on the menu bar.

2   Click on Program Options in the drop-down menu.

3   Click on the proper date in the pop-up calendar that appears the lower right hand corner of Medisoft.

Customizing the Menu and Toolbar

Another Medisoft feature that can improve the efficiency of an office is the ability to customize the menu and toolbars. First, the user can right-click anywhere on an empty spot in the menu bar (Figure 12-19) to turn the tool bar or sidebar off and on or choose the option to **Customize.**

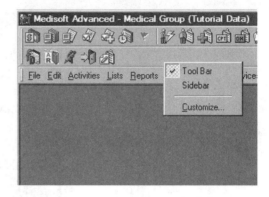

▶ **Figure 12-19   Customizing the Toolbar, Sidebar, and Menu Bar**

If Customize is chosen, a pop-up menu displays with tabs titled Toolbars, Commands, and Options. A whole chapter could be written involving the details of each tab and the quantity of options users are given. The idea of adding this tip is for the user to become familiar with this option, not to master it.

A quick tip is to find a utility that would assist the office and drag it to the toolbar. In Figure 12-20, the calculator was dragged to the toolbar. Now, it is simple to give patients quotes on services while still inside of Medisoft. Always remember, in every utility, there is a Help button to guide you through the learning process.

Setting Program Options

Setting up **Program Options** can literally save hundreds of hours of time over a year's span and again, a whole chapter could be written on it. In this section, we will take a brief look at the utility and what each tab has to offer. Always remember, Help is just a click away.

Program Options can be modified by clicking on File on the menu bar and then Program Options (Figure 12-21). Inside Program Options are eight tabs that allow the user to modify the functions of the program and thus produce a more efficient environment. The following list explains each tab (Figure 12-22).

General: Addresses the general options for the program—backup options, startup options and alert settings to name a few.

Data Entry: Allows the user to change transaction, patient, and deposit entry features along with other shortcuts to auto enter city and state by zip and to use enter to move between fields.

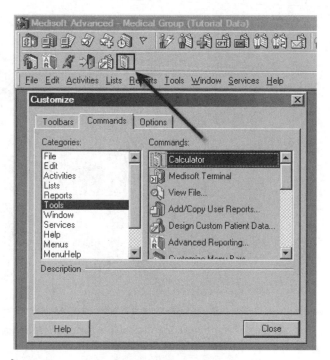

▶ Figure 12-20 **A Look Inside Customize**

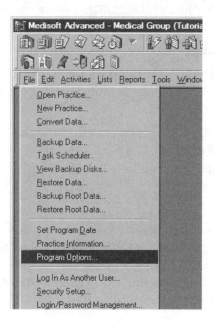

▶ Figure 12-21 **Modifying Program Options**

Payment Application: Sets up default payment codes, Small Balance Write-off, and system defaults for payment applications.

Aging Reports: Sets up the default aging columns for patient and insurance aging.

HIPAA: Allows the program to automatically logoff users after a period of inactive time and turns on warnings for unapproved CPT* and ICD-9-CM codes. This feature should be activated after the CPT* and ICD-9-CM codes are reviewed and checked for HIPAA approval. This is

---

*CPT is a registered trademark of the American Medical Association.

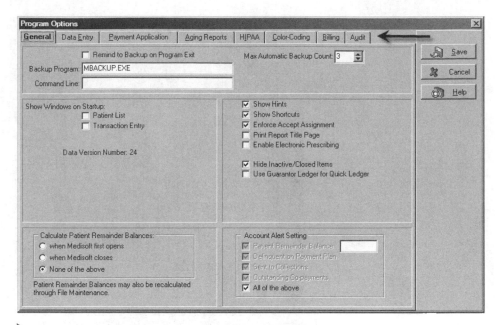

▶ Figure 12-22　**Defining the Tabs in Program Options**

done under the List/Diagnosis Codes or List/Procedure/Payment/ Adjustment Codes.

Color Coding:　Allows transaction and patient color coding.

Billing:　Defines billing parameters for Claims Manager, Statements, Billing Notes, and sets default formats for the receipt, statement, face sheet, and quick list.

Audit:　Allows the user to define the tables that will be audited and the form of auditing that will be done. This is the data that will be sent to the Audit Reports.

Final Draft

Final Draft is word processing software that is interfaced with Medisoft. It allows offices to merge patient data with documents or keep progress notes and records for each patient. It is fully functioning word processing software that includes spell check, mail merge, and document formatting, among many other features.

Access Final Draft by selecting Activities from the menu bar and Final Draft from the dropdown menu, or click on the Final Draft icon (Figure 12-23).

▶ Test Your Knowledge 12-2

Write a detailed explanation of the three types of free Medisoft support detailing where and how they are accessed.

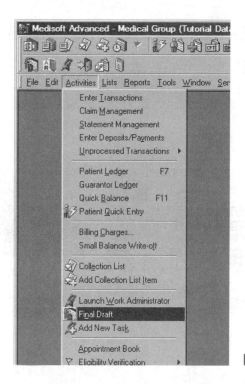

▶ **Figure 12-23 Accessing Final Draft**

Medisoft Quick Tips   One More Time: Free Support for Medisoft

At the close of this book, nothing is more fitting than reviewing one more time where to get free support for Medisoft.

Help in Medisoft   Help is located on the menu bar of Medisoft or by hitting F1 from any place within the program (Figure 12-24).

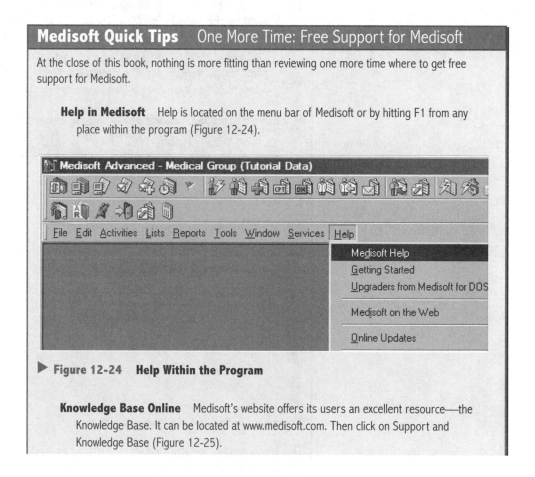

▶ **Figure 12-24 Help Within the Program**

Knowledge Base Online   Medisoft's website offers its users an excellent resource—the Knowledge Base. It can be located at www.medisoft.com. Then click on Support and Knowledge Base (Figure 12-25).

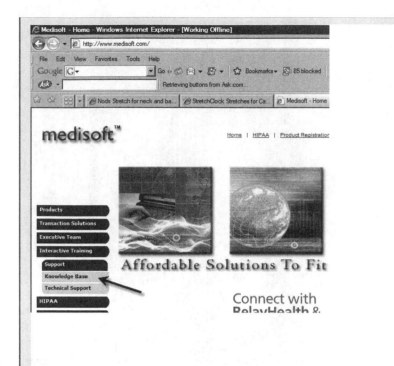

▶ Figure 12-25   **Help at Medisoft's Knowledge Base**

Manual on the Installation CD   Each installation CD comes preloaded with a Medisoft manual. The manual is in an Adobe format, and the installation CD comes with Adobe Reader software to install in case the user does not have it already. After the manual is opened, desired topics can be found in the index at the start of the manual or may be searched for by going to Edit on the menu bar then Search or Find (Figure 12-26).

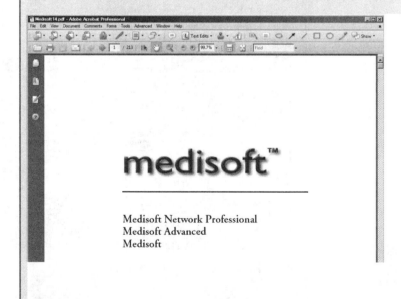

▶ Figure 12-26   **Help in Medisoft's Manual**

Tip: Save the manual on your computer Desktop for easy retrieval and to avoid damaging the installation CD.

CHAPTER REVIEW

Multiple Choice

1. Where are appointments scheduled?
   a. Medisoft
   b. Office Hours
   c. Schedule
   d. All of the above

2. Where are patient Charts and Cases created?
   a. Transaction Entry
   b. List/Patient
   c. Office Hours
   d. All of the above

3. Where are charges entered?
   a. Transaction Entry
   b. Charge Entry
   c. List/Charges
   d. All of the above

4. Where are payments entered?
   a. Transaction Entry
   b. Activities/Enter Deposit/Payment
   c. Payment Entry
   d. Both a and b

5. Which utility bills insurance companies?
   a. Statement Management
   b. Insurance Biller
   c. Claim Management
   d. Collection List

6. Which utility bills patients?
   a. Statement Management
   b. Patient Biller
   c. Claim Management
   d. Collection List

7. Which report is most often used by Medisoft practices to analyze data?
   a. Patient Day Sheet
   b. Practice Analysis
   c. Patient Analysis
   d. Program Analysis

8. Where would you set default payment codes for patients?
   a. Transaction Entry
   b. Patient Entry
   c. Payment Entry
   d. Program Options

9. Where would you add overdue claims and statements to follow-up?
   a. Collection List
   b. Transaction Entry
   c. Follow-up List
   d. All of the above

10. When running File Maintenance, which tab is rarely used?
    a. Purge Data
    b. Rebuild Indexes
    c. Pack Data
    d. Recalculate Balances

11. When using Design Custom Reports and Bills, which Master File would be selected to create labels for the responsible parties?
    a. Patient
    b. Case
    c. Claim
    d. Guarantor

12. Which two reports should have matching daily receipts?
    a. Appointment List and Patient Day Sheet
    b. Patient Day Sheet and Superbill
    c. Deposit Report and Patient Day Sheet
    d. Deposit Report and Superbill

13. To turn on Medisoft to audit the tables, the utility used is
    a. Practice Information.
    b. Work Administrator.
    c. Audit Administrator.
    d. Program Options.

14. To get rid of notes and stickies that have to-do items listed on them, they can be added to
    a. Work Administrator.
    b. Collection List.
    c. Program Options.
    d. Notes and Stickies.

15. Where can you get Medisoft help?
    a. Help within Medisoft
    b. Knowledge Base Online at www.medisoft.com
    c. Manual on the Medisoft Installation CD
    d. All of the above

True/False

Identify each of the following statements as true or false.

1. A patient must be first added to Medisoft before charges can be added.

2. Either the Deposit Report or the Patient Day Sheet will suffice to balance the day.

3. Setting the Program Date changes the date for the entire computer.

4. Work Administrator manages the items in the Collection List.

5. To add a group to Medisoft, click on File and then Group Setup in the drop-down menu.

6. Small Balance Write-off writes off small balances for both insurance companies and patients.

7. Program Options allows a user to set up color coding for Transactions and Patients.

8. File Maintenance should be done annually.

9. Billing charges should be researched before a clinic implements them.

10. Final Draft allows a clinic to create a mail merge letter.

Short Answer

1. At Sunny Life Clinic, charges are entered on Monday and Thursdays. Bob enters them on Monday and Betty on Friday. Explain how you would use Work Administrator to automatically issue these assignments.

2. Describe the process you would go through each day for a checks and balance routine.

3. Explain the function of Final Draft.

Resources

Medisoft: **www.medisoft.com**

This website offers the number one resource for learning and solving Medisoft challenges. After entering this website, click on Support and Knowledge Base.

CMS: **www.cms.gov**

Centers for Medicare and Medicaid Services is an excellent resource for billing information. It is recommended when you are in the billing field to review updates and additions at least monthly. Also, you can subscribe to listservs and be emailed notifications of changes. The site provides the national guidelines for Medicare and Medicaid. You can also locate your local Medicare and Medicaid carriers and visit their sites, which will provide regional insight and information.

Blue Cross Blue Shield and Other Insurance Company Websites: **www .bcbs.com**

The national website for Blue Cross Blue Shield (BCBS) provides a section called Blue Finder for Professionals with general billing information for providers. Use the Blue Finder for Individuals to locate your local BCBS plans and link to their sites for more detailed information. You can use a general Internet search engine to find websites of other major payers for their billing information.

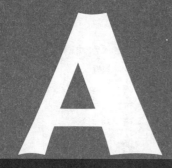

Mock Clinic Simulation

INTRODUCTION

Chapter 12 reviewed all of the content presented in each chapter of *Mastering Medisoft*. The mock clinic exercises in this appendix will test the knowledge you have gained by reading this textbook and applying the practice exercises contained in each chapter. The following exercises will simulate the process of setting up Medisoft in a new clinic, Sunny Life Clinic, and performing tasks from entering the practice information to performing the Medisoft Daily Basics to developing follow-up and backup procedures.

PRACTICE EXERCISE A-1: Creating Sunny Life Clinic

Each computer lab is a little different, and it is assumed that Medisoft is already installed on the computer you will be using. If Medisoft is not installed on the computer, complete instructions are found on your Medisoft CD. Just insert the CD and a pop-up menu will appear on the screen, giving the option to read the installation directions.

Once Medisoft is installed, a new set of data needs to be created. Click on File on the menu bar and New Practice from the drop-down list. If Medisoft was just installed, the program will prompt you to create a new set of data. Either way, the Create a New Set of Data window will appear (Figure A-1). In this box, type the practice name, "Sunny Life Clinic" and the data path name of "Sunny," then press Create. Medisoft will now create a folder inside the MediData folder named Sunny. Sunny will contain all the tables to store the information for Sunny Life Clinic. Numerous tables will be created to manage patient information, diagnosis codes, procedure codes, and insurance companies. The MediData folder is the folder where all the practice data resides. For example, if a clinic has three doctors all with different tax identification numbers (i.e., different business entities), three separate folders would exist under one MediData folder.

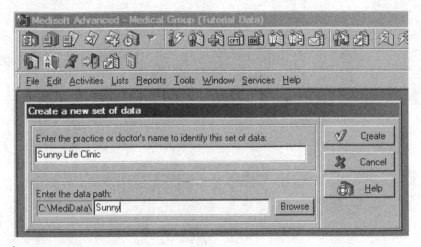

▶ Figure A-1   Create a New Set of Data

PRACTICE EXERCISE A-2:   Entering Practice Information

With the creation of Sunny Life Clinic, the next step is to enter the clinic information (Figure A-2). Enter the following Practice Information and click Save:

Practice Name: Sunny Life Clinic

Street: 5055 E Ford Road

City: Mesa

State: AZ

Zip Code: 85205

Phone: (480) 444-4866

Fax Phone: (480) 444-4867

Type: Medical

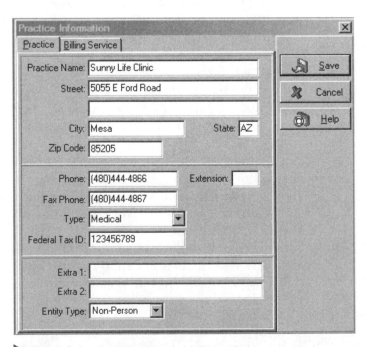

▶ Figure A-2   Entering Practice Information

Federal Tax ID: 12-3456789

Entity Type: Non-Person

Note: Entity Type is an electronic transaction requirement used to populate electronic fields.

PRACTICE EXERCISE A-3: Creating List Items

The next step in creating Sunny Life Clinic is to populate the Lists (Figure A-3). The Lists contain all of the information used by the practice, including provider information, patient information, and procedure codes. If any of the lists were viewed individually, they would appear to be spreadsheets (Figure A-4). Medisoft pulls the bits and pieces of data from the collective spreadsheets to accomplish the needed tasks, i.e., appointment scheduling, reporting, or billing.

For this exercise, open the appropriate list and enter the information listed in each category that follows. Remember, if you get stuck, use your three forms of free support (Help within the program, CD manual, or Knowledge Base). In addition, not all tables will be populated, only the most used and required tables.

Provider List and Class

To enter the provider information, enter the Class under the provider. To do this, choose Lists, Provider, Class, and New and enter:

Class Name: Sunny Life Clinic

Description: Group NPI

National ID: 2222222222

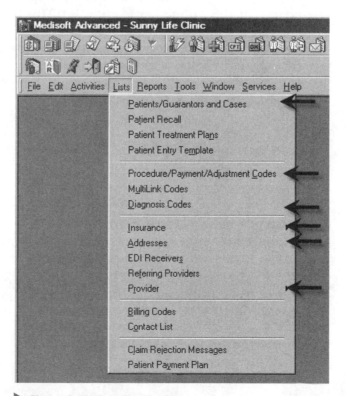

▶ Figure A-3 **Creating the Lists**

Chart Nu...	Last Name	First Name	Middle Ini...	Street 1
AGADW000	Again	Dwight		1742 N. 83rd Ave.
AUSAN000	Austin	Andrew		1999 Allthe Way
BORJO000	Bordon	John		777 Hardway Ln.
BRIEL000	Brimley	Elmo		1234 W. Glendale Ave.
BRIJA000	Brimley	Jay		1234 W. Glendale Ave.
BRISU000	Brimley	Susan		1234 W. Glendale Ave.
CATSA000	Catera	Sammy		7214 Shape Cir.
CLIWA000	Clinger	Wallace		200 Pennsylvania Ave.
DOEJA000	Doe	Jane	S	222 East Jane Street
DOEJO000	Doe	John		222 East Jane Street
DOOJA000	Doogan	James		
GOOCH000	Gooding	Charles		
HARTO000	Hartman	Tonya		1571 Knap Way
JACTH000	Jacks	Theodore		3686 E. Baranca Ct.
JASST000	Jasper	Stephanie	L	
JOHWI000	Johnson	William	J	
JONSU000	Jones	Suzy	Q	2273 Easy Suzy Street
JORBO000	Jordan	Bonita		5055 E University Dr. # T-11
JORJA000	Jordan	Jane	N	5055 E University Dr. # T-11
KARJE000	Karvel	Jessica	C	
KOSCH000	Koseman	Chadwick		3278 E. Joseph Way
LEWMO000	Lewis	Monique		

▶ **Figure A-4 Sample View of a Medisoft Table**

After completing, click Save.

Note: Because of data validation requirements, Medisoft will give an error that the ID number is not valid. This is known. Click OK.

Next, go to the provider information and create a new provider. Enter the following:

Address Tab:

Last Name: Pearce

First Name: Charles

Middle Initial: W

Street: 5055 E Ford Road

City: Mesa   **State:**   AZ   **Zip:**   85205

Phone: (480) 692-3457

Default Pins Tab:

Tax ID: 12-3456789   **National Identifier:** 3333333333

Default Group Tab:

Provider Class: SUN00

After completing, click Save.

Entering Procedure Codes

Next, select Lists, Procedure/Payment/Adjustment Codes. Charges, payments, and adjustments need to be created. Create the following, keeping in mind that the proper Type needs to be selected or the code cannot be used for the intended purpose.

Code 1	Description	Type	Amount
BCBSADJ	Blue Shield Adjustment	Insurance Adjustment	.00
BCBSPMT	Blue Shield Payment	Insurance Payment	.00
BCBSWO	Blue Shield Withhold	Insurance Withhold	.00
CASH	Cash Payment	Cash Payment	.00
CHECK	Check Payment	Check Payment	.00
MEDADJ	Medicare Adjustment	Insurance Payment	.00
MEDPMT	Medicare Payment	Insurance Payment	.00
VITAMIN	Vitamin Packs	Procedure Charge	30.00
(Mark Patient Only Responsible)			
80050	General Health Screen	Procedure Charge	40.00
84702	Pregnancy Test	Procedure Charge	20.00
97010	Hotpack	Procedure Charge	10.00
99201	Office Visit New Patient	Procedure Charge	30.00
99211	Office Visit Est. Patient	Procedure Charge	25.00

Entering Diagnosis Codes

Next, select Lists, Diagnosis Codes and create these new diagnosis codes:

Code 1	Description
250.01	Diabetes Melitus
719.47	Pain Ankle
372.03	Pink Eye
V22.1	Pregnancy
836.1	Tear Torn Knee Lateral

Entering Addresses

Addresses are commonly required in box 32 of the claim form. In this exercise, two addresses will be created. Go to Lists, Addresses and enter the following:

Address 1

Name: Sunny Life Clinic

Street: 5055 E Ford Road

City: Mesa **State:** AZ **Zip:** 85205

Type: Facility

Phone: (480) 444-2366

Fax: (480) 444-2367

National ID: 2222222222

Address 2

Name: Sunny Life Clinic

Street: 13274 Anchor Point Road

City: Mesa   **State:** AZ   **Zip:** 85205

Type: Facility

Phone: (480) 444-2366

Fax: (480) 444-2367

National ID: 2222222222

Tip: Here is an ideal place to use the "Set Default" tab. This allows data to be copied from the first address to the second address. To remove a default, hold the Control Key and click Remove Default.

Entering Insurance Companies

Insurance companies can be added when setting up the clinic or when the patient is entered. In this exercise, add the following insurance companies (Blue Shield and Medicare) prior to the patient entry and then, in patient entry, Aetna insurance will be added "on the fly." Go to Lists, Insurance and Carriers and add:

Insurance 1

Blue Shield

1234 Yankee Doodle Drive Suite 101

St. Paul, AZ 88888

Phone: 888-333-4444

Insurance 2

Medicare

8924 Commerce Drive Unit A

Chandler, AZ 86456

Phone: 888-212-4111

Tip: Make sure the Options tab is completed correctly for insurance type and signatures.

Entering Patients

Upon arriving at the clinic, new patients are given paperwork to complete and sign. For simplicity, we will assume for this exercise that the patient has completed the necessary paperwork, signed an agreement to have the clinic release confidential information, and has assigned the insurance benefits to the clinic. Next, complete Charts and Cases for the following five patients:

Patient 1

Name: David F. Lyle

Address: 1431 University Ave., Mesa, AZ 85205

Phone: 480-444-9666   **Cell:** 480-790-6000

DOB: 07/02/1961

Employer: Self-Employed

Insurance: None – Cash Case

Guarantor: Self   **Facility:** Ford Rd Clinic

Allergies and Notes: Make sure the patient pays in full at time of service.

Patient 2

Name: Marijane S. Anderson

Address: 10799 Jefferson Street, Blaine, AZ 85343

Phone: 480-692-3457   **Cell:** 480-692-2793

DOB: 05/11/1941

Employer: Retired May 1, 2006

Insurance: Medicare   **Policy:** 432-78-9875A
Group: NONE (type letters into field)

Insured: Self

Secondary Insurance: Aetna Insurance

Submit to: 1555 Forest View Lane, Scottsdale, AZ 85208

Phone: 888-997-4567

Policy: 1214-454010   **Group:** YRYSN-00

Guarantor: Self   **Facility:** Ford Rd Clinic

Allergies and Notes: Patient wants records at time of service.

Patient 3

Name: Timothy J. Nelson

Address: 5334 Glenwood Ave. Staples, AZ 85779

Phone: 480-828-0388   **Cell:** 480-330-9537

DOB: 01/27/1962

Employer: Accounting 101 Professionals   **Phone:** 480-888-1040

Insurance: BCBS   **Policy:** 47490713-44   **Group:** YRU03

Insured: Self

Guarantor: Self   **Facility:** Anchor Point Rd Clinic

Copay: $20 per Visit

Patient 4

Name: William J. Nelson

Address: 5334 Glenwood Ave, Staples, AZ 85779

Phone: 480-828-0388   **Cell:** 480-851-0354

DOB: 10/14/1996

Employer: Child

Insurance: BCBS   **Policy:** 47490713-44   **Group:** YRU03

Insured: Timothy J. Nelson

Guarantor: Timothy J. Nelson   **Facility:** Anchor Point Rd Clinic

Copay: $20 per Visit

Patient 5

Name: Jordan J. Nelson

Address: 5334 Glenwood Ave, Staples, AZ 85779

Phone: 480-828-0388   **Cell:** 480-330-1744

DOB: 12/04/1992

Employer: Child

Insurance: BCBS   **Policy:** 47490713-44   **Group:** YRU03

Insured: Timothy J. Nelson

Guarantor: Timothy J. Nelson   **Facility:** Anchor Point Rd Clinic

Copay: $20 per Visit

PRACTICE EXERCISE A-4:   Security Setup

Now that Sunny Life Clinic has been created and the demographics entered, it is time to secure the data. Sunny Life Clinic has two employees and one doctor. Set up security for each.

Doctor

Login Name: Bill

Full Name: Charles W. Pearce

Password: Lucky1995

Question: What school did you attend?   **Answer:** Crookston

Access Level: 1

Employee One

Login Name: Diane

Full Name: Diane Johnson

Password: USPS2000

Question: What's your pet's name?   **Answer:** Dipstick

Access Level: 1

Employee Two

Login Name: Billy

Full Name: William Todd

Password: Sasha1991

Question: What's your mother's maiden name? **Answer:** Anderson

Access Level: 2

It's time to double-check your work. The following items can be printed to proof your work:

User Information

The user information can be printed by clicking on Tools on the toolbar and User Information from the drop-down. After printing, compare the totals of your practice to Figure A-5. If your totals do not match, review the appropriate item under the Lists menu.

User Information Report

5/8/2012

Practice Name:	Sunny Life Clinic
Street 1:	5055 E Ford Road
Street 2:	
City:	Mesa
State:	AZ
Zip Code:	85205
Phone:	(480) 444-4866
Tax ID Number:	123456789

Number of Charts:	5
Number of Insurance Carriers:	3
Number of Addresses:	4
Number of Providers:	1
Number of Referring Providers:	0
Number of Cases:	5
Number of Transactions:	0

Data Storage:	10470197 bytes (10.47 Megabytes)

▶ **Figure A-5   Answers to User Information**

Patient Information

After proofing the user information, proof the patient information. This is done by selecting Reports from the toolbar and Custom Report List from the drop-down menu. Next, select Patient Face Sheet (Figure A-6) and print all available patients. After printing the five patients, compare your report to the information given to be entered in the above exercise, paying close attention to detail.

Sunny Life Clinic
Patient Face Sheet
5/8/2012

Patient Chart #: ANDMA000
Patient Name: Marijane S. Anderson
Street 1: 10799 Jefferson Street
Street 2:
City: Blaine, AZ 85343
Phone: (480)692-3457

D.O.B: 05/11/1941   Age: 67
Sex: Female
SSN:
Mar Status:
S.O.F:
Assigned Provider:

Employer Name:
Street 1:
City:
Phone:

Case Information

Case Desc: Medicare/Aetna
Last Visit: 4/12/2012
Referral:
Guarantor Name: Marijane S. Anderson
Street 1: 10799 Jefferson Street
City: Blaine, AZ 85343
Phone: (480)692-3457
SSN:

Diagnosis 1:
Diagnosis 2:
Diagnosis 3:
Diagnosis 4:

Ins Co #: MED00

Insured 1 Name: Marijane S. Anderson

▶ **Figure A-6 Comparing Patient Face Sheets**

PRACTICE EXERCISE A-5: Schedule Modification and Design Custom Reports and Bills

In this exercise, you will schedule the patients, charge them, and post payments to their accounts.

Scheduling

Sunny Life Clinic has opened for business, and there are five patients on the schedule for April 12, 2012. Enter the following patients in the appropriate time slots and add the pop-up note to the time slot if applicable.

Time	Patient	Resource
9:00	Marijane S. Anderson	Doctor Visit
10:00	David F. Lyle	Doctor Visit
11:00	Timothy J. Nelson	Doctor Visit
12:00	William J. Nelson	Doctor Visit
1:00	Jordan J. Nelson	Lab Test

Tip: The resources need to be added "on the fly" or, in other words, by pressing F8 and adding the resource directly from the entry screen rather than adding it to a list menu. To do this, right-click on the resource entry box and add a new resource.

Confirming the Schedule and Noting the Services

Now, as each patient is seen by the doctor, note the appropriate charges in the Note box of the appointment along with the patient's diagnosis. This will print on the Appointment List for the clerk to enter into Medisoft.

Enter the following procedure and diagnosis codes into Medisoft. If you have Office Hours Professional available, also mark the visit as Checked Out. If you have free Office Hours, this option is not available.

Patient	Procedure and Diagnosis Codes
Marijane S. Anderson	Proc: 99211, 80050, 97010, VITAMIN DX: 719.47
David F. Lyle	Proc: 99201, 80050 DX: 836.1
Timothy J. Nelson	Proc: 99211 DX: 250.01
William J. Nelson	Proc: 99201, VITAMINS DX: 372.03
Jordan J. Nelson	Proc: 84702 DX: V22.1

Modifying the Appointment List Report

Ideally, an appointment list could be printed showing all of the detail in the Notes area of the appointment. This is essential to passing the appointment report to the billing clerk for entering the charges. However, Medisoft allows only a limited amount of space to print the Notes from the appointment. To accommodate the desire to print the entire note, you are now going to modify the Appointment List.

To modify the Appointment List, click on Reports and Design Custom Reports and Bills from the drop-down list. Then, once inside the Medisoft Report Designer, choose File and Open Report. This will give a list of available reports to be modified; choose Appointment List. Resave the report by clicking on File and Save As, then call the report 1 – Good Appointment List.

Next, remove the Phone, Length, and Reason fields from both the Header line and Detail line by clicking on the field and pressing the delete key. Now, move the Notes field over to where the Phone field was. The additional area will now accommodate a much larger note and move the Date, Time, and Name closer to the right and closer together. Finally, go to File on the toolbar and Report Properties and under the General Tab change the Page Orientation to Landscape. Under the Selected Band field, choose detail and make the Band Height .50. Click OK, save the report, and exit. You may need to modify the report several times before getting the desired result. When Designing Custom Reports and Bills, remember it takes practice and patience.

Tip: Double-click on any of the fields inside Design Custom Reports and Bills and experiment with the options, Auto Size, Positions, Font, etc., and display the results.

Printing the Appointment List

Now that the appointments have been entered and a custom report has been designed, it is time to print the appointment list. Go to Reports on the toolbar, Design Custom Reports and Bills, and select the new report; 1 – Good Appointment List. Print the appointment list for April 12, 2012 (Figure A-7). It is now time to double-check your work. Follow these instructions to review your work for accuracy:

Sunny Life Clinic
Appointment List
5/8/2012

Date	Time	Name	Note
4/12/2012	9:00 am	Anderson, Marijane S	Patient wants records at time of service. Proc: 99211, 80050, 97010, VITAMIN DX: 719.47
4/12/2012	10:00 am	Lyle, David F	Make sure the patient pays in full at time of service. Proc: 99201, 80050 DX: 836.1
4/12/2012	1:00 pm	Nelson, Jordan J	Proc: 84702 DX: V22.1
4/12/2012	11:00 am	Nelson, Timothy J	Proc: 99211 DX: 250.01
4/12/2012	12:00 pm	Nelson, William J	Proc: 99201, VITAMINS DX: 372.03

▶ **Figure A-7   1 – Good Appointment List**

Appointment List

After printing the appointment list, compare it to Figure A-7 for accuracy and readability.

PRACTICE EXERCISE A-6:   Charge and Payment Entry

In this exercise, charges and patient payments will be entered into the patient accounts, and they will be proofed.

Charge Entry

Open Enter Transactions from the Activities menu on the toolbar in Medisoft and process the Charges along with the diagnosis codes from the 1 – Good Appointment List printed in the previous exercise.

Patient Payment Entry

Enter the following patient payments into Enter Transactions and Enter Deposit/Payments.

Patient	Payment
David F. Lyle	$20.00 (Cash – Enter into Enter Transactions)
Timothy J. Nelson	$20.00 (Check #123 – Include payments for William and Jordan in this check and process in Enter Deposits/Payments)
William J. Nelson	$5.00 (See note for Timothy J. Nelson)
Jordan J. Nelson	$5.00 (See note for Timothy J. Nelson)

It is now time to double-check your work. Follow the instructions below to review your work for accuracy.

Patient Day Sheet

To check your Charge and Payment Entry, run a Patient Day Sheet under the Reports Menu of the toolbar and Day Sheet option from the drop-down menu. Be careful to enter April 12, 2012, as the Date From and the proper date you created the transactions. After printing the report, compare the individual transactions on the first page (Figure A-8) and the summary on the second page (Figure A-12) to proof your work.

Sunny Life Clinic
Patient Day Sheet
May 08, 2012
4/12/2012

Entry	Date	Document	POS	Description	Provider	Code	Modifiers	Amount
ANDMA000 Anderson, Marijane S								
4	4/12/2012	0805040000	11	Office Visit Est. Patient	CWP	99211		35.00
5	4/12/2012	0805040000	11	General Health Screen	CWP	80050		40.00
6	4/12/2012	0805040000	11	Hotpack	CWP	97010		10.00
8	4/12/2012	0805040000	11	Vitamin Packs	CWP	VITAMIN		30.00

Patient's Charges	Patient's Receipts	Insurance Receipts	Adjustments	Patient Balance
$105.00	$0.00	$0.00	$0.00	$105.00

Entry	Date	Document	POS	Description	Provider	Code	Modifiers	Amount
LYLDA000 Lyle, David F								
7	4/12/2012	0805040000	11	Office Visit New Patient FFS	CWP	99201		30.00
8	4/12/2012	0805040000	11	General Health Screen	CWP	80050		40.00
13	4/12/2012	0805040000	11	Cash Payment	CWP	CASH		-30.00

Patient's Charges	Patient's Receipts	Insurance Receipts	Adjustments	Patient Balance
$70.00	$-20.00	$0.00	$0.00	$50.00

Entry	Date	Document	POS	Description	Provider	Code	Modifiers	Amount
NELJ0000 Nelson, Jordon J								
10	4/12/2012	0805040000	11	Pregnancy Test	CWP	84702		30.00
15	4/12/2012	0805040000	11	#123 Nelson Timothy J	CWP	CHECK		-5.00

Patient's Charges	Patient's Receipts	Insurance Receipts	Adjustments	Patient Balance
$20.00	$-5.00	$0.00	$0.00	$15.00

Entry	Date	Document	POS	Description	Provider	Code	Modifiers	Amount
NELT1000 Nelson, Timothy J								
11	4/12/2012	0805040000	11	Office Visit Est. Patient	CWP	99211		35.00
14	4/12/2012	0805040000	11	#123 Nelson Timothy J	CWP	CHECK		-10.00

Patient's Charges	Patient's Receipts	Insurance Receipts	Adjustments	Patient Balance
$25.00	$-20.00	$0.00	$0.00	$5.00

Entry	Date	Document	POS	Description	Provider	Code	Modifiers	Amount
NELW1000 Nelson, William J								
13	4/12/2012	0805040000	11	Office Visit New Patient FFS	CWP	99201		30.00
16	4/12/2012	0805040000	11	#123 Nelson Timothy J	CWP	CHECK		-5.00

Patient's Charges	Patient's Receipts	Insurance Receipts	Adjustments	Patient Balance
$30.00	$-5.00	$0.00	$0.00	$25.00

▶ **Figure A-8   Patient Day Sheet, Page 1**

PRACTICE EXERCISE A-7:   Claim and Statement Management

On a typical work day, after all the patients are seen, the schedule is reviewed, charges and payments are entered and proofed. The next step is to process your claims and statements.

Claim Management

Go into Claim Management from the Activities menu and print the claims using the Laser CMS (Primary) W/Form. Compare them to your prior information and check the signatures, diagnoses, and procedures (Figure A-9) for accuracy, making sure all the signatures and boxes are completed correctly. If not, correct your work and reprint the claims.

1500	BLUE SHIELD
HEALTH INSURANCE CLAIM FORM	1234 YANKEE DOODLE DRIVE SUITE 101
APPROVED BY NATIONAL UNIFORM CLAIM COMMITTEE 08/05	ST PAUL AZ 88888

CARRIER

PICA ☐☐☐   PICA ☐☐☐

1. MEDICARE ☐ (Medicare #) MEDICAID ☐ (Medicaid #) TRICARE CHAMPUS ☐ (Sponsor's SSN) CHAMPVA ☐ (Member ID#) GROUP HEALTH PLAN ☐ (SSN or ID) FECA BLK LUNG ☐ (SSN) OTHER ☒ (ID)   1a. INSURED'S I.D. NUMBER (For Program in Item 1) 47490713-44

2. PATIENT'S NAME (Last Name, First Name, Middle Initial) NELSON JORDON J   3. PATIENT'S BIRTH DATE MM 12 DD 04 YY 1992 SEX M☐ F☒   4. INSURED'S NAME (Last Name, First Name, Middle Initial) NELSON TIMOTHY J

5. PATIENT'S ADDRESS (No., Street) 5334 GLENWOOD AVE   6. PATIENT RELATIONSHIP TO INSURED Self☐ Spouse☐ Child☒ Other☐   7. INSURED'S ADDRESS (No., Street) 5334 GLENWOOD AVE

CITY STAPLES   STATE AZ   8. PATIENT STATUS Single☒ Married☐ Other☐   CITY STAPLES   STATE AZ

ZIP CODE 85779   TELEPHONE (Include Area Code) (480) 8280388   Employed☐ Full-Time Student☐ Part-Time Student☐   ZIP CODE 85779   TELEPHONE (Include Area Code) (480) 8280388

9. OTHER INSURED'S NAME (Last Name, First Name, Middle Initial)   10. IS PATIENT'S CONDITION RELATED TO: 11. INSURED'S POLICY GROUP OR FECA NUMBER YRU03

a. OTHER INSURED'S POLICY OR GROUP NUMBER   a. EMPLOYMENT? (Current or Previous) YES☐ NO☒   a. INSURED'S DATE OF BIRTH MM 01 DD 27 YY 1962 SEX M☒ F☐

b. OTHER INSURED'S DATE OF BIRTH MM DD YY SEX M☐ F☐   b. AUTO ACCIDENT? YES☐ NO☒ PLACE (State)   b. EMPLOYER'S NAME OR SCHOOL NAME

c. EMPLOYER'S NAME OR SCHOOL NAME   c. OTHER ACCIDENT? YES☐ NO☒   c. INSURANCE PLAN NAME OR PROGRAM NAME

d. INSURANCE PLAN NAME OR PROGRAM NAME   10d. RESERVED FOR LOCAL USE   d. IS THERE ANOTHER HEALTH BENEFIT PLAN? YES☐ NO☒ If yes, return to and complete item 9 a-d.

READ BACK OF FORM BEFORE COMPLETING & SIGNING THIS FORM.
12. PATIENT'S OR AUTHORIZED PERSON'S SIGNATURE I authorize the release of any medical or other information necessary to process this claim. I also request payment of government benefits either to myself or to the party who accepts assignment below.
SIGNED SIGNATURE ON FILE   DATE 05/04/08

13. INSURED'S OR AUTHORIZED PERSON'S SIGNATURE I authorize payment of medical benefits to the undersigned physician or supplier for services described below.
SIGNED SIGNATURE ON FILE

PATIENT AND INSURED INFORMATION

14. DATE OF CURRENT: MM DD YY ILLNESS (First symptom) OR INJURY (Accident) OR PREGNANCY(LMP)   15. IF PATIENT HAS HAD SAME OR SIMILAR ILLNESS. GIVE FIRST DATE MM DD YY   16. DATES PATIENT UNABLE TO WORK IN CURRENT OCCUPATION FROM MM DD YY TO MM DD YY

17. NAME OF REFERRING PROVIDER OR OTHER SOURCE   17a.   17b. NPI   18. HOSPITALIZATION DATES RELATED TO CURRENT SERVICES FROM MM DD YY TO MM DD YY

19. RESERVED FOR LOCAL USE   20. OUTSIDE LAB? YES☐ NO☒ $ CHARGES

21. DIAGNOSIS OR NATURE OF ILLNESS OR INJURY (Relate Items 1, 2, 3 or 4 to Item 24E by Line)
1. V22.1   3.
2.   4.

22. MEDICAID RESUBMISSION CODE   ORIGINAL REF. NO.

23. PRIOR AUTHORIZATION NUMBER

24. A. DATE(S) OF SERVICE						B. PLACE OF SERVICE	C. EMG	D. PROCEDURES, SERVICES, OR SUPPLIES (Explain Unusual Circumstances)		E. DIAGNOSIS POINTER	F. $ CHARGES	G. DAYS OR UNITS	H. EPSDT Family Plan	I. ID. QUAL.	J. RENDERING PROVIDER ID. #
From MM	DD	YY	To MM	DD	YY			CPT/HCPCS	MODIFIER						
1	04	12	12	04	12	12	11		84702		1	20 00	1		NPI	3333333333
2															NPI	
3															NPI	
4															NPI	
5															NPI	
6															NPI	

PHYSICIAN OR SUPPLIER INFORMATION

25. FEDERAL TAX I.D. NUMBER 12 3456789 SSN☐ EIN☒   26. PATIENT'S ACCOUNT NO. NELJ0000 10   27. ACCEPT ASSIGNMENT? (For govt. claims, see back) YES☒ NO☐   28. TOTAL CHARGE $ 20 00   29. AMOUNT PAID $ 30. BALANCE DUE $ 20 00

31. SIGNATURE OF PHYSICIAN OR SUPPLIER INCLUDING DEGREES OR CREDENTIALS (I certify that the statements on the reverse apply to this bill and are made a part thereof.)
SIGNED CHARLES W PEARCE MD 4/12/12   DATE

32. SERVICE FACILITY LOCATION INFORMATION
a. NPI   b.

33. BILLING PROVIDER INFO & PH # (480) 692 3457
SUNNY LIFE CLINIC
13274 ANCHOR POINT ROAD
MESA AZ 85205
a. 2222222222   b.

▶ **Figure A-9 Claim Management**

Statement Management

Prepare the Billing tab of Program Options under File on the toolbar to perform Cycle Billing every 30 days, showing Standard Statement Detail and Remainder Statement Detail only.

Open Statement Management under the Activities menu on the toolbar and create Remainder Statements. Print the Remainder Statements using the form Remainder Statement (0, 30, 60, 90). There should be two statements, one for Marijane Anderson (Figure A-10), and one for David Lyle.

Sunny Life Clinic
5055 E Ford Road
Mesa, AZ 85205
(480)444-4866

Statement Date	Page
5/8/2012	1

Marijane S. Anderson
10799 Jefferson Street
Blaine, AZ 85343

Chart Number
ANDMA000

Date of Last Payment: 4/12/2012	Amount:	-46.40

Patient: Marijane S. Anderson		Chart Number: ANDMA000			Case: Medicare/Aetna		
Dates	Procedure	Procedure	Charge	Amount Paid by Insurance	Paid By Guarantor	Adjustments	Remainder
04/12/12	VITAMIN	Vitamin Packs	30.00	0.00		0.00	30.00

▶ **Figure A-10 Statement Management**

PRACTICE EXERCISE A-8: Insurance Payments and Check and Balance System

Each day, the mail arrives, containing insurance payments and denials, patient checks, and inquiries. Process the mail payments listed below in Enter Deposits/Payments under the Activities menu on the toolbar.

Processing Mail Payments

Patient	Mail Payment and/or Adjustment
Marijane S. Anderson	Medicare Payment CK 666 for DOS 4/12/2012 Pd on 99211 - $16.00 - Adj. $5.00 Pd on 80050 - $24.00 - Adj. $10.00 Pd on 97010 - $6.40 - Adj. $2.00 Total Paid $46.40
Timothy J. Nelson	BCBS Payment Check 333 - Pd $5.00 (DOS 4/12/2012)
William J. Nelson	BCBS Payment Check 334 - Pd $5.00 Adj. $5.00 (DOS 4/12/2012)
Jordan J. Nelson	BCBS Payment Check 335 - Pd $0.00 Adj. $0.00 (DOS 4/12/2012 - Patient owes co-pay)

Check and Balance System

Now that all the appointments, charges and payments are entered into Medisoft, a complete checks and balance can be performed on the system. First, print the deposit slip for April 12, 2012, which could be taken to the bank. Compare it to Figure A-11. Next, run a Patient Day Sheet for April 12, 2012, as done in the prior section. Compare the Deposit Report to the Patient Day Sheet (Figure A-12) to make sure the balances match. If not, identify your errors, correct them, and rerun the reports.

Sunny Life Clinic
Deposit Report
5/8/2012

Description	Check No.	Payor	Checks	Cash	Credit Card	Electronic	Totals
Thursday - April 12, 2012							
	123	Nelson, Timothy J	30.00				30.00
	666	Medicare	46.40				46.40
	333	Blue Shield	5.00				5.00
	334	Blue Shield	5.00				5.00
	335	Blue Shield	0.00				0.00
0805040000		Lyle, David F		20.00			20.00
4/12/2012 Items:	6						
			$86.50	$20.00	$0.00	$0.00	$106.40
Total Deposit Items:	6	Report Totals:	$86.40	$20.00	$0.00	$0.00	$106.40

▶ **Figure A-11 Deposit Report**

On a typical day at the clinic, the claims and statements would not be processed until the mail payments were entered and the checks and balances done. However, for the purpose of this exercise, we had to run the claims and statements first in order for them to generate.

It is now time to double-check your work. Follow the instructions below to review your work for accuracy.

Claim Management

Review Claim Management and see how many claims still need to be processed. There should only be one claim for Chart ANDMA000, and it is for the secondary claim. Print the secondary claim now using the Laser CMS (Secondary) W/Form, compare your work with Figure A-13, and correct if necessary.

Statement Management

Go into Statement Management and create remainder statements again since the insurance payments were posted. Review and print the state-

Sunny Life Clinic
Patient Day Sheet User Match
May 08, 2012
4/12/2012

Total # Patients	5
Total # Procedures	8
Total Procedure Charges	$250.00
Total Global Surgical Procedures	$0.00
Total Product Charges	$0.00
Total Inside Lab Charges	$0.00
Total Outside Lab Charges	$0.00
Total Billing Charges	$0.00
Total Tax Charges	$0.00
Total Charges	$250.00
Total Insurance Payments	-$56.40
Total Cash Copayments	$0.00
Total Check Copayments	$0.00
Total Credit Card Copayments	$0.00
Total Patient Cash Payments	-$20.00
Total Patient Check Payments	-$30.00
Total Credit Card Payments	$0.00
Total Receipts	$106.40
Total Credit Adjustments	$0.00
Total Debit Adjustments	$0.00
Total Insurance Credit Adjustments	$0.00
Total Insurance Debit Adjustments	$0.00
Total Insurance Withholds	$0.00
Total Adjustments	-$22.00
Net Effect on Accounts Receivable	$121.60

Practice Totals:

Total # of Procedures	8
Total Charges	$250.00
Total Payments	$106.40
Total Adjustments	-$22.00
Accounts receivable	$121.60

▶ Figure A-12   **Patient Day Sheet, Summary Page**

ments and compare to Figure A-14. One new statement should be created that was generated after insurance payments were posted. If necessary, go back and correct any errors.

PRACTICE EXERCISE A-9:   **Trending Accounts Receivable and Developing a Follow-up Plan**

Every good accounts receivable management plan includes tracking the days in accounts receivable and developing a follow-up plan.

Calculating the Days in Accounts Receivable

In this exercise, we will pretend that the amount of data in Sunny Life Clinic is for three months. Print a Practice Analysis Report by selecting Reports from the toolbar, Analysis Report from the drop-down menu, and Practice Analysis from the sidebar. Print a complete report of all the transactions in Sunny Life Clinic and calculate the days in AR by figuring that this data covers the last 90 days (Figure A-15). Show your work and round up to the nearest whole day. Your answer should be 44 days in accounts receivable.

1500

HEALTH INSURANCE CLAIM FORM
APPROVED BY NATIONAL UNIFORM CLAIM COMMITTEE 08/05

☐☐☐ PICA

AETNA INSURANCE
1555 FOREST VIEW LANE
SCOTTSDALE, AZ 85208

CARRIER →

1. MEDICARE (Medicare #) ☐ **MEDICAID** (Medicaid #) ☐ **TRICARE CHAMPUS** (Sponsor's SSN) ☐ **CHAMPVA** (Member ID#) ☐ **GROUP HEALTH PLAN** (SSN or ID) ☐ **FECA BLK LUNG** (SSN) ☐ **OTHER** (ID) ☒	**1a. INSURED'S I.D. NUMBER** (For Program in Item 1) 1214-454010	

2. PATIENT'S NAME (Last Name, First Name, Middle Initial)
ANDERSON MARIJANE S

3. PATIENT'S BIRTH DATE MM DD YY **SEX** M ☐ F ☒

4. INSURED'S NAME (Last Name, First Name, Middle Initial)
ANDERSON MARIJANE S

5. PATIENT'S ADDRESS (No., Street)
10799 JEFFERSON STREET

6. PATIENT RELATIONSHIP TO INSURED
Self ☒ Spouse ☐ Child ☐ Other ☐

4. INSURED'S ADDRESS (No., Street)
10799 JEFFERSON STREET

CITY BLAINE **STATE** AZ

8. PATIENT STATUS
Single ☐ Married ☐ Other ☐

CITY BLAINE **STATE** AZ

ZIP CODE 85343 **TELEPHONE** (Include Area Code) (480) 6923457

Employed ☐ Full-Time Student ☐ Part-Time Student ☐

ZIP CODE 85343 **TELEPHONE** (Include Area Code) (480) 6923457

9. OTHER INSURED'S NAME (Last Name, First Name, Middle Initial)
ANDERSON MARIJANE S

10. IS PATIENT'S CONDITION RELATED TO:

11. INSURED'S POLICY GROUP OR FECA NUMBER
YRYSN-00

a. OTHER INSURED'S POLICY OR GROUP NUMBER
432789875A

a. EMPLOYMENT? (Current or Previous)
YES ☐ NO ☒

a. INSURED'S DATE OF BIRTH MM DD YY 05 11 1941 **SEX** M ☐ F ☒

b. OTHER INSURED'S DATE OF BIRTH MM DD YY **SEX** M ☐ F ☒

b. AUTO ACCIDENT? PLACE (State)
YES ☐ NO ☒

b. EMPLOYER'S NAME OR SCHOOL NAME

c. EMPLOYER'S NAME OR SCHOOL NAME

c. OTHER ACCIDENT?
YES ☐ NO ☒

c. INSURANCE PLAN NAME OR PROGRAM NAME
AETNA INSURANCE

d. INSURANCE PLAN NAME OR PROGRAM NAME
MEDICARE

10d. RESERVED FOR LOCAL USE

d. IS THERE ANOTHER HEALTH BENEFIT PLAN?
YES ☒ NO ☐ If yes, return to and complete item 9 a-d.

READ BACK OF FORM BEFORE COMPLETING & SIGNING THIS FORM.
12. PATIENT'S OR AUTHORIZED PERSON'S SIGNATURE I authorize the release of any medical or other information necessary to process this claim. I also request payment of government benefits either to myself or to the party who accepts assignment below.

SIGNED SIGNATURE ON FILE DATE 05/04/08

13. INSURED'S OR AUTHORIZED PERSON'S SIGNATURE I authorize payment of medical benefits to the undersigned physician or supplier for services described below.

SIGNED SIGNATURE ON FILE

PATIENT AND INSURED INFORMATION →

14. DATE OF CURRENT: MM DD YY ◄ ILLNESS (First symptom) OR INJURY (Accident) OR PREGNANCY(LMP)

15. IF PATIENT HAS HAD SAME OR SIMILAR ILLNESS. GIVE FIRST DATE MM DD YY

16. DATES PATIENT UNABLE TO WORK IN CURRENT OCCUPATION FROM MM DD YY TO MM DD YY

17. NAME OF REFERRING PROVIDER OR OTHER SOURCE
17a.
17b. NPI

18. HOSPITALIZATION DATES RELATED TO CURRENT SERVICES FROM MM DD YY TO MM DD YY

19. RESERVED FOR LOCAL USE

20. OUTSIDE LAB? YES ☐ NO ☒ $ CHARGES

21. DIAGNOSIS OR NATURE OF ILLNESS OR INJURY (Relate Items 1, 2, 3 or 4 to Item 24E by Line)
1. 719 . 47
2. ____
3. ____
4. ____

22. MEDICAID RESUBMISSION CODE ORIGINAL REF. NO.

23. PRIOR AUTHORIZATION NUMBER

24. A. DATE(S) OF SERVICE From MM DD YY To MM DD YY	B. PLACE OF SERVICE	C. EMG	D. PROCEDURES, SERVICES, OR SUPPLIES (Explain Unusual Circumstances) CPT/HCPCS MODIFIER	E. DIAGNOSIS POINTER	F. $ CHARGES	G. DAYS OR UNITS	H. EPSDT Family Plan	I. ID. QUAL.	J. RENDERING PROVIDER ID. #
1	04 12 12 04 12 12	11		99211	1	25 00	1		NPI	3333333333
2	04 12 12 04 12 12	11		80050	1	40 00	1		NPI	3333333333
3	04 12 12 04 12 12	11		97010	1	10 00	1		NPI	3333333333
4									NPI	
5									NPI	
6									NPI	

25. FEDERAL TAX I.D. NUMBER SSN EIN 123456789 ☒

26. PATIENT'S ACCOUNT NO. ANDMA000

27. ACCEPT ASSIGNMENT? (For govt. claims, see back) YES ☒ NO ☐

28. TOTAL CHARGE $ 75 00

29. AMOUNT PAID $

30. BALANCE DUE $ 75 00

31. SIGNATURE OF PHYSICIAN OR SUPPLIER INCLUDING DEGREES OR CREDENTIALS (I certify that the statements on the reverse apply to this bill and are made a part thereof.)
CHARLES W PEARCE MD
SIGNED DATE 05/04/08

32. SERVICE FACILITY LOCATION INFORMATION
a. NPI b.

33. BILLING PROVIDER INFO & PH # ( )
SUNNY LIFE CLINIC
13274 ANCHOR POINT ROAD
MESA, AZ 85205
a. 2222222222 b.

PHYSICIAN OR SUPPLIER INFORMATION →

NUCC Instruction Manual available at: www.nucc.org **PLEASE PRINT OR TYPE** APPROVED OMB-0938-0999 FORM CMS-1500 (08-05)

▶ **Figure A-13 Reviewing Claim Management**

Sunny Life Clinic
5055 E Ford Road
Mesa, AZ 85205
(480)444-4866

Statement Date	Page
5/8/2012	1

Timothy J. Nelson
5334 Glenwood Ave
Staples, AZ 85779

Chart Number
NELTI000

Date of Last Payment: 4/12/2012	Amount:	-5.00

Patient: William J. Nelson   Chart Number: NELWI000   Case: BCBS

Dates	Procedure	Procedure	Charge	Amount Paid by Insurance	Paid By Guarantor	Adjustments	Remained
04/12/12	99201	Office Visit New Patient FFS	30.00	-5.00	-5.00	-5.00	$5.00

Patient: Jordan J. Nelson   Chart Number: NELJO000   Case: BCBS

Dates	Procedure	Procedure	Charge	Amount Paid by Insurance	Paid By Guarantor	Adjustments	Remained
04/12/12	84702	Pregnancy Test	20.00	0.00	-5.00	0.00	15.00

▶ **Figure A-14   Reviewing Statement Management**

Sunny Life Clinic
Practice Analysis
From 1/1/1900 to 12/31/2050

Code	Modifers Description	Amount	Units	Average	Costs	Net
	Total Procedure Charges					$250.00
	Total Global Surgical Procedures					$0.00
	Total Product Charges					$0.00
	Total Inside Lab Charges					$0.00
	Total Outside Lab Charges					$0.00
	Total Billing Charges					$0.00
	Total Tax Charges					$0.00
	Total Charges					$250.00
	Total Insurance Payments					-$56.40
	Total Cash Copayments					$0.00
	Total Check Copayments					$0.00
	Total Credit Card Copayments					$0.00
	Total Patient Cash Payments					-$20.00
	Total Patient Check Payments					-$30.00
	Total Credit Card Payments					$0.00
	Total Payments					-$106.40
	Total Deductibles					$0.00
	Total Debit Adjustments					$0.00
	Total Credit Adjustments					$0.00
	Total Insurance Debit Adjustments					$0.00
	Total Insurance Credit Adjustments					-$22.00
	Total Insurance Withholds					$0.00
	Total Adjustments					-$22.00
	Net Effect in Accounts Receivable					$121.60

▶ **Figure A-15   AR Trending**

Write a Follow-up Plan

You have been asked by your supervisor to write a follow-up plan for the clinic. Write a detailed plan of how self-pay, non-contract, and contract insurance balances will be handled by the clinic and processed within Medisoft.

ESSAY QUESTIONS

In this last section, there is no visual way to check the work inside Medisoft when it is completed. The remaining exercises must be completed by writing a step-by-step procedure for each task.

1. **Back up Medisoft.** Write a step-by-step procedure on how to back up Medisoft assuming the backup will be saved on the E drive. Write a detailed plan on how Sunny Life Clinic will rotate backup media and utilize a backup plan.

2. **File Maintenance.** Write a step-by-step procedure on how to complete File Maintenance in Medisoft, assuming that Purge Data will not be done. Write a detailed plan for how Sunny Life Clinic will perform maintenance on a regular schedule.

3. **Billing Charges.** Write a step-by-step plan to assess whether your office could legally assess billing charges, the office policy used to implement billing charges, and how you would utilize Medisoft to access billing charges.

4. **Reporting Systems.** Describe a reporting system for Sunny Life Clinic that includes daily reports, monthly reports, quarterly reports, and yearly reports. Define the reports to be produced for each category and the reasons these reports will be useful to the owners of Sunny Life Clinic.

5. **Linking Insurance Companies with Payment and Adjustment Codes.** Describe how the insurance payment and adjustment codes can be associated with the insurance so they do not have to be selected each time in Enter Deposit/Payments.

B

Source Documents

Sunny Life Clinic
REGISTRATION FORM
(Please Print)

Today's Date: 09/04/2008	PCP:

PATIENT INFORMATION

| Patient's last name: Johnson | First: William | Middle: Jon | ☒ Mr. ☐ Miss
☐ Mrs. ☐ Ms. | Marital status: Single

Single ☒ Mar ☐ Div ☐ Sep ☐ Wid ☐ | | |

Is this your legal name? ☒ Yes ☐ No	If not, what is your legal name?	(Former name):	Birth date: 10/14/1986	Age: 22	Sex: ☒ M ☐ F

Street address: 8459 College Road	Social Security no.: 473-12-4578	Home phone no.: (812) 851-0354

P.O. box: PO Box 1	City: Moorhead	State: MN	ZIP Code: 56601

Occupation: Computer Programmer	Employer: Microsoft	Employer phone no.: (812) 828-0388

Chose clinic because/referred to clinic by (Please check one box):	☐ Dr.	☒ Insurance plan	☐ Hospital

☐ Family	☐ Friend	☐ Close to home/work	☐ Yellow Pages	☐ Other

Other family members seen here:

INSURANCE INFORMATION

(Please give your insurance card to the receptionist.)

Person responsible for bill: Self – Same as Above	Birth date:	Insurance Information Blue Shield 88 W Bell Rd, Phoenix, AZ 85027	Home phone no.: ( )

| Is this person a patient here? ☐ Yes ☐ No | | | |

Occupation:	Employer:	Employer address:	Employer phone no.: ( )

| Is this patient covered by insurance? ☒ Yes ☐ No | | | |

Please indicate primary insurance	☐ Medicare	☒ Blue Shield	☐ Medicaid	☐ Champus	☐ Group
☐ FECA	☐ HMO	☐ PPO	☐ Capitated Insurance	☐ Other	

Subscriber's name: William Johnson	Sex: ☒ M ☐ F	Subscriber's S.S. no.: Same	Birth date:	Group no.: MICRO55	Policy no.: 014578945	Co-payment: $ 20.00

| Patient's relationship to subscriber: | ☒ Self | ☐ Spouse | ☐ Child | ☐ Other | | |

Name of secondary insurance (if applicable):	Subscriber's name:	Sex: ☐ M ☐ F	Group no.:	Policy no.:

Patient's relationship to subscriber:	☐ Self	☐ Spouse	☐ Child	☐ Other	Birth Date:

CONTACT INFORMATION IN CASE OF EMERGENCY

Name of local friend or relative (not living at same address): Timothy J. Johnson	Relationship to patient: Father	Home phone no.: (812) 330-9537	Work phone no.: ( )

The above information is true to the best of my knowledge. I authorize release of any medical information or other information necessary to process this claim. I also request payment of government benefits either to myself or to the party who accepts assignment below. I further understand that I am ultimately responsible for payment of services rendered by Sunny Life Clinic.

_____ _____
Patient/Guardian signature *Date*

Sunny Life Clinic
REGISTRATION FORM
(Please Print)

Today's Date: 09/08/2008	PCP:

PATIENT INFORMATION

Patient's last name: Lyle	First: David	Middle: F.	☒ Mr. ☐ Miss ☐ Mrs. ☐ Ms.	Marital status: Married Single ☐ Mar ☒ Div ☐ Sep ☐ Wid ☐

Is this your legal name? ☒ Yes ☐ No	If not, what is your legal name?	(Former name):	Birth date: 07/02/1951	Age: 57	Sex: ☒ M ☐ F

Street address: 2003 Harley Street	Social Security no.: 473-12-4579	Home phone no.: (216) 790-6000

P.O. box:	City: Gilbert	State: AZ	ZIP Code: 85234

Occupation: Secretary	Employer: B Softouch Inc.	Employer phone no.: (216) 432-2366

Chose clinic because/referred to clinic by (Please check one box):	☐ Dr.	☐ Insurance plan	☐ Hospital
☐ Family	☐ Friend	☐ Close to home/work	☒ Yellow Pages	☐ Other

Other family members seen here:

INSURANCE INFORMATION
(Please give your insurance card to the receptionist.)

Person responsible for bill: Self – Same As Above	Birth date:	Insurance Information None	Home phone no.: (216) 790-6000

Is this person a patient here? ☒ Yes ☐ No

Occupation:	Employer:	Employer address:	Employer phone no.:

Is this patient covered by insurance? ☐ Yes ☒ No

Please indicate primary insurance	☐ Medicare	☐ Blue Shield	☐ Medicaid	☐ Champus	☐ Group
☐ FECA	☐ HMO	☐ PPO	☐ Capitated Insurance	☐ Other	

Subscriber's name:	Sex: ☐ M ☐ F	Subscriber's S.S. no.:	Birth date:	Group no.:	Policy no.:	Co-payment:

Patient's relationship to subscriber:	☐ Self	☐ Spouse	☐ Child	☐ Other

Name of secondary insurance (if applicable):	Subscriber's name	Sex: ☐ M ☐ F	Group no.:	Policy no.:

Patient's relationship to subscriber:	☐ Self	☐ Spouse	☐ Child	☐ Other	Birth Date:

CONTACT INFORMATION IN CASE OF EMERGENCY

Name of local friend or relative (not living at same address): Joseph D. Lyle	Relationship to patient: Brother	Home phone no.: (216) 070-1954	Work phone no.: ( )

The above information is true to the best of my knowledge. I authorize release of any medical information or other information necessary to process this claim. I also request payment of government benefits either to myself or to the party who accepts assignment below. I further understand that I am ultimately responsible for payment of services rendered by Sunny Life Clinic.

Patient/Guardian signature   _Date_

Sunny Life Clinic
REGISTRATION FORM
(Please Print)

Today's Date: 09/04/2008	PCP:

PATIENT INFORMATION

Patient's last name: Jordan	First: Jane	Middle: N.	☐ Mr. ☐ Miss ☐ Mrs. ☒ Ms.	Marital status: Single Single ☒ Mar ☐ Div ☐ Sep ☐ Wid ☐

Is this your legal name? ☒ Yes ☐ No	If not, what is your legal name?	(Former name):	Birth date: 12/04/1990	Age: 18	Sex: ☐ M ☒ F

Street address: 5055 E University Drive # T11	Social Security no.: 476-12-4578	Home phone no.: (812) 330-1744

P.O. box:	City: Mesa	State: AZ	ZIP Code: 85205

Occupation: YMCA Life Guard	Employer: YMCA	Employer phone no.: (812) 174-4330

Chose clinic because/referred to clinic by (Please check one box):   ☐ Dr.   ☐ Insurance plan   ☐ Hospital

☒ Family   ☐ Friend   ☐ Close to home/work   ☐ Yellow Pages   ☐ Other

Other family members seen here:

INSURANCE INFORMATION

(Please give your insurance card to the receptionist.)

Person responsible for bill: Bonita Jordan	Birth date: 05/01/1965	Insurance Information Garden Grove Insurance 65 Honolulu Dr., Honolulu, HI 96816	Home phone no.: (812) 330-1744

Is this person a patient here?   ☒ Yes   ☐ No

Occupation: Medical Assistant	Employer: Sunny Life Clinic	Employer address: 5222 Baseline Rd, Gilbert, 85234	Employer phone no.: (800) 333-4747

Is this patient covered by insurance?   ☒ Yes   ☐ No

Please indicate primary insurance   ☐ Medicare   ☐ Blue Shield   ☐ Medicaid   ☐ Champus   ☒ Group

☐ FECA   ☐ HMO   ☐ PPO   ☐ Capitated Insurance   ☐ Other

Subscriber's name: Sex: Bonita Jordan ☐ M ☒ F	Subscriber's S.S. no.: 469-12-4567	Birth date: 05/01/1965	Group no.: SLC89	Policy no.: 469-12-4567	Co-payment: $ 10.00

Patient's relationship to subscriber: ☐ Self   ☐ Spouse   ☒ Child   ☐ Other

Name of secondary insurance (if applicable):	Subscriber's name:	Sex: ☐ M ☐ F	Group no.:	Policy no.:

Patient's relationship to subscriber: ☐ Self   ☐ Spouse   ☐ Child   ☐ Other   Birth Date:

CONTACT INFORMATION IN CASE OF EMERGENCY

Name of local friend or relative (not living at same address): Marijane Sanderson	Relationship to patient: Grandmother	Home phone no.: (812) 692-3457	Work phone no.: ( )

The above information is true to the best of my knowledge. I authorize release of any medical information or other information necessary to process this claim. I also request payment of government benefits either to myself or to the party who accepts assignment below. I further understand that I am ultimately responsible for payment of services rendered by Sunny Life Clinic.

Patient/Guardian signature   _Date_

C

Patient Superbills: Source Documents 1024–1046

Happy Valley Medical Clinic
5222 E. Baseline Rd.
Gilbert, AZ 85234
(800)333-4747

Date: 9/4/2008

Doc - JM

AGADW000   Again, Dwight   9/4/2008   9:15:00 AM

EXAM	FEE	PROCEDURES		FEE	LABORATORY		FEE
New Patient		Anoscopy	46600		Aerobic Culture	87070	
Problem Focused	99201	Arthrocentesis/Aspiration/Injection			Amylase	82150	
Expanded Problem, Focused	99202	Small Joint	*20600		B12	82607	
Detailed	99203	Interm Joint	*20605		CBC & Diff	85025	
Comprehensive	99204	Major Joint	*20610		CHEM 20	80019	
Comprehensive/High Complex	99204	Audiometry	92552		Chlamydia Screen	86317	
Initial Visit/Procedure	99025	Cast Application			Cholesterol	82465	
Well Exam Infant (up to 12 mos.)	99318	Location Long Short			Digoxin	80162	
Well Exam 1 – 4 yrs.	99382	Catherization	*53670		Electrolytes	80005	
Well Exam 5 – 11 yrs.	99383	Circumcision	54150		Ferritin	82728	
Well Exam 12 – 17 yrs.	99384	Colposcopy	*57452		Folate	82746	
Well Exam 18 – 39 yrs.	99385	Colposcopy w /Biopsy	*57454		GC Screen	87070	
Well Exam 40 – 64 yrs.	99386	Cryosurgery Premalignant Lesion			Glucose	(82947) *Dx 2*	
		Location(s):			Glucose 1 HR	82950	
Established Patient		Cryosurgery Warts			Glycosylated HGB (A1C)	83036	
Minimum	99211 *Dx*	Location(s):			HCT	85014	
Problem Focused	(99212) *1-2*	Curettement Lesion w /Biopsy	CTF		HDL	83718	
Expanded Problem Focused	99213	Curettement Lesion w o/ Biopsy			Hep BSAG	86278	
Detailed	99214	Single	*11050		Hepatitis Profile	80059	
Comprehensive/High Complex	99215	2 – 4	*11051		HGB & HCT	85014	
Well Exam Infant (up to 12 mos.)	99391	> 4	*11052		HIV	86311	
Well Exam 1 – 4 yrs.	99392	Diaphram Fitting	*57170		Iron & TBC 83540	83550	
Well Exam 5 – 11 yrs.	99393	Ear Irrigation	69210		Kidney Profile	80007	
Well Exam 12 – 17 yrs.	99394	ECG	93000		Lead	83655	
Well Exam 18 – 39 yrs.	99395	Endometrial Biopsy	*58100		Liver Profile	82977	
Well Exam 40 – 64 yrs.	99396	Exc. Lesion w /Biopsy	CTF		Mono Test	86308	
		w /o Biopsy			Pap Smear	88155	
Obstetrics		Location Size			Pregnancy Test	84703	
Total OB Care	59400	Exc. Skin Tags (1 – 15)	*11200		Prenatal Profile	80055	
Obstetrical Visit	99212	Each Additional 10	*11201		Pro Time	85610	
Injections		Fracture Treatment			PSA	84153	
Administration Sub. / IM	90782	Loc			RPR	86592	
Drug		w /Reduc w /o Reduc			Sed. Rate	85651	
Dosage		Fracture Treatment F/U	99024		Stool Culture	87045	
Allergy	95155	I & D Abscess Single/Simple	*10060		Stool O & P	87177	
Cocci Skin Test	86490	Multiple or Comp	*10061		Strep Screen	(86403) *Dx 1*	
DPT	90701	I & D Pilonidal Cyst Simple	*10080		Theophylline	80198	
Haemophilus	90737	Pilonidal Cyst Complex	10081		Thyroid Profile	80091	
Influenza	90724	IV Therapy – To One Hour	90780		TSH	84443	
MMR	90707	Each Additional Hour	*90781		Urinalysis	81000	
OPV	90712	Laceration Repair			Urine Culture	87088	
Pneumovax	90732	Location Size Sim/Comp			Drawing Fee	36415	
TB Skin Test	86585	Laryngoscopy	31505		Specimen Collection	99000	
TD	90718	Oximetry	94760				
Unlisted Immun	90749	Punch Biopsy	CTF				
		Rhythm Strip	93040				
		Treadmill	93015				
		Trigger Point or Tendon Sheath Inj.	*20550				
		Tympanometry	92567				

Diagnosis / ICD – 9   *Tonsillitus 463.0, Diabetes 250.01*

I acknowledge receipt of medical services and authorize the release of any medical information necessary to process this claim for healthcare payment only. I ☐ do ☐ do not authorize payment to the provider Patient Signature	Tax ID Number:	Total Estimated Charges: Payment Amount: *$20.00*

		Happy Valley Medical Clinic				
1025		5222 E. Baseline Rd.			Date: 9/4/2008	
Doc - REL		Gilbert, AZ 85234 (800)333-4747				

AUSAN000   Austin, Andrew   9/4/2008   10:15:00 AM

EXAM	FEE	PROCEDURES	FEE	LABORATORY		FEE
New Patient		Anoscopy	46600	Aerobic Culture	87070	
Problem Focused	99201	Arthrocentesis/Aspiration/Injection		Amylase	82150	
Expanded Problem, Focused	99202	Small Joint	*20600	B12	82607	
Detailed	99203	Interm Joint	*20605	CBC & Diff	85025	
Comprehensive	99204	Major Joint	*20610	CHEM 20	80019	
Comprehensive/High Complex	99204	Audiometry	92552	Chlamydia Screen	86317	
Initial Visit/Procedure	99025	Cast Application		Cholesterol	82465	
Well Exam Infant (up to 12 mos.)	99318	Location Long Short		Digoxin	80162	
Well Exam 1 – 4 yrs.	99382	Catherization	*53670	Electrolytes	80005	
Well Exam 5 – 11 yrs.	99383	Circumcision	54150	Ferritin	82728	
Well Exam 12 – 17 yrs.	99384	Colposcopy	*57452	Folate	82746	
Well Exam 18 – 39 yrs.	99385	Colposcopy w /Biopsy	*57454	GC Screen	87070	
Well Exam 40 – 64 yrs.	99386	Cryosurgery Premalignant Lesion		Glucose	82947	
		Location(s):		Glucose 1 HR	82950	
Established Patient		Cryosurgery Warts		Glycosylated HGB (A1C)	83036	
Minimum	99211	Location(s):		HCT	85014	
Problem Focused	(99212) *Dx 1*	Curettement Lesion w /Biopsy	CTF	HDL	83718	
Expanded Problem Focused	99213	Curettement Lesion w o/ Biopsy		Hep BSAG	86278	
Detailed	99214	Single	*11050	Hepatitis Profile	80059	
Comprehensive/High Complex	99215	2 – 4	*11051	HGB & HCT	85014	
Well Exam Infant (up to 12 mos.)	99391	> 4	*11052	HIV	86311	
Well Exam 1 – 4 yrs.	99392	Diaphram Fitting	*57170	Iron & TBC	83540	83550
Well Exam 5 – 11 yrs.	99393	Ear Irrigation	69210	Kidney Profile	80007	
Well Exam 12 – 17 yrs.	99394	ECG	93000	Lead	83655	
Well Exam 18 – 39 yrs.	99395	Endometrial Biopsy	*58100	Liver Profile	82977	
Well Exam 40 – 64 yrs.	99396	Exc. Lesion w /Biopsy	CTF	Mono Test	86308	
		w /o Biopsy		Pap Smear	88155	
Obstetrics		Location Size		Pregnancy Test	84703	
Total OB Care	59400	Exc. Skin Tags (1 – 15)	*11200	Prenatal Profile	80055	
Obstetrical Visit	99212	Each Additional 10	*11201	Pro Time	85610	
Injections		Fracture Treatment		PSA	84153	
Administration Sub. / IM	90782	Loc		RPR	86592	
Drug		w /Reduc	w /o Reduc	Sed. Rate	85651	
Dosage		Fracture Treatment F/U	99024	Stool Culture	87045	
Allergy	95155	I & D Abscess Single/Simple	*10060	Stool O & P	87177	
Cocci Skin Test	86490	Multiple or Comp	*10061	Strep Screen	86403	
DPT	90701	I & D Pilonidal Cyst Simple	*10080	Theophylline	80198	
Haemophilus	90737	Pilonidal Cyst Complex	10081	Thyroid Profile	80091	
Influenza	90724	IV Therapy – To One Hour	90780	TSH	84443	
MMR	90707	Each Additional Hour	*90781	Urinalysis	81000	
OPV	90712	Laceration Repair		Urine Culture	87088	
Pneumovax	90732	Location Size Sim/Comp		Drawing Fee	36415	
TB Skin Test	86585	Laryngoscopy	31505	Specimen Collection	99000	
TD	90718	Oximetry	94760			
Unlisted Immun	90749	Punch Biopsy	CTF			
		Rhythm Strip	93040			
Chest X-Ray	*71020* *Dx 1*	Treadmill	93015			
		Trigger Point or Tendon Sheath Inj.	*20550			
		Tympanometry	92567			

Diagnosis / ICD – 9 *Bronchitis 490.0*		Total Estimated Charges:	
I acknowledge receipt of medical services and authorize the release of any medical information necessary to process this claim for healthcare payment only. I ☐ do ☐ do not authorize payment to the provider Patient Signature	Tax ID Number:	Payment Amount:	*$10.00*

Happy Valley Medical Clinic
5222 E. Baseline Rd.
Gilbert, AZ 85234
(800)333-4747

Date: 9/4/2008

Doc - MM

BORJO000	Bordon, John	9/4/2008	2:00:00 PM

EXAM	FEE	PROCEDURES	FEE	LABORATORY	FEE
New Patient		Anoscopy	46600	Aerobic Culture	87070	
Problem Focused	99201	Arthrocentesis/Aspiration/Injection		Amylase	82150	
Expanded Problem, Focused	99202	Small Joint	*20600	B12	82607	
Detailed	99203	Interm Joint	*20605	CBC & Diff	85025	
Comprehensive	99204	Major Joint	*20610	CHEM 20	80019	
Comprehensive/High Complex	99204	Audiometry	92552	Chlamydia Screen	86317	
Initial Visit/Procedure	99025	Cast Application		Cholesterol	82465	
Well Exam Infant (up to 12 mos.)	99318	Location Long Short		Digoxin	80162	
Well Exam 1 – 4 yrs.	99382	Catherization	*53670	Electrolytes	80005	
Well Exam 5 – 11 yrs.	99383	Circumcision	54150	Ferritin	82728	
Well Exam 12 – 17 yrs.	99384	Colposcopy	*57452	Folate	82746	
Well Exam 18 – 39 yrs.	99385	Colposcopy w /Biopsy	*57454	GC Screen	87070	
Well Exam 40 – 64 yrs.	99386	Cryosurgery Premalignant Lesion		Glucose	82947	
		Location(s):		Glucose 1 HR	82950	
Established Patient		Cryosurgery Warts		Glycosylated HGB (A1C)	83036	
Minimum	(99211) *Dx 1*	Location(s):		HCT	85014	
Problem Focused	99212	Curettement Lesion w /Biopsy	CTF	HDL	83718	
Expanded Problem Focused	99213	Curettement Lesion w o/ Biopsy		Hep BSAG	86278	
Detailed	99214	Single	*11050	Hepatitis Profile	80059	
Comprehensive/High Complex	99215	2 – 4	*11051	HGB & HCT	85014	
Well Exam Infant (up to 12 mos.)	99391	> 4	*11052	HIV	86311	
Well Exam 1 – 4 yrs.	99392	Diaphram Fitting	*57170	Iron & TBC 83540	83550	
Well Exam 5 – 11 yrs.	99393	Ear Irrigation	69210	Kidney Profile	80007	
Well Exam 12 – 17 yrs.	99394	ECG	93000	Lead	83655	
Well Exam 18 – 39 yrs.	99395	Endometrial Biopsy	*58100	Liver Profile	82977	
Well Exam 40 – 64 yrs.	99396	Exc. Lesion w /Biopsy	CTF	Mono Test	86308	
		w /o Biopsy		Pap Smear	88155	
Obstetrics		Location Size		Pregnancy Test	84703	
Total OB Care	59400	Exc. Skin Tags (1 – 15)	*11200	Prenatal Profile	80055	
Obstetrical Visit	99212	Each Additional 10	*11201	Pro Time	85610	
Injections		Fracture Treatment		PSA	84153	
Administration Sub. / IM	90782	Loc		RPR	86592	
Drug		w /Reduc w /o Reduc		Sed. Rate	85651	
Dosage		Fracture Treatment F/U	99024	Stool Culture	87045	
Allergy	95155	I & D Abscess Single/Simple	*10060	Stool O & P	87177	
Cocci Skin Test	86490	Multiple or Comp	*10061	Strep Screen	86403	
DPT	90701	I & D Pilonidal Cyst Simple	*10080	Theophylline	80198	
Haemophilus	90737	Pilonidal Cyst Complex	10081	Thyroid Profile	80091	
Influenza	90724	IV Therapy – To One Hour	90780	TSH	84443	
MMR	90707	Each Additional Hour	*90781	Urinalysis	81000	
OPV	90712	Laceration Repair		Urine Culture	87088	
Pneumovax	90732	Location Size Sim/Comp		Drawing Fee	36415	
TB Skin Test	86585	Laryngoscopy	31505	Specimen Collection	99000	
TD	90718	Oximetry	94760			
Unlisted Immun	90749	Punch Biopsy	CTF			
		Rhythm Strip	93040			
		Treadmill	93015			
		Trigger Point or Tendon Sheath Inj.	*20550			
		Tympanometry	92567			

Diagnosis / ICD – 9   *Low Back Pain 724.2*

I acknowledge receipt of medical services and authorize the release of any medical information necessary to process this claim for healthcare payment only. I ☐ do ☐ do not authorize payment to the provider Patient Signature	**Tax ID Number:**

Total Estimated Charges:
Payment Amount:

Doc - WH

Happy Valley Medical Clinic
5222 E. Baseline Rd.
Gilbert, AZ 85234
(800)333-4747

Date: 9/4/2008

BRIEL000	Brimley, Elmo	9/4/2008	8:00:00 AM

EXAM	FEE	PROCEDURES		FEE	LABORATORY		FEE
New Patient		Anoscopy	46600		Aerobic Culture	87070	
Problem Focused	99201	Arthrocentesis/Aspiration/Injection			Amylase	82150	
Expanded Problem, Focused	99202	Small Joint	*20600		B12	82607	
Detailed	99203	Interm Joint	*20605		CBC & Diff	85025	
Comprehensive	99204	Major Joint	*20610		CHEM 20	80019	
Comprehensive/High Complex	99204	Audiometry	92552		Chlamydia Screen	86317	
Initial Visit/Procedure	99025	Cast Application			Cholesterol	82465	
Well Exam Infant (up to 12 mos.)	99318	Location Long Short			Digoxin	80162	
Well Exam 1 – 4 yrs.	99382	Catherization	*53670		Electrolytes	80005	
Well Exam 5 – 11 yrs.	99383	Circumcision	54150		Ferritin	82728	
Well Exam 12 – 17 yrs.	99384	Colposcopy	*57452		Folate	82746	
Well Exam 18 – 39 yrs.	99385	Colposcopy w /Biopsy	*57454		GC Screen	87070	
Well Exam 40 – 64 yrs.	99386	Cryosurgery Premalignant Lesion			Glucose	82947	
		Location(s):			Glucose 1 HR	82950	
Established Patient		Cryosurgery Warts			Glycosylated HGB (A1C)	83036	
Minimum	99211	Location(s):			HCT	85014	
Problem Focused	99212	Curettement Lesion w /Biopsy	CTF		HDL	83718	
Expanded Problem Focused	99213	Curettement Lesion w o/ Biopsy			Hep BSAG	86278	
Detailed	99214	Single	*11050		Hepatitis Profile	80059	
Comprehensive/High Complex	99215	2 – 4	*11051		HGB & HCT	85014	
Well Exam Infant (up to 12 mos.)	99391	> 4	*11052		HIV	86311	
Well Exam 1 – 4 yrs.	99392	Diaphram Fitting	*57170		Iron & TBC	83540	83550
Well Exam 5 – 11 yrs.	99393	Ear Irrigation	69210		Kidney Profile	80007	
Well Exam 12 – 17 yrs.	99394	ECG	93000		Lead	83655	
Well Exam 18 – 39 yrs.	99395	Endometrial Biopsy	*58100		Liver Profile	82977	
Well Exam 40 – 64 yrs.	99396	Exc. Lesion w /Biopsy	CTF		Mono Test	86308	
		w /o Biopsy			Pap Smear	88155	
Obstetrics		Location Size			Pregnancy Test	84703	
Total OB Care	59400	Exc. Skin Tags (1 – 15)	*11200		Prenatal Profile	80055	
Obstetrical Visit	99212	Each Additional 10	*11201		Pro Time	85610	
Injections		Fracture Treatment			PSA	84153	
Administration Sub. / IM	90782	Loc			RPR	86592	
Drug		w /Reduc w /o Reduc			Sed. Rate	85651	
Dosage		Fracture Treatment F/U	99024		Stool Culture	87045	
Allergy	95155	I & D Abscess Single/Simple	*10060		Stool O & P	87177	
Cocci Skin Test	86490	Multiple or Comp	*10061		Strep Screen	86403	
DPT	90701	I & D Pilonidal Cyst Simple	*10080		Theophylline	80198	
Haemophilus	90737	Pilonidal Cyst Complex	10081		Thyroid Profile	80091	
Influenza	90724	IV Therapy – To One Hour	90780		TSH	84443	
MMR	90707	Each Additional Hour	*90781		Urinalysis	81000	
OPV	90712	Laceration Repair			Urine Culture	87088	
Pneumovax	90732	Location Size Sim/Comp			Drawing Fee	36415	
TB Skin Test	86585	Laryngoscopy	31505		Specimen Collection	99000	
TD	90718	Oximetry	94760				
Unlisted Immun	90749	Punch Biopsy	CTF				
		Rhythm Strip	93040				
MultiLink Diabet	*Dx 1*	Treadmill	93015				
		Trigger Point or Tendon Sheath Inj.	*20550				
		Tympanometry	92567				

Diagnosis / ICD – 9 *Diabetes 250.01*

I acknowledge receipt of medical services and authorize the release of any medical information necessary to process this claim for healthcare payment only.

I ☐ do ☐ do not authorize payment to the provider

Patient Signature

Tax ID Number:

Total Estimated Charges:

Payment Amount: CK# 463 $10.00

		1028		Happy Valley Medical Clinic				Date: 9/4/2008	

1028

Doc - JM

Happy Valley Medical Clinic
5222 E. Baseline Rd.
Gilbert, AZ 85234
(800)333-4747

Date: 9/4/2008

BRIJA000   Brimley, Jay   9/4/2008   8:30:00 AM

EXAM	FEE	PROCEDURES		FEE	LABORATORY		FEE
New Patient		Anoscopy		46600	Aerobic Culture	87070	
Problem Focused	99201	Arthrocentesis/Aspiration/Injection			Amylase	82150	
Expanded Problem, Focused	99202	Small Joint		*20600	B12	82607	
Detailed	99203	Interm Joint		*20605	CBC & Diff	85025	
Comprehensive	99204	Major Joint		*20610	CHEM 20	80019	
Comprehensive/High Complex	99204	Audiometry		92552	Chlamydia Screen	86317	
Initial Visit/Procedure	99025	Cast Application			Cholesterol	82465	
Well Exam Infant (up to 12 mos.)	99318	Location Long Short			Digoxin	80162	
Well Exam 1 – 4 yrs.	99382	Catherization		*53670	Electrolytes	80005	
Well Exam 5 – 11 yrs.	99383	Circumcision		54150	Ferritin	82728	
Well Exam 12 – 17 yrs.	99384	Colposcopy		*57452	Folate	82746	
Well Exam 18 – 39 yrs.	99385	Colposcopy w /Biopsy		*57454	GC Screen	87070	
Well Exam 40 – 64 yrs.	99386	Cryosurgery Premalignant Lesion			Glucose	82947	
		Location(s):			Glucose 1 HR	82950	
Established Patient		Cryosurgery Warts			Glycosylated HGB (A1C)	83036	
Minimum	(99211) *Dx 1*	Location(s):			HCT	85014	
Problem Focused	99212	Curettement Lesion w /Biopsy		CTF	HDL	83718	
Expanded Problem Focused	99213	Curettement Lesion w o/ Biopsy			Hep BSAG	86278	
Detailed	99214	Single		*11050	Hepatitis Profile	80059	
Comprehensive/High Complex	99215	2 – 4		*11051	HGB & HCT	85014	
Well Exam Infant (up to 12 mos.)	99391	> 4		*11052	HIV	86311	
Well Exam 1 – 4 yrs.	99392	Diaphram Fitting		*57170	Iron & TBC 83540	83550	
Well Exam 5 – 11 yrs.	99393	Ear Irrigation		69210	Kidney Profile	80007	
Well Exam 12 – 17 yrs.	99394	ECG		93000	Lead	83655	
Well Exam 18 – 39 yrs.	99395	Endometrial Biopsy		*58100	Liver Profile	82977	
Well Exam 40 – 64 yrs.	99396	Exc. Lesion w /Biopsy		CTF	Mono Test	86308	
		w /o Biopsy			Pap Smear	88155	
Obstetrics		Location Size			Pregnancy Test	84703	
Total OB Care	59400	Exc. Skin Tags (1 – 15)		*11200	Prenatal Profile	80055	
Obstetrical Visit	99212	Each Additional 10		*11201	Pro Time	85610	
Injections		Fracture Treatment			PSA	84153	
Administration Sub. / IM	90782	Loc			RPR	86592	
Drug		w /Reduc	w /o Reduc		Sed. Rate	85651	
Dosage		Fracture Treatment F/U		99024	Stool Culture	87045	
Allergy	95155	I & D Abscess Single/Simple		*10060	Stool O & P	87177	
Cocci Skin Test	86490	Multiple or Comp		*10061	Strep Screen	86403	
DPT	90701	I & D Pilonidal Cyst Simple		*10080	Theophylline	80198	
Haemophilus	90737	Pilonidal Cyst Complex		10081	Thyroid Profile	80091	
Influenza	90724	IV Therapy – To One Hour		90780	TSH	84443	
MMR	90707	Each Additional Hour		*90781	Urinalysis	81000	
OPV	90712	Laceration Repair			Urine Culture	87088	
Pneumovax	90732	Location Size Sim/Comp			Drawing Fee	36415	
TB Skin Test	86585	Laryngoscopy		31505	Specimen Collection	99000	
TD	90718	Oximetry		94760			
Unlisted Immun	90749	Punch Biopsy		CTF			
		Rhythm Strip		93040			
X-Ray Chest 4 view	*71030* *Dx 1*	Treadmill		93015			
		Trigger Point or Tendon Sheath Inj.		*20550			
		Tympanometry		92567			

Diagnosis / ICD – 9   *Lead Miner's Lung 503*

	Total Estimated Charges:

I acknowledge receipt of medical services and authorize the release of any medical information necessary to process this claim for healthcare payment only.

I ☐ do ☐ do not   authorize payment to the provider

Patient Signature

Tax ID Number:

Total
Estimated
Charges:

Payment
Amount:

Doc - JM

Happy Valley Medical Clinic
5222 E. Baseline Rd.
Gilbert, AZ 85234
(800)333-4747

Date: 9/4/2008

BRISU000   Brimley, Susan   9/4/2008   8:15:00 AM

EXAM	FEE	PROCEDURES	FEE	LABORATORY	FEE
New Patient		Anoscopy	46600	Aerobic Culture	87070	
Problem Focused	99201	Arthrocentesis/Aspiration/Injection		Amylase	82150	
Expanded Problem, Focused	99202	Small Joint	*20600	B12	82607	
Detailed	99203	Interm Joint	*20605	CBC & Diff	85025	
Comprehensive	99204	Major Joint	*20610	CHEM 20	80019	
Comprehensive/High Complex	99204	Audiometry	92552	Chlamydia Screen	86317	
Initial Visit/Procedure	99025	Cast Application		Cholesterol	82465	
Well Exam Infant (up to 12 mos.)	99318	Location Long Short		Digoxin	80162	
Well Exam 1 – 4 yrs.	99382	Catherization	*53670	Electrolytes	80005	
Well Exam 5 – 11 yrs.	99383	Circumcision	54150	Ferritin	82728	
Well Exam 12 – 17 yrs.	99384	Colposcopy	*57452	Folate	82746	
Well Exam 18 – 39 yrs.	99385	Colposcopy w /Biopsy	*57454	GC Screen	87070	
Well Exam 40 – 64 yrs.	99386	Cryosurgery Premalignant Lesion		Glucose	82947	
		Location(s):		Glucose 1 HR	82950	
Established Patient		Cryosurgery Warts		Glycosylated HGB (A1C)	83036	
Minimum	99211	Location(s):		HCT	85014	
Problem Focused _Mod = 25_	(99212) _Dx 2_	Curettement Lesion w /Biopsy	CTF	HDL	83718	
Expanded Problem Focused	99213	Curettement Lesion w o/ Biopsy		Hep BSAG	86278	
Detailed	99214	Single	*11050	Hepatitis Profile	80059	
Comprehensive/High Complex	99215	2 – 4	*11051	HGB & HCT	85014	
Well Exam Infant (up to 12 mos.)	99391	> 4	*11052	HIV	86311	
Well Exam 1 – 4 yrs.	99392	Diaphram Fitting	*57170	Iron & TBC 83540	83550	
Well Exam 5 – 11 yrs.	99393	Ear Irrigation	69210	Kidney Profile	80007	
Well Exam 12 – 17 yrs.	99394	ECG	93000	Lead	83655	
Well Exam 18 – 39 yrs.	99395	Endometrial Biopsy	*58100	Liver Profile	82977	
Well Exam 40 – 64 yrs.	99396	Exc. Lesion w /Biopsy	CTF	Mono Test	86308	
		w /o Biopsy		Pap Smear	88155	
Obstetrics		Location Size		Pregnancy Test	84703 _Dx 1_	
Total OB Care	59400	Exc. Skin Tags (1 – 15)	*11200	Prenatal Profile	80055	
Obstetrical Visit	(99212) _Dx 1_	Each Additional 10	*11201	Pro Time	85610	
Injections		Fracture Treatment		PSA	84153	
Administration Sub. / IM	90782	Loc		RPR	86592	
Drug		w /Reduc w /o Reduc		Sed. Rate	85651	
Dosage		Fracture Treatment F/U	99024	Stool Culture	87045	
Allergy	95155	I & D Abscess Single/Simple	*10060	Stool O & P	87177	
Cocci Skin Test	86490	Multiple or Comp	*10061	Strep Screen	86403	
DPT	90701	I & D Pilonidal Cyst Simple	*10080	Theophylline	80198	
Haemophilus	90737	Pilonidal Cyst Complex	10081	Thyroid Profile	80091	
Influenza	90724	IV Therapy – To One Hour	90780	TSH	84443	
MMR	90707	Each Additional Hour	*90781	Urinalysis	81000	
OPV	90712	Laceration Repair		Urine Culture	87088	
Pneumovax	90732	Location Size Sim/Comp		Drawing Fee	36415	
TB Skin Test	86585	Laryngoscopy	31505	Specimen Collection	99000	
TD	90718	Oximetry	94760			
Unlisted Immun	90749	Punch Biopsy	CTF			
		Rhythm Strip	93040			
		Treadmill	93015			
X-Ray Chest	_71020_ _Dx 2_	Trigger Point or Tendon Sheath Inj.	*20550			
		Tympanometry	92567			

Diagnosis / ICD – 9   _Pregnancy V22.1, Chronic Bronchitis 491.0_

I acknowledge receipt of medical services and authorize the release of any medical information necessary to process this claim for healthcare payment only.

I ☐ do ☐ do not authorize payment to the provider

Patient Signature

Tax ID Number:

Total Estimated Charges:

Payment Amount: _CK# $10.00_
_553_

1030

Doc - JM

Happy Valley Medical Clinic
5222 E. Baseline Rd.
Gilbert, AZ 85234
(800)333-4747

Date: 9/4/2008

CATSA000   Catera, Sammy   9/4/2008   10:00:00 AM

EXAM	FEE	PROCEDURES	FEE	LABORATORY		FEE
New Patient		Anoscopy	46600	Aerobic Culture	87070	
Problem Focused	99201	Arthrocentesis/Aspiration/Injection		Amylase	82150	
Expanded Problem, Focused	99202	Small Joint	*20600	B12	82607	
Detailed	99203	Interm Joint	*20605	CBC & Diff	85025	
Comprehensive	99204	Major Joint	*20610	CHEM 20	80019	
Comprehensive/High Complex	99204	Audiometry	92552	Chlamydia Screen	86317	
Initial Visit/Procedure	99025	Cast Application		Cholesterol	82465	
Well Exam Infant (up to 12 mos.)	99318	Location Long Short		Digoxin	80162	
Well Exam 1 – 4 yrs.	99382	Catherization	*53670	Electrolytes	80005	
Well Exam 5 – 11 yrs.	99383	Circumcision	54150	Ferritin	82728	
Well Exam 12 – 17 yrs.	99384	Colposcopy	*57452	Folate	82746	
Well Exam 18 – 39 yrs.	99385	Colposcopy w /Biopsy	*57454	GC Screen	87070	
Well Exam 40 – 64 yrs.	99386	Cryosurgery Premalignant Lesion		Glucose	82947	
		Location(s):		Glucose 1 HR	82950	
Established Patient		Cryosurgery Warts		Glycosylated HGB (A1C)	83036	
Minimum	99211	Location(s):		HCT	85014	
Problem Focused	(99212) Dx 1	Curettement Lesion w /Biopsy	CTF	HDL	83718	
Expanded Problem Focused	99213	Curettement Lesion w o/ Biopsy		Hep BSAG	86278	
Detailed	99214	Single	*11050	Hepatitis Profile	80059	
Comprehensive/High Complex	99215	2 – 4	*11051	HGB & HCT	85014	
Well Exam Infant (up to 12 mos.)	99391	> 4	*11052	HIV	86311	
Well Exam 1 – 4 yrs.	99392	Diaphram Fitting	*57170	Iron & TBC	83540	83550
Well Exam 5 – 11 yrs.	99393	Ear Irrigation	69210	Kidney Profile	80007	
Well Exam 12 – 17 yrs.	99394	ECG	93000	Lead	83655	
Well Exam 18 – 39 yrs.	99395	Endometrial Biopsy	*58100	Liver Profile	82977	
Well Exam 40 – 64 yrs.	99396	Exc. Lesion w /Biopsy	CTF	Mono Test	86308	
		w /o Biopsy		Pap Smear	88155	
Obstetrics		Location Size		Pregnancy Test	84703	
Total OB Care	59400	Exc. Skin Tags (1 – 15)	*11200	Prenatal Profile	80055	
Obstetrical Visit	99212	Each Additional 10	*11201	Pro Time	85610	
Injections		Fracture Treatment		PSA	84153	
Administration Sub. / IM	90782	Loc		RPR	86592	
Drug		w /Reduc w /o Reduc		Sed. Rate	85651	
Dosage		Fracture Treatment F/U	99024	Stool Culture	87045	
Allergy	95155	I & D Abscess Single/Simple	*10060	Stool O & P	87177	
Cocci Skin Test	86490	Multiple or Comp	*10061	Strep Screen	86403	
DPT	90701	I & D Pilonidal Cyst Simple	*10080	Theophylline	80198	
Haemophilus	90737	Pilonidal Cyst Complex	10081	Thyroid Profile	80091	
Influenza	90724	IV Therapy – To One Hour	90780	TSH	84443	
MMR	90707	Each Additional Hour	*90781	Urinalysis	81000	
OPV	90712	Laceration Repair		Urine Culture	87088	
Pneumovax	90732	Location Size Sim/Comp		Drawing Fee	36415	
TB Skin Test	86585	Laryngoscopy	31505	Specimen Collection	99000	
TD	90718	Oximetry	94760			
Unlisted Immun	90749	Punch Biopsy	CTF			
		Rhythm Strip	93040			
		Treadmill	93015			
		Trigger Point or Tendon Sheath Inj.	*20550			
		Tympanometry	92567			

Diagnosis / ICD – 9   *Gastric Ulcer 531.90*

I acknowledge receipt of medical services and authorize the release of any medical information necessary to process this claim for healthcare payment only.

I ☐ do ☐ do not authorize payment to the provider

Patient Signature

Tax ID Number:

Total Estimated Charges:

Payment Amount:

1031	Happy Valley Medical Clinic	Date: 9/4/2008
Doc - REL	5222 E. Baseline Rd. Gilbert, AZ 85234 (800)333-4747	

CLIWA000	Clinger, Wallace	9/4/2008	2:45:00 PM

EXAM	FEE	PROCEDURES	FEE	LABORATORY	FEE
New Patient		Anoscopy	46600	Aerobic Culture	87070	
Problem Focused	99201	Arthrocentesis/Aspiration/Injection		Amylase	82150	
Expanded Problem, Focused	99202	Small Joint	*20600	B12	82607	
Detailed	99203	Interm Joint	*20605	CBC & Diff	85025	
Comprehensive	99204	Major Joint	*20610	CHEM 20	80019	
Comprehensive/High Complex	99204	Audiometry	92552	Chlamydia Screen	86317	
Initial Visit/Procedure	99025	Cast Application		Cholesterol	82465	
Well Exam Infant (up to 12 mos.)	99318	Location Long Short		Digoxin	80162	
Well Exam 1 – 4 yrs.	99382	Catherization	*53670	Electrolytes	80005	
Well Exam 5 – 11 yrs.	99383	Circumcision	54150	Ferritin	82728	
Well Exam 12 – 17 yrs.	99384	Colposcopy	*57452	Folate	82746	
Well Exam 18 – 39 yrs.	99385	Colposcopy w /Biopsy	*57454	GC Screen	87070	
Well Exam 40 – 64 yrs.	99386	Cryosurgery Premalignant Lesion		Glucose	82947	
		Location(s):		Glucose 1 HR	82950	
Established Patient		Cryosurgery Warts		Glycosylated HGB (A1C)	83036	
Minimum	99211	Location(s):		HCT	85014	
Problem Focused	99212	Curettement Lesion w /Biopsy	CTF	HDL	83718	
Expanded Problem Focused	99213	Curettement Lesion w o/ Biopsy		Hep BSAG	86278	
Detailed	99214	Single	*11050	Hepatitis Profile	80059	
Comprehensive/High Complex	99215	2 – 4	*11051	HGB & HCT	85014	
Well Exam Infant (up to 12 mos.)	99391	> 4	*11052	HIV	86311	
Well Exam 1 – 4 yrs.	99392	Diaphram Fitting	*57170	Iron & TBC	83540	83550
Well Exam 5 – 11 yrs.	99393	Ear Irrigation	69210	Kidney Profile	80007	
Well Exam 12 – 17 yrs.	99394	ECG	93000	Lead	83655	
Well Exam 18 – 39 yrs.	99395	Endometrial Biopsy	*58100	Liver Profile	82977	
Well Exam 40 – 64 yrs.	99396	Exc. Lesion w /Biopsy	CTF	Mono Test	86308	
		w /o Biopsy		Pap Smear	88155	
Obstetrics		Location Size		Pregnancy Test	84703	
Total OB Care	59400	Exc. Skin Tags (1 – 15)	*11200	Prenatal Profile	80055	
Obstetrical Visit	99212	Each Additional 10	*11201	Pro Time	85610	
Injections		Fracture Treatment		PSA	84153	
Administration Sub. / IM	90782	Loc		RPR	86592	
Drug		w /Reduc w /o Reduc		Sed. Rate	85651	
Dosage		Fracture Treatment F/U	99024	Stool Culture	87045	
Allergy	95155	I & D Abscess Single/Simple	*10060	Stool O & P	87177	
Cocci Skin Test	86490	Multiple or Comp	*10061	Strep Screen	86403	
DPT	90701	I & D Pilonidal Cyst Simple	*10080	Theophylline	80198	
Haemophilus	90737	Pilonidal Cyst Complex	10081	Thyroid Profile	80091	
Influenza	90724	IV Therapy – To One Hour	90780	TSH	84443	
MMR	90707	Each Additional Hour	*90781	Urinalysis	81000	
OPV	90712	Laceration Repair		Urine Culture	87088	
Pneumovax	90732	Location Size Sim/Comp		Drawing Fee	36415	
TB Skin Test	86585	Laryngoscopy	31505	Specimen Collection	99000	
TD	90718	Oximetry	94760			
Unlisted Immun	90749	Punch Biopsy	CTF			
		Rhythm Strip	93040			
		Treadmill	93015			
MultiLink - Trucke	*Dx 1*	Trigger Point or Tendon Sheath Inj.	*20550			
		Tympanometry	92567			

Diagnosis / ICD – 9 *Exam Routine Health V70.0*		Total Estimated Charges:	
I acknowledge receipt of medical services and authorize the release of any medical information necessary to process this claim for healthcare payment only. I ☐ do ☐ do not authorize payment to the provider Patient Signature	Tax ID Number:	Payment Amount:	*$15.00*

Happy Valley Medical Clinic
5222 E. Baseline Rd.
Gilbert, AZ 85234
(800)333-4747

Date: 9/4/2008

Doc - REL

| DOOJA000 | Doogan, James | 9/4/2008 | 4:15:00 PM |

EXAM	FEE	PROCEDURES	FEE	LABORATORY	FEE
New Patient		Anoscopy	46600	Aerobic Culture	87070	
Problem Focused	99201	Arthrocentesis/Aspiration/Injection		Amylase	82150	
Expanded Problem, Focused	99202	Small Joint	*20600	B12	82607	
Detailed	99203	Interm Joint	*20605	CBC & Diff	85025	
Comprehensive	99204	Major Joint	*20610	CHEM 20	80019	
Comprehensive/High Complex	99204	Audiometry	92552	Chlamydia Screen	86317	
Initial Visit/Procedure	99025	Cast Application		Cholesterol	82465	
Well Exam Infant (up to 12 mos.)	99318	Location Long Short		Digoxin	80162	
Well Exam 1 – 4 yrs.	99382	Catherization	*53670	Electrolytes	80005	
Well Exam 5 – 11 yrs.	99383	Circumcision	54150	Ferritin	82728	
Well Exam 12 – 17 yrs.	99384	Colposcopy	*57452	Folate	82746	
Well Exam 18 – 39 yrs.	99385	Colposcopy w /Biopsy	*57454	GC Screen	87070	
Well Exam 40 – 64 yrs.	99386	Cryosurgery Premalignant Lesion		Glucose	82947	
		Location(s):		Glucose 1 HR	82950	
Established Patient		Cryosurgery Warts		Glycosylated HGB (A1C)	83036	
Minimum	(99211) *Dx 1*	Location(s):		HCT	85014	
Problem Focused	99212	Curettement Lesion w /Biopsy	CTF	HDL	83718	
Expanded Problem Focused	99213	Curettement Lesion w o/ Biopsy		Hep BSAG	86278	
Detailed	99214	Single	*11050	Hepatitis Profile	80059	
Comprehensive/High Complex	99215	2 – 4	*11051	HGB & HCT	85014	
Well Exam Infant (up to 12 mos.)	99391	> 4	*11052	HIV	86311	
Well Exam 1 – 4 yrs.	99392	Diaphram Fitting	*57170	Iron & TBC 83540	83550	
Well Exam 5 – 11 yrs.	99393	Ear Irrigation	69210	Kidney Profile	80007	
Well Exam 12 – 17 yrs.	99394	ECG	93000	Lead	83655	
Well Exam 18 – 39 yrs.	99395	Endometrial Biopsy	*58100	Liver Profile	82977	
Well Exam 40 – 64 yrs.	99396	Exc. Lesion w /Biopsy	CTF	Mono Test	86308	
		w /o Biopsy		Pap Smear	88155	
Obstetrics		Location Size		Pregnancy Test	84703	
Total OB Care	59400	Exc. Skin Tags (1 – 15)	*11200	Prenatal Profile	80055	
Obstetrical Visit	99212	Each Additional 10	*11201	Pro Time	85610	
Injections		Fracture Treatment		PSA	84153	
Administration Sub. / IM	90782	Loc		RPR	86592	
Drug		w /Reduc w /o Reduc		Sed. Rate	85651	
Dosage		Fracture Treatment F/U	99024	Stool Culture	87045	
Allergy	95155	I & D Abscess Single/Simple	*10060	Stool O & P	87177	
Cocci Skin Test	86490	Multiple or Comp	*10061	Strep Screen	86403	
DPT	90701	I & D Pilonidal Cyst Simple	*10080	Theophylline	80198	
Haemophilus	90737	Pilonidal Cyst Complex	10081	Thyroid Profile	80091	
Influenza	90724	IV Therapy – To One Hour	90780	TSH	84443	
MMR	90707	Each Additional Hour	*90781	Urinalysis	81000	
OPV	90712	Laceration Repair		Urine Culture	87088	
Pneumovax	90732	Location Size Sim/Comp		Drawing Fee	36415	
TB Skin Test	86585	Laryngoscopy	31505	Specimen Collection	99000	*Dx 1*
TD	90718	Oximetry	94760			
Unlisted Immun	90749	Punch Biopsy	CTF			
		Rhythm Strip	93040			
		Treadmill	93015			
		Trigger Point or Tendon Sheath Inj.	*20550			
		Tympanometry	92567			

Diagnosis / ICD – 9   *Food Poisoning 005.9*

| Total Estimated Charges: |
| Payment Amount: |

Tax ID Number:

I acknowledge receipt of medical services and authorize the release of any medical information necessary to process this claim for healthcare payment only.

I ☐ do ☐ do not authorize payment to the provider

Patient Signature

	1033	Happy Valley Medical Clinic 5222 E. Baseline Rd. Gilbert, AZ 85234 (800)333-4747	Date: 9/4/2008
	Doc - WH		

GOOCH000	Gooding, Charles	9/4/2008	2:15:00 PM

EXAM	FEE	PROCEDURES	FEE	LABORATORY	FEE
New Patient		Anoscopy	46600	Aerobic Culture	87070	
Problem Focused	99201	Arthrocentesis/Aspiration/Injection		Amylase	82150	
Expanded Problem, Focused	99202	Small Joint	*20600	B12	82607	
Detailed	99203	Interm Joint	*20605	CBC & Diff	85025	
Comprehensive	99204	Major Joint	*20610	CHEM 20	80019	
Comprehensive/High Complex	99204	Audiometry	92552	Chlamydia Screen	86317	
Initial Visit/Procedure	99025	Cast Application		Cholesterol	82465	
Well Exam Infant (up to 12 mos.)	99318	Location Long Short		Digoxin	80162	
Well Exam 1 – 4 yrs.	99382	Catherization	*53670	Electrolytes	80005	
Well Exam 5 – 11 yrs.	99383	Circumcision	54150	Ferritin	82728	
Well Exam 12 – 17 yrs.	99384	Colposcopy	*57452	Folate	82746	
Well Exam 18 – 39 yrs.	99385	Colposcopy w /Biopsy	*57454	GC Screen	87070	
Well Exam 40 – 64 yrs.	99386	Cryosurgery Premalignant Lesion		Glucose	82947	
		Location(s):		Glucose 1 HR	82950	
Established Patient		Cryosurgery Warts		Glycosylated HGB (A1C)	83036	
Minimum	99211	Location(s):		HCT	85014	
Problem Focused	99212 *Dx*	Curettement Lesion w /Biopsy	CTF	HDL	83718	
Expanded Problem Focused	(99213) *1+2*	Curettement Lesion w o/ Biopsy		Hep BSAG	86278	
Detailed	99214	Single	*11050	Hepatitis Profile	80059	
Comprehensive/High Complex	99215	2 – 4	*11051	HGB & HCT	85014	
Well Exam Infant (up to 12 mos.)	99391	> 4	*11052	HIV	86311	
Well Exam 1 – 4 yrs.	99392	Diaphram Fitting	*57170	Iron & TBC	83540	83550
Well Exam 5 – 11 yrs.	99393	Ear Irrigation	69210	Kidney Profile	80007	
Well Exam 12 – 17 yrs.	99394	ECG	93000	Lead	83655	
Well Exam 18 – 39 yrs.	99395	Endometrial Biopsy	*58100	Liver Profile	82977	
Well Exam 40 – 64 yrs.	99396	Exc. Lesion w /Biopsy	CTF	Mono Test	86308	
		w /o Biopsy		Pap Smear	88155	
Obstetrics		Location Size		Pregnancy Test	84703	
Total OB Care	59400	Exc. Skin Tags (1 – 15)	*11200	Prenatal Profile	80055	
Obstetrical Visit	99212	Each Additional 10	*11201	Pro Time	85610	
Injections		Fracture Treatment		PSA	84153	
Administration Sub. / IM	90782	Loc		RPR	86592	
Drug		w /Reduc w /o Reduc		Sed. Rate	85651	
Dosage		Fracture Treatment F/U	99024	Stool Culture	87045	
Allergy	95155	I & D Abscess Single/Simple	*10060	Stool O & P	87177	
Cocci Skin Test	86490	Multiple or Comp	*10061	Strep Screen	(86403) *Dx 2*	
DPT	90701	I & D Pilonidal Cyst Simple	*10080	Theophylline	80198	
Haemophilus	90737	Pilonidal Cyst Complex	10081	Thyroid Profile	80091	
Influenza	90724	IV Therapy – To One Hour	90780	TSH	84443	
MMR	90707	Each Additional Hour	*90781	Urinalysis	81000	
OPV	90712	Laceration Repair		Urine Culture	87088	
Pneumovax	90732	Location Size Sim/Comp		Drawing Fee	36415	
TB Skin Test	86585	Laryngoscopy	31505	Specimen Collection	99000	
TD	90718	Oximetry	94760			
Unlisted Immun	90749	Punch Biopsy	CTF			
		Rhythm Strip	93040			
		Treadmill	93015			
		Trigger Point or Tendon Sheath Inj.	*20550			
		Tympanometry	92567			

Diagnosis / ICD – 9   *Chicken Pox 052.9, Strep 034.0*

I acknowledge receipt of medical services and authorize the release of any medical information necessary to process this claim for healthcare payment only.	Tax ID Number:
I ☐ do ☐ do not authorize payment to the provider	
Patient Signature	

Total Estimated Charges:	
Payment Amount:	*$10.00*

1034	Happy Valley Medical Clinic	Date: 9/4/2008
Doc - WH	5222 E. Baseline Rd. Gilbert, AZ 85234 (800)333-4747	

JACTH000	Jacks, Theodore	9/4/2008	3:15:00 PM

EXAM	FEE	PROCEDURES	FEE	LABORATORY	FEE
New Patient		Anoscopy	46600	Aerobic Culture	87070	
Problem Focused	99201	Arthrocentesis/Aspiration/Injection		Amylase	82150	
Expanded Problem, Focused	99202	Small Joint	*20600	B12	82607	
Detailed	99203	Interm Joint	*20605	CBC & Diff	85025	
Comprehensive	99204	Major Joint	*20610	CHEM 20	80019	
Comprehensive/High Complex	99204	Audiometry	92552	Chlamydia Screen	86317	
Initial Visit/Procedure	99025	Cast Application		Cholesterol	82465	
Well Exam Infant (up to 12 mos.)	99318	Location Long Short		Digoxin	80162	
Well Exam 1 – 4 yrs.	99382	Catherization	*53670	Electrolytes	80005	
Well Exam 5 – 11 yrs.	99383	Circumcision	54150	Ferritin	82728	
Well Exam 12 – 17 yrs.	99384	Colposcopy	*57452	Folate	82746	
Well Exam 18 – 39 yrs.	99385	Colposcopy w /Biopsy	*57454	GC Screen	87070	
Well Exam 40 – 64 yrs.	99386	Cryosurgery Premalignant Lesion		Glucose	82947	
		Location(s):		Glucose 1 HR	82950	
Established Patient		Cryosurgery Warts		Glycosylated HGB (A1C)	83036	
Minimum	99211	*Dx* Location(s):		HCT	85014	
Problem Focused	(99212) *1+2*	Curettement Lesion w /Biopsy	CTF	HDL	83718	
Expanded Problem Focused	99213	Curettement Lesion w o/ Biopsy		Hep BSAG	86278	
Detailed	99214	Single	*11050	Hepatitis Profile	80059	
Comprehensive/High Complex	99215	2 – 4	*11051	HGB & HCT	85014	
Well Exam Infant (up to 12 mos.)	99391	> 4	*11052	HIV	86311	
Well Exam 1 – 4 yrs.	99392	Diaphram Fitting	*57170	Iron & TBC	83540	83550
Well Exam 5 – 11 yrs.	99393	Ear Irrigation	69210	Kidney Profile	80007	
Well Exam 12 – 17 yrs.	99394	ECG	93000	Lead	83655	
Well Exam 18 – 39 yrs.	99395	Endometrial Biopsy	*58100	Liver Profile	82977	
Well Exam 40 – 64 yrs.	99396	Exc. Lesion w /Biopsy	CTF	Mono Test	86308	
		w /o Biopsy		Pap Smear	88155	
Obstetrics		Location Size		Pregnancy Test	84703	
Total OB Care	59400	Exc. Skin Tags (1 – 15)	*11200	Prenatal Profile	80055	
Obstetrical Visit	99212	Each Additional 10	*11201	Pro Time	85610	
Injections		Fracture Treatment		PSA	84153	
Administration Sub. / IM	90782	Loc		RPR	86592	
Drug		w /Reduc w /o Reduc		Sed. Rate	85651	
Dosage		Fracture Treatment F/U	99024	Stool Culture	87045	
Allergy	95155	I & D Abscess Single/Simple	*10060	Stool O & P	87177	
Cocci Skin Test	86490	Multiple or Comp	*10061	Strep Screen	86403	
DPT	90701	I & D Pilonidal Cyst Simple	*10080	Theophylline	80198	
Haemophilus	90737	Pilonidal Cyst Complex	10081	Thyroid Profile	80091	
Influenza	90724	IV Therapy – To One Hour	90780	TSH	84443	
MMR	90707	Each Additional Hour	*90781	Urinalysis	81000	
OPV	90712	Laceration Repair		Urine Culture	87088	
Pneumovax	90732	Location Size Sim/Comp		Drawing Fee	36415	
TB Skin Test	86585	Laryngoscopy	31505	Specimen Collection	99000	
TD	90718	Oximetry	94760			
Unlisted Immun	90749	Punch Biopsy	CTF			
		Rhythm Strip	93040			
		Treadmill	93015			
X- Ray Chest 2 view	*71020* *2*	Trigger Point or Tendon Sheath Inj.	*20550			
		Tympanometry	92567			

Diagnosis / ICD – 9 *Fatigue 780.7, Breathing Diff. 786.09*

I acknowledge receipt of medical services and authorize the release of any medical information necessary to process this claim for healthcare payment only. I ☐ do ☐ do not authorize payment to the provider Patient Signature	Tax ID Number:	**Total Estimated Charges:** Payment Amount: *CK* *$5.00* *56510*

Happy Valley Medical Clinic
5222 E. Baseline Rd.
Gilbert, AZ 85234
(800)333-4747

Date: 9/4/2008

Doc - JM

JASST000   Jasper, Stephanie L   9/4/2008   3:00:00 PM

EXAM	FEE	PROCEDURES	FEE	LABORATORY	FEE
New Patient		Anoscopy	46600	Aerobic Culture	87070	
Problem Focused	99201	Arthrocentesis/Aspiration/Injection		Amylase	82150	
Expanded Problem, Focused	99202	Small Joint	*20600	B12	82607	
Detailed	99203	Interm Joint	*20605	CBC & Diff	85025	
Comprehensive	99204	Major Joint	*20610	CHEM 20	80019	
Comprehensive/High Complex	99204	Audiometry	92552	Chlamydia Screen	86317	
Initial Visit/Procedure	99025	Cast Application		Cholesterol	82465	
Well Exam Infant (up to 12 mos.)	99318	Location Long Short		Digoxin	80162	
Well Exam 1 – 4 yrs.	99382	Catherization	*53670	Electrolytes	80005	
Well Exam 5 – 11 yrs.	99383	Circumcision	54150	Ferritin	82728	
Well Exam 12 – 17 yrs.	99384	Colposcopy	*57452	Folate	82746	
Well Exam 18 – 39 yrs.	99385	Colposcopy w /Biopsy	*57454	GC Screen	87070	
Well Exam 40 – 64 yrs.	99386	Cryosurgery Premalignant Lesion		Glucose	82947	
		Location(s):		Glucose 1 HR	82950	
Established Patient		Cryosurgery Warts		Glycosylated HGB (A1C)	83036	
Minimum	99211	Location(s):		HCT	85014	
Problem Focused	99212	Curettement Lesion w /Biopsy	CTF	HDL	83718	
Expanded Problem Focused	(99213) Dx 1	Curettement Lesion w o/ Biopsy		Hep BSAG	86278	
Detailed	99214	Single	*11050	Hepatitis Profile	80059	
Comprehensive/High Complex	99215	2 – 4	*11051	HGB & HCT	85014	
Well Exam Infant (up to 12 mos.)	99391	> 4	*11052	HIV	86311	
Well Exam 1 – 4 yrs.	99392	Diaphram Fitting	*57170	Iron & TBC	83540	83550
Well Exam 5 – 11 yrs.	99393	Ear Irrigation	69210	Kidney Profile	80007	
Well Exam 12 – 17 yrs.	99394	ECG	93000	Lead	83655	
Well Exam 18 – 39 yrs.	99395	Endometrial Biopsy	*58100	Liver Profile	82977	
Well Exam 40 – 64 yrs.	99396	Exc. Lesion w /Biopsy	CTF	Mono Test	86308	
		w /o Biopsy		Pap Smear	88155	
Obstetrics		Location Size		Pregnancy Test	84703	
Total OB Care	59400	Exc. Skin Tags (1 – 15)	*11200	Prenatal Profile	80055	
Obstetrical Visit	99212	Each Additional 10	*11201	Pro Time	85610	
Injections		Fracture Treatment		PSA	84153	
Administration Sub. / IM	90782	Loc		RPR	86592	
Drug		w /Reduc w /o Reduc		Sed. Rate	85651	
Dosage		Fracture Treatment F/U	99024	Stool Culture	87045	
Allergy	95155	I & D Abscess Single/Simple	*10060	Stool O & P	87177	
Cocci Skin Test	86490	Multiple or Comp	*10061	Strep Screen	86403	
DPT	90701	I & D Pilonidal Cyst Simple	*10080	Theophylline	80198	
Haemophilus	90737	Pilonidal Cyst Complex	10081	Thyroid Profile	80091	
Influenza	90724	IV Therapy – To One Hour	90780	TSH	84443	
MMR	90707	Each Additional Hour	*90781	Urinalysis	81000	
OPV	90712	Laceration Repair		Urine Culture	87088	
Pneumovax	90732	Location Size Sim/Comp		Drawing Fee	36415	
TB Skin Test	86585	Laryngoscopy	31505	Specimen Collection	99000	
TD	90718	Oximetry	94760			
Unlisted Immun	90749	Punch Biopsy	CTF			
		Rhythm Strip	93040			
		Treadmill	93015			
X-Ray	73130 Dx 1	Trigger Point or Tendon Sheath Inj.	*20550			
		Tympanometry	92567			

Diagnosis / ICD – 9   *Broken Arm-Fractured Rad 813.81*

I acknowledge receipt of medical services and authorize the release of any medical information necessary to process this claim for healthcare payment only. I ☐ do ☐ do not authorize payment to the provider Patient Signature	Tax ID Number:	Total Estimated Charges:
		Payment Amount: *$15.00*

Date of Accident 9/4/08

Doc - REL

Happy Valley Medical Clinic
5222 E. Baseline Rd.
Gilbert, AZ 85234
(800)333-4747

Date: 9/4/2008

JOHWI000	Johnson, WIlliam J	9/4/2008	8:45:00 AM

EXAM	FEE	PROCEDURES	FEE	LABORATORY	FEE
New Patient		Anoscopy	46600	Aerobic Culture	87070	
Problem Focused	99201	Arthrocentesis/Aspiration/Injection		Amylase	82150	
Expanded Problem, Focused	99202	Small Joint	*20600	B12	82607	
Detailed	(99203) Dx 1	Interm Joint	*20605	CBC & Diff	85025	
Comprehensive	99204	Major Joint	*20610	CHEM 20	80019	
Comprehensive/High Complex	99204	Audiometry	92552	Chlamydia Screen	86317	
Initial Visit/Procedure	99025	Cast Application		Cholesterol	82465	
Well Exam Infant (up to 12 mos.)	99318	Location Long Short		Digoxin	80162	
Well Exam 1 – 4 yrs.	99382	Catherization	*53670	Electrolytes	80005	
Well Exam 5 – 11 yrs.	99383	Circumcision	54150	Ferritin	82728	
Well Exam 12 – 17 yrs.	99384	Colposcopy	*57452	Folate	82746	
Well Exam 18 – 39 yrs.	99385	Colposcopy w /Biopsy	*57454	GC Screen	87070	
Well Exam 40 – 64 yrs.	99386	Cryosurgery Premalignant Lesion		Glucose	82947	
		Location(s):		Glucose 1 HR	82950	
Established Patient		Cryosurgery Warts		Glycosylated HGB (A1C)	83036	
Minimum	99211	Location(s):		HCT	85014	
Problem Focused	99212	Curettement Lesion w /Biopsy	CTF	HDL	83718	
Expanded Problem Focused	99213	Curettement Lesion w o/ Biopsy		Hep BSAG	86278	
Detailed	99214	Single	*11050	Hepatitis Profile	80059	
Comprehensive/High Complex	99215	2 – 4	*11051	HGB & HCT	85014	
Well Exam Infant (up to 12 mos.)	99391	> 4	*11052	HIV	86311	
Well Exam 1 – 4 yrs.	99392	Diaphram Fitting	*57170	Iron & TBC 83540	83550	
Well Exam 5 – 11 yrs.	99393	Ear Irrigation	69210	Kidney Profile	80007	
Well Exam 12 – 17 yrs.	99394	ECG	93000	Lead	83655	
Well Exam 18 – 39 yrs.	99395	Endometrial Biopsy	*58100	Liver Profile	82977	
Well Exam 40 – 64 yrs.	99396	Exc. Lesion w /Biopsy	CTF	Mono Test	86308	
		w /o Biopsy		Pap Smear	88155	
Obstetrics		Location Size		Pregnancy Test	84703	
Total OB Care	59400	Exc. Skin Tags (1 – 15)	*11200	Prenatal Profile	80055	
Obstetrical Visit	99212	Each Additional 10	*11201	Pro Time	85610	
Injections		Fracture Treatment		PSA	84153	
Administration Sub. / IM	90782	Loc		RPR	86592	
Drug		w /Reduc w /o Reduc		Sed. Rate	85651	
Dosage		Fracture Treatment F/U	99024	Stool Culture	87045	
Allergy	95155	I & D Abscess Single/Simple	*10060	Stool O & P	87177	
Cocci Skin Test	86490	Multiple or Comp	*10061	Strep Screen	86403	
DPT	90701	I & D Pilonidal Cyst Simple	*10080	Theophylline	80198	
Haemophilus	90737	Pilonidal Cyst Complex	10081	Thyroid Profile	80091	
Influenza	90724	IV Therapy – To One Hour	90780	TSH	84443	
MMR	90707	Each Additional Hour	*90781	Urinalysis	81000	
OPV	90712	Laceration Repair		Urine Culture	87088	
Pneumovax	90732	Location Size Sim/Comp		Drawing Fee	36415	
TB Skin Test	86585	Laryngoscopy	31505	Specimen Collection	99000	
TD	90718	Oximetry	94760			
Unlisted Immun	90749	Punch Biopsy	CTF			
		Rhythm Strip	93040			
		Treadmill	93015			
MRI -	74246 Dx 1	Trigger Point or Tendon Sheath Inj.	*20550			
		Tympanometry	92567			

Diagnosis / ICD – 9 *Gallstones 535.5*

I acknowledge receipt of medical services and authorize the release of any medical information necessary to process this claim for healthcare payment only.

I ☐ do ☐ do not authorize payment to the provider

Patient Signature

Tax ID Number:

Total Estimated Charges:

Payment Amount: *CK* $20.00
60011

1037	Happy Valley Medical Clinic	Date: 9/4/2008
Doc - JM	5222 E. Baseline Rd. Gilbert, AZ 85234 (800)333-4747	

JONSU000   Jones, Suzy Q   9/4/2008   10:45:00 AM

EXAM	FEE	PROCEDURES	FEE	LABORATORY	FEE
New Patient		Anoscopy	46600	Aerobic Culture	87070	
Problem Focused	99201	Arthrocentesis/Aspiration/Injection		Amylase	82150	
Expanded Problem, Focused	99202	Small Joint	*20600	B12	82607	
Detailed	99203	Interm Joint	*20605	CBC & Diff	85025	
Comprehensive	99204	Major Joint	*20610	CHEM 20	80019	
Comprehensive/High Complex	99204	Audiometry	92552	Chlamydia Screen	86317	
Initial Visit/Procedure	99025	Cast Application		Cholesterol	(82465) Dx 1
Well Exam Infant (up to 12 mos.)	99318	Location Long Short		Digoxin	80162	
Well Exam 1 – 4 yrs.	99382	Catherization	*53670	Electrolytes	80005	
Well Exam 5 – 11 yrs.	99383	Circumcision	54150	Ferritin	82728	
Well Exam 12 – 17 yrs.	99384	Colposcopy	*57452	Folate	82746	
Well Exam 18 – 39 yrs.	99385	Colposcopy w /Biopsy	*57454	GC Screen	87070	
Well Exam 40 – 64 yrs.	99386	Cryosurgery Premalignant Lesion		Glucose	82947	
		Location(s):		Glucose 1 HR	82950	
Established Patient		Cryosurgery Warts		Glycosylated HGB (A1C)	83036	
Minimum	(99211) Dx 1	Location(s):		HCT	85014	
Problem Focused	99212	Curettement Lesion w /Biopsy	CTF	HDL	83718	
Expanded Problem Focused	99213	Curettement Lesion w o/ Biopsy		Hep BSAG	86278	
Detailed	99214	Single	*11050	Hepatitis Profile	80059	
Comprehensive/High Complex	99215	2 – 4	*11051	HGB & HCT	85014	
Well Exam Infant (up to 12 mos.)	99391	> 4	*11052	HIV	86311	
Well Exam 1 – 4 yrs.	99392	Diaphram Fitting	*57170	Iron & TBC 83540	83550	
Well Exam 5 – 11 yrs.	99393	Ear Irrigation	69210	Kidney Profile	80007	
Well Exam 12 – 17 yrs.	99394	ECG	93000	Lead	83655	
Well Exam 18 – 39 yrs.	99395	Endometrial Biopsy	*58100	Liver Profile	82977	
Well Exam 40 – 64 yrs.	99396	Exc. Lesion w /Biopsy	CTF	Mono Test	86308	
		w /o Biopsy		Pap Smear	88155	
Obstetrics		Location Size		Pregnancy Test	84703	
Total OB Care	59400	Exc. Skin Tags (1 – 15)	*11200	Prenatal Profile	80055	
Obstetrical Visit	99212	Each Additional 10	*11201	Pro Time	85610	
Injections		Fracture Treatment		PSA	84153	
Administration Sub. / IM	90782	Loc		RPR	86592	
Drug		w /Reduc w /o Reduc		Sed. Rate	85651	
Dosage		Fracture Treatment F/U	99024	Stool Culture	87045	
Allergy	95155	I & D Abscess Single/Simple	*10060	Stool O & P	87177	
Cocci Skin Test	86490	Multiple or Comp	*10061	Strep Screen	86403	
DPT	90701	I & D Pilonidal Cyst Simple	*10080	Theophylline	80198	
Haemophilus	90737	Pilonidal Cyst Complex	10081	Thyroid Profile	80091	
Influenza	90724	IV Therapy – To One Hour	90780	TSH	84443	
MMR	90707	Each Additional Hour	*90781	Urinalysis	81000	
OPV	90712	Laceration Repair		Urine Culture	87088	
Pneumovax	90732	Location Size Sim/Comp		Drawing Fee	36415	
TB Skin Test	86585	Laryngoscopy	31505	Specimen Collection	99000	
TD	90718	Oximetry	94760			
Unlisted Immun	90749	Punch Biopsy	CTF			
		Rhythm Strip	93040			
		Treadmill	93015			
		Trigger Point or Tendon Sheath Inj.	*20550			
		Tympanometry	92567			

Diagnosis / ICD – 9   *Heart Disease 422.9*

I acknowledge receipt of medical services and authorize the release of any medical information necessary to process this claim for healthcare payment only. I ☐ do ☐ do not authorize payment to the provider Patient Signature	Tax ID Number:	Total Estimated Charges:
		Payment Amount: $10.00

Doc - JM

Happy Valley Medical Clinic
5222 E. Baseline Rd.
Gilbert, AZ 85234
(800)333-4747

Date: 9/4/2008

JORJA000   Jordan, Jane N   9/4/2008   1:15:00 PM

EXAM		FEE	PROCEDURES		FEE	LABORATORY		FEE
New Patient			Anoscopy		46600	Aerobic Culture	87070	
Problem Focused		99201	*Dx* Arthrocentesis/Aspiration/Injection			Amylase	82150	
Expanded Problem, Focused		(99202) *1-2*	Small Joint		*20600	B12	82607	
Detailed		99203	Interm Joint		*20605	CBC & Diff	85025	
Comprehensive		99204	Major Joint		*20610	CHEM 20	80019	
Comprehensive/High Complex		99204	Audiometry		92552	Chlamydia Screen	(86317) *Dx 2*	
Initial Visit/Procedure		99025	Cast Application			Cholesterol	82465	
Well Exam Infant (up to 12 mos.)		99318	Location Long Short			Digoxin	80162	
Well Exam 1 – 4 yrs.		99382	Catherization		*53670	Electrolytes	80005	
Well Exam 5 – 11 yrs.		99383	Circumcision		54150	Ferritin	82728	
Well Exam 12 – 17 yrs.		99384	Colposcopy		*57452	Folate	82746	
Well Exam 18 – 39 yrs.		99385	Colposcopy w /Biopsy		*57454	GC Screen	87070	
Well Exam 40 – 64 yrs.		99386	Cryosurgery Premalignant Lesion			Glucose	82947	
			Location(s):			Glucose 1 HR	82950	
Established Patient			Cryosurgery Warts			Glycosylated HGB (A1C)	83036	
Minimum		99211	Location(s):			HCT	85014	
Problem Focused		99212	Curettement Lesion w /Biopsy		CTF	HDL	83718	
Expanded Problem Focused		99213	Curettement Lesion w o/ Biopsy			Hep BSAG	86278	
Detailed		99214	Single		*11050	Hepatitis Profile	80059	
Comprehensive/High Complex		99215	2 – 4		*11051	HGB & HCT	85014	
Well Exam Infant (up to 12 mos.)		99391	> 4		*11052	HIV	86311	
Well Exam 1 – 4 yrs.		99392	Diaphram Fitting		*57170	Iron & TBC 83540	83550	
Well Exam 5 – 11 yrs.		99393	Ear Irrigation		69210	Kidney Profile	80007	
Well Exam 12 – 17 yrs.		99394	ECG		93000	Lead	83655	
Well Exam 18 – 39 yrs.		99395	Endometrial Biopsy		*58100	Liver Profile	82977	
Well Exam 40 – 64 yrs.		99396	Exc. Lesion w /Biopsy		CTF	Mono Test	86308	
			w /o Biopsy			Pap Smear	88155	
Obstetrics			Location Size			Pregnancy Test	84703	
Total OB Care		59400	Exc. Skin Tags (1 – 15)		*11200	Prenatal Profile	80055	
Obstetrical Visit		99212	Each Additional 10		*11201	Pro Time	85610	
Injections			Fracture Treatment			PSA	84153	
Administration Sub. / IM		90782	Loc			RPR	86592	
Drug			w /Reduc		w /o Reduc	Sed. Rate	85651	
Dosage			Fracture Treatment F/U		99024	Stool Culture	87045	
Allergy		95155	I & D Abscess Single/Simple		*10060	Stool O & P	87177	
Cocci Skin Test		86490	Multiple or Comp		*10061	Strep Screen	86403	
DPT		90701	I & D Pilonidal Cyst Simple		*10080	Theophylline	80198	
Haemophilus		90737	Pilonidal Cyst Complex		10081	Thyroid Profile	80091	
Influenza		90724	IV Therapy – To One Hour		90780	TSH	84443	
MMR		90707	Each Additional Hour		*90781	Urinalysis	81000	
OPV		90712	Laceration Repair			Urine Culture	87088	
Pneumovax		90732	Location Size Sim/Comp			Drawing Fee	36415	
TB Skin Test		86585	Laryngoscopy		31505	Specimen Collection	99000	
TD		90718	Oximetry		94760			
Unlisted Immun		90749	Punch Biopsy		CTF			
			Rhythm Strip		93040			
			Treadmill		93015			
X-Ray Ankle		*73610* *Dx 1*	Trigger Point or Tendon Sheath Inj.		*20550			
			Tympanometry		92567			

Diagnosis / ICD – 9   *Achilles Tend 726.71, Exam V70.0*

Total Estimated Charges:	
Payment Amount:	

I acknowledge receipt of medical services and authorize the release of any medical information necessary to process this claim for healthcare payment only.

I ☐ do ☐ do not authorize payment to the provider

Patient Signature

Tax ID Number:

1039			Happy Valley Medical Clinic			Date: 9/4/2008	
Doc - JM			5222 E. Baseline Rd. Gilbert, AZ 85234 (800)333-4747				

KARJE000	Karvel, Jessica C	9/4/2008	4:00:00 PM

EXAM	FEE	PROCEDURES		FEE	LABORATORY		FEE
New Patient		Anoscopy	46600		Aerobic Culture	87070	
Problem Focused	99201	Arthrocentesis/Aspiration/Injection			Amylase	82150	
Expanded Problem, Focused	99202	Small Joint	*20600		B12	82607	
Detailed	99203	Interm Joint	*20605		CBC & Diff	85025	
Comprehensive	99204	Major Joint	*20610		CHEM 20	80019	
Comprehensive/High Complex	99204	Audiometry	92552		Chlamydia Screen	86317	
Initial Visit/Procedure	99025	Cast Application			Cholesterol	82465	
Well Exam Infant (up to 12 mos.)	99318	Location Long Short			Digoxin	80162	
Well Exam 1 – 4 yrs.	99382	Catherization	*53670		Electrolytes	80005	
Well Exam 5 – 11 yrs.	99383	Circumcision	54150		Ferritin	82728	
Well Exam 12 – 17 yrs.	99384	Colposcopy	*57452		Folate	82746	
Well Exam 18 – 39 yrs.	99385	Colposcopy w /Biopsy	*57454		GC Screen	87070	
Well Exam 40 – 64 yrs.	99386	Cryosurgery Premalignant Lesion			Glucose	82947	
		Location(s):			Glucose 1 HR	82950	
Established Patient		Cryosurgery Warts			Glycosylated HGB (A1C)	83036	
Minimum	(99211) *Dx 1*	Location(s):			HCT	85014	
Problem Focused	99212	Curettement Lesion w /Biopsy	CTF		HDL	83718	
Expanded Problem Focused	99213	Curettement Lesion w o/ Biopsy			Hep BSAG	86278	
Detailed	99214	Single	*11050		Hepatitis Profile	80059	
Comprehensive/High Complex	99215	2 – 4	*11051		HGB & HCT	85014	
Well Exam Infant (up to 12 mos.)	99391	> 4	*11052		HIV	86311	
Well Exam 1 – 4 yrs.	99392	Diaphram Fitting	*57170		Iron & TBC	83540	83550
Well Exam 5 – 11 yrs.	99393	Ear Irrigation	69210		Kidney Profile	80007	
Well Exam 12 – 17 yrs.	99394	ECG	93000		Lead	83655	
Well Exam 18 – 39 yrs.	99395	Endometrial Biopsy	*58100		Liver Profile	82977	
Well Exam 40 – 64 yrs.	99396	Exc. Lesion w /Biopsy	CTF		Mono Test	86308	
		w /o Biopsy			Pap Smear	88155	
Obstetrics		Location Size			Pregnancy Test	84703	
Total OB Care	59400	Exc. Skin Tags (1 – 15)	*11200		Prenatal Profile	80055	
Obstetrical Visit	99212	Each Additional 10	*11201		Pro Time	85610	
Injections		Fracture Treatment			PSA	84153	
Administration Sub. / IM	90782	Loc			RPR	86592	
Drug		w /Reduc w /o Reduc			Sed. Rate	85651	
Dosage		Fracture Treatment F/U	99024		Stool Culture	87045	
Allergy	95155	I & D Abscess Single/Simple	*10060		Stool O & P	87177	
Cocci Skin Test	86490	Multiple or Comp	*10061		Strep Screen	86403	
DPT	90701	I & D Pilonidal Cyst Simple	*10080		Theophylline	80198	
Haemophilus	90737	Pilonidal Cyst Complex	10081		Thyroid Profile	80091	
Influenza	90724	IV Therapy – To One Hour	90780		TSH	84443	
MMR	90707	Each Additional Hour	*90781		Urinalysis	81000	
OPV	90712	Laceration Repair			Urine Culture	87088	
Pneumovax	90732	Location Size Sim/Comp			Drawing Fee	36415	
TB Skin Test	86585	Laryngoscopy	31505		Specimen Collection	99000	
TD	90718	Oximetry	94760				
Unlisted Immun	90749	Punch Biopsy	CTF				
		Rhythm Strip	93040				
		Treadmill	93015				
		Trigger Point or Tendon Sheath Inj.	*20550				
		Tympanometry	92567				

Diagnosis / ICD – 9 *Poison Ivy 692.6*

I acknowledge receipt of medical services and authorize the release of any medical information necessary to process this claim for healthcare payment only. I ☐ do ☐ do not authorize payment to the provider Patient Signature	Tax ID Number:	Total Estimated Charges: Payment Amount: *CK* *$10.00* *126*

Doc - REL

Happy Valley Medical Clinic
5222 E. Baseline Rd.
Gilbert, AZ 85234
(800)333-4747

Date: 9/4/2008

LYLDA000   Lyle, David F   9/4/2008   10:30:00 AM

EXAM	FEE	PROCEDURES	FEE	LABORATORY	FEE
New Patient		Anoscopy	46600	Aerobic Culture	87070
Problem Focused	(99201) Dx 1	Arthrocentesis/Aspiration/Injection		Amylase	82150
Expanded Problem, Focused	99202	Small Joint	*20600	B12	82607
Detailed	99203	Interm Joint	*20605	CBC & Diff	85025
Comprehensive	99204	Major Joint	*20610	CHEM 20	80019
Comprehensive/High Complex	99204	Audiometry	92552	Chlamydia Screen	86317
Initial Visit/Procedure	99025	Cast Application		Cholesterol	82465
Well Exam Infant (up to 12 mos.)	99318	Location Long Short		Digoxin	80162
Well Exam 1 – 4 yrs.	99382	Catherization	*53670	Electrolytes	80005
Well Exam 5 – 11 yrs.	99383	Circumcision	54150	Ferritin	82728
Well Exam 12 – 17 yrs.	99384	Colposcopy	*57452	Folate	82746
Well Exam 18 – 39 yrs.	99385	Colposcopy w /Biopsy	*57454	GC Screen	87070
Well Exam 40 – 64 yrs.	99386	Cryosurgery Premalignant Lesion		Glucose	82947
		Location(s):		Glucose 1 HR	82950
Established Patient		Cryosurgery Warts		Glycosylated HGB (A1C)	83036
Minimum	99211	Location(s):		HCT	85014
Problem Focused	99212	Curettement Lesion w /Biopsy	CTF	HDL	83718
Expanded Problem Focused	99213	Curettement Lesion w o/ Biopsy		Hep BSAG	86278
Detailed	99214	Single	*11050	Hepatitis Profile	80059
Comprehensive/High Complex	99215	2 – 4	*11051	HGB & HCT	85014
Well Exam Infant (up to 12 mos.)	99391	> 4	*11052	HIV	86311
Well Exam 1 – 4 yrs.	99392	Diaphram Fitting	*57170	Iron & TBC 83540	83550
Well Exam 5 – 11 yrs.	99393	Ear Irrigation	69210	Kidney Profile	80007
Well Exam 12 – 17 yrs.	99394	ECG	93000	Lead	83655
Well Exam 18 – 39 yrs.	99395	Endometrial Biopsy	*58100	Liver Profile	82977
Well Exam 40 – 64 yrs.	99396	Exc. Lesion w /Biopsy	CTF	Mono Test	86308
		w /o Biopsy		Pap Smear	88155
Obstetrics		Location Size		Pregnancy Test	84703
Total OB Care	59400	Exc. Skin Tags (1 – 15)	*11200	Prenatal Profile	80055
Obstetrical Visit	99212	Each Additional 10	*11201	Pro Time	85610
Injections		Fracture Treatment		PSA	84153
Administration Sub. / IM	90782	Loc		RPR	86592
Drug		w /Reduc w /o Reduc		Sed. Rate	85651
Dosage		Fracture Treatment F/U	99024	Stool Culture	87045
Allergy	95155	I & D Abscess Single/Simple	*10060	Stool O & P	87177
Cocci Skin Test	86490	Multiple or Comp	*10061	Strep Screen	86403
DPT	90701	I & D Pilonidal Cyst Simple	*10080	Theophylline	80198
Haemophilus	90737	Pilonidal Cyst Complex	10081	Thyroid Profile	80091
Influenza	90724	IV Therapy – To One Hour	90780	TSH	84443
MMR	90707	Each Additional Hour	*90781	Urinalysis	81000
OPV	90712	Laceration Repair		Urine Culture	87088
Pneumovax	90732	Location Size Sim/Comp		Drawing Fee	36415
TB Skin Test	86585	Laryngoscopy	31505	Specimen Collection	99000
TD	90718	Oximetry	94760		
Unlisted Immun	90749	Punch Biopsy	CTF		
		Rhythm Strip	93040		
		Treadmill	93015		
		Trigger Point or Tendon Sheath Inj.	*20550		
		Tympanometry	92567		

Diagnosis / ICD – 9   *Headache Migrain 346.9*

I acknowledge receipt of medical services and authorize the release of any medical information necessary to process this claim for healthcare payment only.

I ☐ do ☐ do not authorize payment to the provider

Patient Signature

Tax ID Number:

Total Estimated Charges:

Payment Amount: *$15.00*

Doc - WH

Happy Valley Medical Clinic
5222 E. Baseline Rd.
Gilbert, AZ 85234
(800)333-4747

Date: 9/4/2008

PALTI000   Palmdale, Timothy   9/4/2008   4:45:00 PM

EXAM	FEE	PROCEDURES	FEE	LABORATORY	FEE
New Patient		Anoscopy 46600		Aerobic Culture 87070	
Problem Focused	99201	Arthrocentesis/Aspiration/Injection		Amylase 82150	
Expanded Problem, Focused	99202	Small Joint *20600		B12 82607	
Detailed	99203	Interm Joint *20605		CBC & Diff 85025	
Comprehensive	99204	Major Joint *20610		CHEM 20 80019	
Comprehensive/High Complex	99204	Audiometry 92552		Chlamydia Screen 86317	
Initial Visit/Procedure	99025	Cast Application		Cholesterol 82465	
Well Exam Infant (up to 12 mos.)	99318	Location Long Short		Digoxin 80162	
Well Exam 1 – 4 yrs.	99382	Catherization *53670		Electrolytes 80005	
Well Exam 5 – 11 yrs.	99383	Circumcision 54150		Ferritin 82728	
Well Exam 12 – 17 yrs.	99384	Colposcopy *57452		Folate 82746	
Well Exam 18 – 39 yrs.	99385	Colposcopy w /Biopsy *57454		GC Screen 87070	
Well Exam 40 – 64 yrs.	99386	Cryosurgery Premalignant Lesion		Glucose 82947	
		Location(s):		Glucose 1 HR 82950	
Established Patient		Cryosurgery Warts		Glycosylated HGB (A1C) 83036	
Minimum	99211	Location(s):		HCT 85014	
Problem Focused	99212	Dx Curettement Lesion w /Biopsy CTF		HDL 83718	
Expanded Problem Focused	(99213) 1-2	Curettement Lesion w o/ Biopsy		Hep BSAG 86278	
Detailed	99214	Single *11050		Hepatitis Profile 80059	
Comprehensive/High Complex	99215	2 – 4 *11051		HGB & HCT 85014	
Well Exam Infant (up to 12 mos.)	99391	> 4 *11052		HIV 86311	
Well Exam 1 – 4 yrs.	99392	Diaphram Fitting *57170		Iron & TBC 83540 83550	
Well Exam 5 – 11 yrs.	99393	Ear Irrigation 69210		Kidney Profile 80007	
Well Exam 12 – 17 yrs.	99394	ECG 93000		Lead 83655	
Well Exam 18 – 39 yrs.	99395	Endometrial Biopsy *58100		Liver Profile 82977	
Well Exam 40 – 64 yrs.	99396	Exc. Lesion w /Biopsy CTF		Mono Test 86308	
		w /o Biopsy		Pap Smear 88155	
Obstetrics		Location Size		Pregnancy Test 84703	
Total OB Care	59400	Exc. Skin Tags (1 – 15) *11200		Prenatal Profile 80055	
Obstetrical Visit	99212	Each Additional 10 *11201		Pro Time 85610	
Injections		Fracture Treatment		PSA 84153	
Administration Sub. / IM	90782	Loc		RPR 86592	
Drug		w /Reduc w /o Reduc		Sed. Rate 85651	
Dosage		Fracture Treatment F/U 99024		Stool Culture 87045	
Allergy	95155	I & D Abscess Single/Simple *10060		Stool O & P 87177	
Cocci Skin Test	86490	Multiple or Comp *10061		Strep Screen 86403	
DPT	90701	I & D Pilonidal Cyst Simple *10080		Theophylline 80198	
Haemophilus	90737	Pilonidal Cyst Complex 10081		Thyroid Profile 80091	
Influenza	90724	IV Therapy – To One Hour 90780		TSH 84443	
MMR	90707	Each Additional Hour *90781		Urinalysis 81000	
OPV	90712	Laceration Repair		Urine Culture 87088	
Pneumovax	90732	Location Size Sim/Comp		Drawing Fee 36415	
TB Skin Test	86585	Laryngoscopy 31505		Specimen Collection 99000	
TD	90718	Oximetry 94760			
Unlisted Immun	90749	Punch Biopsy CTF			
		Rhythm Strip 93040			
		Treadmill 93015			
Chest x-ray	7.2052	Dx 2 Trigger Point or Tendon Sheath Inj. *20550			
		Tympanometry 92567			

Diagnosis / ICD – 9   *Scoliosis 737.30, Bronch. 490.0*

Total Estimated Charges:

I acknowledge receipt of medical services and authorize the release of any medical information necessary to process this claim for healthcare payment only.

Tax ID Number:

Payment Amount: *$10.00*

I ☐ do ☐ do not   authorize payment to the provider

Patient Signature

Happy Valley Medical Clinic
5222 E. Baseline Rd.
Gilbert, AZ 85234
(800)333-4747

Date: 9/4/2008

Doc - REL

PETAN000	Peters, Anthony	9/4/2008	1:00:00 PM

EXAM	FEE	PROCEDURES	FEE	LABORATORY	FEE
New Patient		Anoscopy	46600	Aerobic Culture	87070
Problem Focused	99201	Arthrocentesis/Aspiration/Injection		Amylase	82150
Expanded Problem, Focused	99202	Small Joint	*20600	B12	82607
Detailed	99203	Interm Joint	*20605	CBC & Diff	85025
Comprehensive	99204	Major Joint	*20610	CHEM 20	80019
Comprehensive/High Complex	99204	Audiometry	92552	Chlamydia Screen	86317
Initial Visit/Procedure	99025	Cast Application		Cholesterol	82465
Well Exam Infant (up to 12 mos.)	99318	Location Long Short		Digoxin	80162
Well Exam 1 – 4 yrs.	99382	Catherization	*53670	Electrolytes	80005
Well Exam 5 – 11 yrs.	99383	Circumcision	54150	Ferritin	82728
Well Exam 12 – 17 yrs.	99384	Colposcopy	*57452	Folate	82746
Well Exam 18 – 39 yrs.	99385	Colposcopy w /Biopsy	*57454	GC Screen	87070
Well Exam 40 – 64 yrs.	99386	Cryosurgery Premalignant Lesion		Glucose	82947
		Location(s):		Glucose 1 HR	82950
Established Patient		Cryosurgery Warts		Glycosylated HGB (A1C)	83036
Minimum	99211	Location(s):		HCT	85014
Problem Focused	(99212) Dx 1	Curettement Lesion w /Biopsy	CTF	HDL	83718
Expanded Problem Focused	99213	Curettement Lesion w o/ Biopsy		Hep BSAG	86278
Detailed	99214	Single	*11050	Hepatitis Profile	80059
Comprehensive/High Complex	99215	2 – 4	*11051	HGB & HCT	85014
Well Exam Infant (up to 12 mos.)	99391	> 4	*11052	HIV	86311
Well Exam 1 – 4 yrs.	99392	Diaphram Fitting	*57170	Iron & TBC 83540	83550
Well Exam 5 – 11 yrs.	99393	Ear Irrigation	69210	Kidney Profile	80007
Well Exam 12 – 17 yrs.	99394	ECG	93000	Lead	83655
Well Exam 18 – 39 yrs.	99395	Endometrial Biopsy	*58100	Liver Profile	82977
Well Exam 40 – 64 yrs.	99396	Exc. Lesion w /Biopsy	CTF	Mono Test	86308
		w /o Biopsy		Pap Smear	88155
Obstetrics		Location Size		Pregnancy Test	84703
Total OB Care	59400	Exc. Skin Tags (1 – 15)	*11200	Prenatal Profile	80055
Obstetrical Visit	99212	Each Additional 10	*11201	Pro Time	85610
Injections		Fracture Treatment		PSA	84153
Administration Sub. / IM	90782	Loc		RPR	86592
Drug		w /Reduc w /o Reduc		Sed. Rate	85651
Dosage		Fracture Treatment F/U	99024	Stool Culture	87045
Allergy	95155	I & D Abscess Single/Simple	*10060	Stool O & P	87177
Cocci Skin Test	86490	Multiple or Comp	*10061	Strep Screen	86403
DPT	90701	I & D Pilonidal Cyst Simple	*10080	Theophylline	80198
Haemophilus	90737	Pilonidal Cyst Complex	10081	Thyroid Profile	80091
Influenza	90724	IV Therapy – To One Hour	90780	TSH	84443
MMR	90707	Each Additional Hour	*90781	Urinalysis	81000
OPV	90712	Laceration Repair		Urine Culture	87088
Pneumovax	90732	Location Size Sim/Comp		Drawing Fee	36415
TB Skin Test	86585	Laryngoscopy	31505	Specimen Collection	99000
TD	90718	Oximetry	94760		
Unlisted Immun	90749	Punch Biopsy	CTF		
		Rhythm Strip	93040		
		Treadmill	93015		
		Trigger Point or Tendon Sheath Inj.	*20550		
		Tympanometry	92567		

Diagnosis / ICD – 9 *Dermatitis 692.9*

I acknowledge receipt of medical services and authorize the release of any medical information necessary to process this claim for healthcare payment only.

I ☐ do ☐ do not authorize payment to the provider

Patient Signature

Tax ID Number:

Total
Estimated
Charges:

Payment
Amount: *$5.00*

1043	Happy Valley Medical Clinic 5222 E. Baseline Rd. Gilbert, AZ 85234 (800)333-4747	Date: 9/4/2008
Doc - WH		

PETZA000   Peters, Zach   9/4/2008   1:30:00 PM

EXAM	FEE	PROCEDURES	FEE	LABORATORY	FEE
New Patient		Anoscopy	46600	Aerobic Culture	87070	
Problem Focused	99201	Arthrocentesis/Aspiration/Injection		Amylase	82150	
Expanded Problem, Focused	99202	Small Joint	*20600	B12	82607	
Detailed	99203	Interm Joint	*20605	CBC & Diff	85025	
Comprehensive	99204	Major Joint	*20610	CHEM 20	80019	
Comprehensive/High Complex	99204	Audiometry	92552	Chlamydia Screen	86317	
Initial Visit/Procedure	99025	Cast Application		Cholesterol	82465	
Well Exam Infant (up to 12 mos.)	99318	Location Long Short		Digoxin	80162	
Well Exam 1 – 4 yrs.	99382	Catherization	*53670	Electrolytes	80005	
Well Exam 5 – 11 yrs.	99383	Circumcision	54150	Ferritln	82728	
Well Exam 12 – 17 yrs.	99384	Colposcopy	*57452	Folate	82746	
Well Exam 18 – 39 yrs.	99385	Colposcopy w /Biopsy	*57454	GC Screen	87070	
Well Exam 40 – 64 yrs.	99386	Cryosurgery Premalignant Lesion		Glucose	82947	
		Location(s):		Glucose 1 HR	82950	
Established Patient		Cryosurgery Warts		Glycosylated HGB (A1C)	83036	
Minimum	99211	Location(s):		HCT	85014	
Problem Focused	99212	Curettement Lesion w /Biopsy	CTF	HDL	83718	
Expanded Problem Focused	99213	Curettement Lesion w o/ Biopsy		Hep BSAG	86278	
Detailed	(99214) *Dx. 1*	Single	*11050	Hepatitis Profile	80059	
Comprehensive/High Complex	99215	2 – 4	*11051	HGB & HCT	85014	
Well Exam Infant (up to 12 mos.)	99391	> 4	*11052	HIV	86311	
Well Exam 1 – 4 yrs.	99392	Diaphram Fitting	*57170	Iron & TBC 83540	83550	
Well Exam 5 – 11 yrs.	99393	Ear Irrigation	69210	Kidney Profile	80007	
Well Exam 12 – 17 yrs.	99394	ECG	93000	Lead	83655	
Well Exam 18 – 39 yrs.	99395	Endometrial Biopsy	*58100	Liver Profile	82977	
Well Exam 40 – 64 yrs.	99396	Exc. Lesion w /Biopsy	CTF	Mono Test	86308	
		w /o Biopsy		Pap Smear	88155	
Obstetrics		Location Size		Pregnancy Test	84703	
Total OB Care	59400	Exc. Skin Tags (1 – 15)	*11200	Prenatal Profile	80055	
Obstetrical Visit	99212	Each Additional 10	*11201	Pro Time	85610	
Injections		Fracture Treatment		PSA	84153	
Administration Sub. / IM	90782	Loc		RPR	86592	
Drug		w /Reduc w /o Reduc		Sed. Rate	85651	
Dosage		Fracture Treatment F/U	99024	Stool Culture	87045	
Allergy	95155	I & D Abscess Single/Simple	*10060	Stool O & P	87177	
Cocci Skin Test	86490	Multiple or Comp	*10061	Strep Screen	86403	
DPT	90701	I & D Pilonidal Cyst Simple	*10080	Theophylline	80198	
Haemophilus	90737	Pilonidal Cyst Complex	10081	Thyroid Profile	80091	
Influenza	90724	IV Therapy – To One Hour	90780	TSH	84443	
MMR	90707	Each Additional Hour	*90781	Urinalysis	81000	
OPV	90712	Laceration Repair		Urine Culture	87088	
Pneumovax	90732	Location Size Sim/Comp		Drawing Fee	36415	
TB Skin Test	86585	Laryngoscopy	31505	Specimen Collection	99000	
TD	90718	Oximetry	94760			
Unlisted Immun	90749	Punch Biopsy	CTF			
		Rhythm Strip	93040			
		Treadmill	93015			
		Trigger Point or Tendon Sheath Inj.	*20550			
		Tympanometry	92567			

Diagnosis / ICD – 9

Allergic Bronch. 493.9

I acknowledge receipt of medical services and authorize the release of any medical information necessary to process this claim for healthcare payment only. I ☐ do ☐ do not authorize payment to the provider Patient Signature	Tax ID Number:

Total Estimated Charges:

Payment Amount: *CK $5.50*
967

Doc - MM

Happy Valley Medical Clinic
5222 E. Baseline Rd.
Gilbert, AZ 85234
(800)333-4747

Date: 9/4/2008

SHEJA000   Shepherd, Jarem   9/4/2008   9:30:00 AM

EXAM	FEE	PROCEDURES	FEE	LABORATORY	FEE
New Patient		Anoscopy	46600	Aerobic Culture	87070
Problem Focused	99201	Arthrocentesis/Aspiration/Injection		Amylase	82150
Expanded Problem, Focused	99202	Small Joint	*20600	B12	82607
Detailed	99203	Interm Joint	*20605	CBC & Diff	85025
Comprehensive	99204	Major Joint	*20610	CHEM 20	80019
Comprehensive/High Complex	99204	Audiometry	92552	Chlamydia Screen	86317
Initial Visit/Procedure	99025	Cast Application		Cholesterol	82465
Well Exam Infant (up to 12 mos.)	99318	Location Long Short		Digoxin	80162
Well Exam 1 – 4 yrs.	99382	Catherization	*53670	Electrolytes	80005
Well Exam 5 – 11 yrs.	99383	Circumcision	54150	Ferritin	82728
Well Exam 12 – 17 yrs.	99384	Colposcopy	*57452	Folate	82746
Well Exam 18 – 39 yrs.	99385	Colposcopy w /Biopsy	*57454	GC Screen	87070
Well Exam 40 – 64 yrs.	99386	Cryosurgery Premalignant Lesion		Glucose	82947
		Location(s):		Glucose 1 HR	82950
Established Patient		Cryosurgery Warts		Glycosylated HGB (A1C)	83036
Minimum	99211	Location(s):		HCT	85014
Problem Focused	(99212) Dx 1	Curettement Lesion w /Biopsy	CTF	HDL	83718
Expanded Problem Focused	99213	Curettement Lesion w o/ Biopsy		Hep BSAG	86278
Detailed	99214	Single	*11050	Hepatitis Profile	80059
Comprehensive/High Complex	99215	2 – 4	*11051	HGB & HCT	85014
Well Exam Infant (up to 12 mos.)	99391	> 4	*11052	HIV	86311
Well Exam 1 – 4 yrs.	99392	Diaphram Fitting	*57170	Iron & TBC 83540	83550
Well Exam 5 – 11 yrs.	99393	Ear Irrigation	69210	Kidney Profile	80007
Well Exam 12 – 17 yrs.	99394	ECG	93000	Lead	83655
Well Exam 18 – 39 yrs.	99395	Endometrial Biopsy	*58100	Liver Profile	82977
Well Exam 40 – 64 yrs.	99396	Exc. Lesion w /Biopsy	CTF	Mono Test	86308
		w /o Biopsy		Pap Smear	88155
Obstetrics		Location Size		Pregnancy Test	84703
Total OB Care	59400	Exc. Skin Tags (1 – 15)	*11200	Prenatal Profile	80055
Obstetrical Visit	99212	Each Additional 10	*11201	Pro Time	85610
Injections		Fracture Treatment		PSA	84153
Administration Sub. / IM	90782	Loc		RPR	86592
Drug		w /Reduc w /o Reduc		Sed. Rate	85651
Dosage		Fracture Treatment F/U	99024	Stool Culture	87045
Allergy	95155	I & D Abscess Single/Simple	*10060	Stool O & P	87177
Cocci Skin Test	86490	Multiple or Comp	*10061	Strep Screen	86403
DPT	90701	I & D Pilonidal Cyst Simple	*10080	Theophylline	80198
Haemophilus	90737	Pilonidal Cyst Complex	10081	Thyroid Profile	80091
Influenza	90724	IV Therapy – To One Hour	90780	TSH	84443
MMR	90707	Each Additional Hour	*90781	Urinalysis	81000
OPV	90712	Laceration Repair		Urine Culture	87088
Pneumovax	90732	Location Size Sim/Comp		Drawing Fee	36415
TB Skin Test	86585	Laryngoscopy	31505	Specimen Collection	99000
TD	90718	Oximetry	94760		
Unlisted Immun	90749	Punch Biopsy	CTF		
		Rhythm Strip	93040		
		Treadmill	93015		
		Trigger Point or Tendon Sheath Inj.	*20550		
		Tympanometry	92567		

Diagnosis / ICD – 9   *Back Spasm 847.2*

I acknowledge receipt of medical services and authorize the release of any medical information necessary to process this claim for healthcare payment only.

I ☐ do ☐ do not authorize payment to the provider

Patient Signature

Tax ID Number:

Total Estimated Charges:

Payment Amount: *$10.00*

1045	Happy Valley Medical Clinic	Date: 9/4/2008
Doc - JM	5222 E. Baseline Rd. Gilbert, AZ 85234 (800)333-4747	

SIMTA000	Simpson, Tanus J	9/4/2008	2:30:00 PM

EXAM	FEE	PROCEDURES	FEE	LABORATORY	FEE
New Patient		Anoscopy	46600	Aerobic Culture	87070
Problem Focused	99201	Arthrocentesis/Aspiration/Injection		Amylase	82150
Expanded Problem, Focused	99202	Small Joint	*20600	B12	82607
Detailed	99203	Interm Joint	*20605	CBC & Diff	85025
Comprehensive	99204	Major Joint	*20610	CHEM 20	80019
Comprehensive/High Complex	99204	Audiometry	92552	Chlamydia Screen	86317
Initial Visit/Procedure	99025	Cast Application		Cholesterol	82465
Well Exam Infant (up to 12 mos.)	99318	Location Long Short		Digoxin	80162
Well Exam 1 – 4 yrs.	99382	Catherization	*53670	Electrolytes	80005
Well Exam 5 – 11 yrs.	99383	Circumcision	54150	Ferritin	82728
Well Exam 12 – 17 yrs.	99384	Colposcopy	*57452	Folate	82746
Well Exam 18 – 39 yrs.	99385	Colposcopy w /Biopsy	*57454	GC Screen	87070
Well Exam 40 – 64 yrs.	99386	Cryosurgery Premalignant Lesion		Glucose	82947
		Location(s):		Glucose 1 HR	82950
Established Patient		Cryosurgery Warts		Glycosylated HGB (A1C)	83036
Minimum	99211	Location(s):		HCT	85014
Problem Focused	99212	Curettement Lesion w /Biopsy	CTF	HDL	83718
Expanded Problem Focused	99213	Curettement Lesion w o/ Biopsy		Hep BSAG	86278
Detailed	99214	Single	*11050	Hepatitis Profile	80059
Comprehensive/High Complex	99215	2 – 4	*11051	HGB & HCT	85014
Well Exam Infant (up to 12 mos.)	99391	> 4	*11052	HIV	86311
Well Exam 1 – 4 yrs.	99392	Diaphram Fitting	*57170	Iron & TBC 83540	83550
Well Exam 5 – 11 yrs.	99393	Ear Irrigation	69210	Kidney Profile	80007
Well Exam 12 – 17 yrs.	99394	ECG	93000	Lead	83655
Well Exam 18 – 39 yrs.	99395	Endometrial Biopsy	*58100	Liver Profile	82977
Well Exam 40 – 64 yrs.	99396	Exc. Lesion w /Biopsy	CTF	Mono Test	86308
		w /o Biopsy		Pap Smear	88155
Obstetrics		Location Size		Pregnancy Test	84703
Total OB Care	59400	Exc. Skin Tags (1 – 15)	*11200	Prenatal Profile	80055
Obstetrical Visit	99212	Each Additional 10	*11201	Pro Time	85610
Injections		Fracture Treatment		PSA	84153
Administration Sub. / IM	90782	Loc		RPR	86592
Drug		w /Reduc w /o Reduc		Sed. Rate	85651
Dosage		Fracture Treatment F/U	99024	Stool Culture	87045
Allergy	95155	I & D Abscess Single/Simple	*10060	Stool O & P	87177
Cocci Skin Test	86490	Multiple or Comp	*10061	Strep Screen	86403
DPT	90701	I & D Pilonidal Cyst Simple	*10080	Theophylline	80198
Haemophilus	90737	Pilonidal Cyst Complex	10081	Thyroid Profile	80091
Influenza	90724	IV Therapy – To One Hour	90780	TSH	84443
MMR	90707	Each Additional Hour	*90781	Urinalysis	81000
OPV	90712	Laceration Repair		Urine Culture	87088
Pneumovax	90732	Location Size Sim/Comp		Drawing Fee	36415
TB Skin Test	86585	Laryngoscopy	31505	Specimen Collection	99000
TD	90718	Oximetry	94760		
Unlisted Immun	90749	Punch Biopsy	CTF		
		Rhythm Strip	93040		
		Treadmill	93015		
MultiLink Cath	Dx 1	Trigger Point or Tendon Sheath Inj.	*20550		
		Tympanometry	92567		

Diagnosis / ICD – 9	*Arthritis 716.9*		Total Estimated Charges:	
I acknowledge receipt of medical services and authorize the release of any medical information necessary to process this claim for healthcare payment only. I ☐ do ☐ do not authorize payment to the provider Patient Signature		Tax ID Number:	Payment Amount:	*$10.75*

	Happy Valley Medical Clinic		Date: 9/4/2008
Doc - REL	5222 E. Baseline Rd.		
	Gilbert, AZ 85234		
	(800)333-4747		

ZIMAN000	Zimmerman, Anthony	9/4/2008	4:30:00 PM

EXAM	FEE	PROCEDURES	FEE	LABORATORY	FEE
New Patient		Anoscopy	46600	Aerobic Culture	87070
Problem Focused	99201	Arthrocentesis/Aspiration/Injection		Amylase	82150
Expanded Problem, Focused	99202	Small Joint	*20600	B12	82607
Detailed	99203	Interm Joint	*20605	CBC & Diff	85025
Comprehensive	99204	Major Joint	*20610	CHEM 20	80019
Comprehensive/High Complex	99204	Audiometry	92552	Chlamydia Screen	86317
Initial Visit/Procedure	99025	Cast Application		Cholesterol	82465
Well Exam Infant (up to 12 mos.)	99318	Location Long Short		Digoxin	80162
Well Exam 1 – 4 yrs.	99382	Catherization	*53670	Electrolytes	80005
Well Exam 5 – 11 yrs.	99383	Circumcision	54150	Ferritin	82728
Well Exam 12 – 17 yrs.	99384	Colposcopy	*57452	Folate	82746
Well Exam 18 – 39 yrs.	99385	Colposcopy w /Biopsy	*57454	GC Screen	87070
Well Exam 40 – 64 yrs.	99386	Cryosurgery Premalignant Lesion		Glucose	82947
		Location(s):		Glucose 1 HR	82950
Established Patient		Cryosurgery Warts		Glycosylated HGB (A1C)	83036
Minimum	99211	Location(s):		HCT	85014
Problem Focused	99212 *Dx*	Curettement Lesion w /Biopsy	CTF	HDL	83718
Expanded Problem Focused	(99213) *1+2*	Curettement Lesion w o/ Biopsy		Hep BSAG	86278
Detailed	99214	Single	*11050	Hepatitis Profile	80059
Comprehensive/High Complex	99215	2 – 4	*11051	HGB & HCT	85014
Well Exam Infant (up to 12 mos.)	99391	> 4	*11052	HIV	86311
Well Exam 1 – 4 yrs.	99392	Diaphram Fitting	*57170	Iron & TBC	83540	83550
Well Exam 5 – 11 yrs.	99393	Ear Irrigation	69210	Kidney Profile	80007
Well Exam 12 – 17 yrs.	99394	ECG	93000	Lead	83655
Well Exam 18 – 39 yrs.	99395	Endometrial Biopsy	*58100	Liver Profile	82977
Well Exam 40 – 64 yrs.	99396	Exc. Lesion w /Biopsy	CTF	Mono Test	86308
		w /o Biopsy		Pap Smear	88155
Obstetrics		Location Size		Pregnancy Test	84703
Total OB Care	59400	Exc. Skin Tags (1 – 15)	*11200	Prenatal Profile	80055
Obstetrical Visit	99212	Each Additional 10	*11201	Pro Time	85610
Injections		Fracture Treatment		PSA	84153
Administration Sub. / IM	90782	Loc		RPR	86592
Drug		w /Reduc w /o Reduc		Sed. Rate	85651
Dosage		Fracture Treatment F/U	99024	Stool Culture	87045
Allergy	95155	I & D Abscess Single/Simple	*10060	Stool O & P	87177
Cocci Skin Test	86490	Multiple or Comp	*10061	Strep Screen	86403
DPT	90701	I & D Pilonidal Cyst Simple	*10080	Theophylline	80198
Haemophilus	90737	Pilonidal Cyst Complex	10081	Thyroid Profile	80091
Influenza	90724	IV Therapy – To One Hour	90780	TSH	84443
MMR	90707	Each Additional Hour	*90781	Urinalysis	81000
OPV	90712	Laceration Repair		Urine Culture	87088
Pneumovax	90732	Location Size Sim/Comp		Drawing Fee	36415
TB Skin Test	86585	Laryngoscopy	31505	Specimen Collection	(99000) *Dx 1*
TD	90718	Oximetry	94760		
Unlisted Immun	90749	Punch Biopsy	CTF		
		Rhythm Strip	93040		
		Treadmill	93015		
X-Ray	*71020* *Dx 2*	Trigger Point or Tendon Sheath Inj.	*20550		
		Tympanometry	92567		

Diagnosis / ICD – 9		Total Estimated Charges:	
Psoriasis 696.1, Low Back Pain 724.2			
I acknowledge receipt of medical services and authorize the release of any medical information necessary to process this claim for healthcare payment only.	Tax ID Number:		
I ☐ do ☐ do not authorize payment to the provider		Payment Amount:	
Patient Signature			

HIPAA Regulations

The Health Insurance Portability and Accountability Act (Public Law 104–191), or HIPAA, was passed in 1996. There is much involved in HIPAA, but the part that is the most important to the medical office specialist (MOS) is the Administrative Simplification subsection, or Title II. The Administrative Simplification subsection (Title II, Subtitle F) (hereafter referred to simply as HIPAA) has four distinct components:

1. Transactions and code sets

2. Uniform identifiers

3. Privacy

4. Security

HIPAA regulates health plans, clearinghouses, and healthcare providers as "covered entities" with regard to these four areas.

TRANSACTIONS AND CODE SETS

HIPAA standardized the formats for electronic data interchange (EDI) by requiring specific transaction standards. These standards are currently used for eight types of electronic health transactions between covered entities: (1) health plan eligibility, (2) enrollment and disenrollment in a health plan, (3) health claims, (4) payments for care and health plan premiums, (5) claim status, (6) First Report of Injury reports, (7) coordination of benefits, and (8) related transactions.

Historically, medical providers and insurance plans used many different electronic formats to exchange, or transact, medical claims and related business. Implementing a national standard will result in the use of one format, thereby simplifying, improving, and making transactions more efficient nationwide. This standardization of formats was the first part of the Administrative Simplification subsection to be implemented. This section also requires standardized code sets such as the HCPCS, CPT-4®, ICD-9-CM, and other codes to be used.*

UNIFORM IDENTIFIERS

HIPAA also established uniform identifier standards, which will be used on all claims and other data transmissions. These standard identifiers include the following:

- The *National Provider Identifier* (NPI) is assigned to doctors, nurses, and other healthcare providers. The use of the NPI has been in effect since May 2007 for Medicare providers.

- The federal *Employer Identification Number* is used to identify employer-sponsored health insurance. The EIN, or tax identification number, is used.

- The *National Health Plan Identifier* is a unique identification number that will be assigned to each insurance plan, and to the organizations that administer insurance plans, such as payers and third-party administrators.

PRIVACY STANDARDS

The HIPAA privacy standards are designed to protect a patient's identifiable health information from unauthorized disclosure or use in any form, while permitting the practice to deliver the best healthcare possible. To comply with the law that became effective April 14, 2003, privacy activities in the average medical office might include these:

- Providing a copy of the office privacy policy informing patients about their privacy rights and how their information can be used.

- Asking the patient to acknowledge receiving a copy of the policy or signing a consent form.

- Obtaining signed authorization forms and in some cases tracking the disclosures of patient health information when it is to be given to a person or organization outside the practice for purposes other than treatment, billing, or payment.

- Adopting clear privacy procedures for its practice.

- Training employees so that they understand the privacy procedures.

- Designating an individual to be responsible for seeing that the privacy procedures are adopted and followed.

- Securing patient records containing individually identifiable health information so that they are not readily available to those who do not need them.

The privacy and security rules use two acronyms that the medical office specialist should learn: PHI, which stands for protected health informa-

*CPT is a registered trademark of the American Medical Association.

tion, and EPHI, which stands for protected health information in an electronic format.

One Example of Implementation

Before HIPAA's privacy rule went into effect, medical practices routinely kept a sign-in sheet or registration sheet at the receptionist's desk. Multiple lines on this sheet allowed each patient arriving for an appointment to sign his or her name. This not only let patients see how many others had arrived before them that day but also gave them the name of each patient who had arrived before them. To protect the privacy of all patients, covered entities now use a single-page sign-in sheet or registration sheet. One patient writes his or her name on the sheet and it is then torn off or removed from the pad. Some practices use self-stick labels to serve the same purpose and save paper.

When the privacy rule initially was issued, it required providers to obtain patient "consent" to use and disclose PHI for purposes of treatment, payment, and healthcare operations, except in emergencies. The rule was almost immediately revised to make consent optional. In general, the practice can use PHI for almost anything related to treating the patient, running the medical practice, and getting paid for services. This means doctors, nurses, and other staff can share the patient's chart within the practice.

Authorization differs from consent in that it does require the patient's permission to disclose PHI. Some examples of instances that would require an authorization would include sending the results of an employment physical to an employer or sending immunization records or the results of an athletic physical to a school.

The authorization form must include the date signed, an expiration date, to whom the information may be disclosed, what information is permitted to be disclosed, and for what purpose the information may be used. The authorization must be signed by the patient or a representative appointed by the patient. Unlike the open concept of consent, authorizations are not global. A new authorization is signed each time there is a different purpose or need for the patient's information to be disclosed.

Practices are permitted to disclose PHI without a patient's authorization or consent when it is requested by an authorized government agency. Generally such requests are for legal (law enforcement, subpoena, court orders, etc.) public health purposes or for enforcement of the privacy rule itself. Providers also are permitted to disclose PHI concerning on-the-job injuries to workers' compensation insurers, state administrators, and other entities to the extent required by state law.

Whether the practice has disclosed PHI based on a signed authorization or to comply with a government agency, the patient is entitled to know about it. The privacy rule gives individuals the right to receive a report of all disclosures made for purposes other than treatment, payment, or operations. Therefore, in most cases the medical office must track the disclosure and keep the records for at least 6 years.

Most healthcare providers and health plans use the services of a variety of other persons or businesses. HIPAA's privacy rule allows covered providers and health plans to disclose protected health information to these "business associates." The privacy rule requires a covered entity to obtain a written agreement from its business associate, which states that the business associate will appropriately safeguard the protected health information it receives or creates on behalf of the covered entity.

Congress provided civil and criminal penalties for covered entities that misuse personal health information. The privacy rule is enforced by the Department of Health and Human Services' Office for Civil Rights (OCR).

SECURITY STANDARDS

Whereas the privacy rule applies to all forms of patients' protected health information, whether electronic, written, or oral, the security rule covers only protected health information that is in electronic form.

Security standards were designed to provide guidelines to all types of covered entities, while affording them flexibility regarding how to implement the standards. Covered entities may use appropriate security measures that enable them to reasonably implement a standard. Security standards were designed to be "technology neutral." That is, the rule does not prescribe the use of specific technologies, so that the healthcare community will not be bound by specific systems or software that may become obsolete.

The security standards are divided into the categories of administrative, physical, and technical safeguards:

- **Administrative safeguards.** In general, these are the administrative functions that should be implemented to meet the security standards. These include assignment or delegation of security responsibility to an individual and security training requirements.

- **Physical safeguards.** In general, these are the mechanisms required to protect electronic systems—their equipment and the data they hold—from threats, environmental hazards, and unauthorized intrusion. They include restricting access to EPHI and retaining off-site computer backups.

- **Technical safeguards.** In general, these are primarily the automated processes used to protect data and control access to data. They include using authentication controls to verify that the person signing onto a computer is authorized to access that EPHI, or encrypting and decrypting data as it is being stored or transmitted.

Computer passwords and software security levels are some examples of technical safeguards. Not everyone in an organization needs access to EPHI. Software program security levels establish which user may or may not access certain information in the software program. For EPHI, the registrar may need to enter insurance and demographic information on the patient, but may not need access to actual medical record documentation areas. A locked filing cabinet or locked room containing the filing cabinets for paper medical charts is another security measure.

The original security rule also proposed a standard for electronic signatures. The final rule, however, covered only security standards. In 2000, President Clinton signed into federal law the Electronic Signatures in Global and National Commerce Act, which made digital signatures as binding as their paper-based counterparts. Although the law made digital signatures valid for commerce, HIPAA does not require the use of electronic signatures. Electronic signature standards will eventually be necessary to achieve a completely paperless health electronic record (HER). A rule for electronic signature standards may be proposed at a later date. For now, a valid electronic signature must meet three criteria:

1. **Message integrity.** The recipient must be able to confirm that the document has not been altered since it was signed.

2. **Nonrepudiation.** The signer must not be able to deny signing the document.

3. **User authentication.** The recipient must be able to confirm that the signature was in fact "signed" by the real person.

Digital signatures meet all three of these criteria. Digital signatures use a branch of mathematics called cryptography and PKI, which stands for Public Key Infrastructure. Each PKI user has two "keys," a private key for signing documents and a public key for verifying his or her signature. A computer software program performs a mathematical calculation on the entire contents of the electronic document to be signed. The result is a unique "message digest," which is then encrypted using the private key.

The digital signature is then attached to or sent with the document. When the recipient wishes to validate the signature, a similar computer program regenerates the "message digest" and decodes the digital signature with the public key. Comparing the two, the program determines if the message digest is identical to that which was originally sent. In this way digital signatures not only confirm that you are the signer but also that the document has not been altered since it was signed.

COMPLIANCE

Continued, ongoing training is required for HIPAA compliance. A one-time introduction is not sufficient. A medical office or facility will assign a designated person to the role as a Compliance Officer. A Compliance Officer is responsible for reviewing office policies and procedures to assure that all applicable HIPAA laws, rules, and regulations are being followed. HIPAA regulations may change over time, so it is important for the Compliance Officer to be up to date on current regulations and conduct training seminars throughout the year. In a small and medium size facility the Office Manager is usually assigned this responsibility. A large facility or hospital may assign a staff member to act as the Compliance Officer. In a hospital setting it is common for there to be a Director of Compliance who reviews policies and procedures with a compliance committee. It is imperative that each medical office and facility commit to comply day-to-day with the ethical and legal standards established in the applicable laws and regulations.[*]

[*]Source: Vines, Deborah; Braceland, Ann; Rollins, Elizabeth; Miller, Susan. *Comprehensive Health Insurance: Billing, Coding, and Reimbursement.* © 2008 Pearson Education, Inc. Upper Saddle River, NJ. Reprinted with permission.

Glossary

accounts receivable (AR) money owed to the clinic for services provided.

adjudicate the process an insurance company uses to process a claim and determine the applicable benefits.

adjustment a transaction, other than a charge or payment, that is entered into a Case either adding to or subtracting from the outstanding balance.

Adjustment Code a code used in deposit/payment entry to post a write-off amount on a patient's account; may be insurance- or patient-related adjustment.

Alert a claim status used to indicate that there are special circumstances surrounding the claim and the office is monitoring the progress.

AMA American Medical Association

ANSI American National Standards Institute

appointment time assigned in the schedule for patients to be seen at the clinic.

Assignment of Benefits a form signed by the insured whereby he or she directs the insurance company to send payment directly to the provider.

Assignment List the pop-up window that displays after the Work Administrator utility is launched.

assignments tasks performed by users in Work Administrator.

audit/edit report feedback from the clearinghouse to the provider documenting the progress of individual claims that have been submitted. This report documents changes to be made or additional information to be submitted on a claim.

Audit Records a report feature that allows the user to audit patient records, track user logins, and view permission settings.

backup a second copy of the original data in case the first copy is destroyed.

Backup Data the Medisoft process of creating a duplicate copy of a dataset.

backup mediums any form of data storage device such as RW-CDs, zip disks, flash drives, and external hard drives.

Backup Root Data the process of creating a duplicate copy of the Medisoft shared files and registration files.

Bands a tab inside Report Properties that allows the user to define the height of the header, detail, and footer sections of the report or bill.

BCBS Blue Cross Blue Shield

beneficiary patient covered under a health insurance plan.

billing charge interest or finance charge added to a patient's account.

Billing Code a unique identifying code created by the user inside the Chart to identify a patient for the purpose of filtering statements, claims, and reports.

birthday rule determines which insurance is primary when two policies are valid for a child. The plan of the parent whose birthday comes first in the calendar year is usually primary.

break time assigned in the schedule where patients will not be seen.

capitation plan contract that a provider signs with a carrier agreeing to treat a certain number of members in the carrier's plan. The carrier then pays the provider based on a designated fee each month for each member in that plan.

Case a grouping of transactions associated to the patient's chart information that is linked to a common billing scenario such as diagnosis, insurance, facility, or provider.

Case Description a field inside the Case that defines the different information for the Case, such as insurance coverage, diagnosis, provider, or facility.

Case Indicator a unique identifying code created by the user inside the Case to identify a patient for the purpose of filtering statements, claims, and reports.

Cash Case a patient Case whereby there is no insurance coverage for the services and only the patient will be billed.

Centers for Disease Control and Prevention (CDC) the government agency that promotes health and quality of life by preventing and controlling disease, injury, and disability.

Centers for Medicare and Medicaid Services (CMS) a government agency formerly known as HCFA. CMS is part of the U.S. Department of Health and Human Services and is responsible for administering Medicare and Medicaid.

Challenge a claim status used to indicate that the insurance company has processed the claim and the office intends to dispute it.

charge a transaction added to a Case for services rendered, adding to the patient's balance.

claim name for a bill that is sent to the insurance company.

claim footer the bottom portion of the Format Grid in an insurance form.

claim header the top portion of the Format Grid in an insurance form.

Claim Management the utility inside Medisoft that allows the user to submit primary, secondary, or tertiary claims to insurance companies, along with tracking the status of each claim.

Claims Manager a separate, add-on program sold by Medisoft to manage electronic transactions.

claim status explains the current position of a claim, i.e., sent, paid, or rejected.

clean claim a claim that has no data errors when submitted to an insurance carrier.

clearinghouse a company that receives claims from multiple providers, evaluates them, and batches them for electronic submission to multiple insurance carriers.

clinic follow-up policies procedures defined by the office to collect self-pay, non-contract, and contract accounts.

CMS-1500 form the standard claim form used by physicians and other healthcare professionals to bill for services rendered.

code set defined by HIPAA as an approved collection of codes used in the healthcare industry to communicate information, e.g., diagnosis, procedure, or place of service.

Collection List a utility inside Medisoft that assists users in follow-up activities.

comment a transaction added to the Case giving the user further clarification about the account.

contract insurance category the section of accounts receivable that has been billed to a contracted insurance company.

Copayment Code a Medisoft code used in deposit/payment entry to apply a patient co-pay to a patient's account.

courtesy billing billing that occurs when clinics request that patients pay for their services on the day of service, and the clinics give the patients a claim form to submit to their insurance. The insurance will then process this and reimburse the patient as specified in the patient's policy.

covered entity an organization subject to the HIPAA law—e.g., insurance companies, clearinghouses, hospitals, and clinics.

CPT* code Current Procedural Terminology code; a five-digit code used to describe what procedures were performed.

*CPT is a registered trademark of the American Medical Association.

create claims the process used within Claim Management to search for transactions that have not been billed and create claims for them.

Current Procedural Terminology (CPT)* a five-digit coding system designed by the American Medical Association (AMA) to report the service or supply received by the patient.

Custom Case data Case information that is added to the screen and customized by the Medisoft user.

Customize feature that allows user to customize the menu, toolbars, and sidebars.

Custom Patient data patient information that is added to the screen and customized by the Medisoft user.

Custom Report List a feature in Medisoft that allows the user to open and print existing reports.

daily backup backup made each day Medisoft is used.

daily Medisoft tasks the six typical Medisoft tasks performed daily at offices.

data field the information contained within the Medisoft tables and items that are selected on the Format Grid.

Data Field Properties the pop-up window associated with each data field that allows the user to define and modify the field.

Data Filters a tab inside of Report Properties that allows the user to establish criteria used to generate the report.

data path location in the computer to find desired data.

days in accounts receivable the average number of days it takes for a clinic to receive its money, calculated as the total AR divided by the average daily revenue.

Deductible Code the Medisoft code used to record the deductible transaction into the patient's account.

Deposit Code a code assigned in Medisoft to each deposit that allows the deposit report to be sorted by the desired code.

Deposit List the utility in Medisoft Advanced and Network Professional that allows the user to record payments, adjustments, and comments; also referred to as Enter Deposits/Payments.

Deposit Report report inside of Enter Deposit/Payments that prints the deposits for a range of dates allowing filters for different payment options.

Design Custom Reports and Bills (DCRB) a utility in Medisoft that allows the user to customize new or existing reports.

detail the middle section of a report.

Detail File companion or sub-file to the Master File.

diagnosis the disease, condition, illness, or accident that is the reason for services provided.

diagnosis codes ICD-9-CM codes that identify a patient's injury and/or illness or reason for routine or preventive services.

dirty claim a claim that is incorrect or is missing information when submitted to an insurance carrier.

Done a claim status used to indicate the insurance has completed processing the claim.

EDI comments notes that provide additional information to the insurance company as to the services provided.

Edit Rule pop-up window under Task Rules List that allows the assignments to be created based on the criteria specified.

Edit Task allows the user to process the work by marking the work done and documenting the details.

EDI transactions data transmitted electronically in a specific format that is used by providers, insurance companies, and clearinghouses to communicate healthcare information including eligibility, claims, claims status, and remittance.

Electronic Data Interchange (EDI) the process of exchanging data electronically between healthcare covered entities: the clinic, the clearinghouse, and the insurance company.

*CPT is a registered trademark of the American Medical Association.

electronic statements statements sent electronically to a clearinghouse to be printed, stuffed, stamped, and mailed by the clearinghouse.

eligibility verifying insurance coverage for a patient.

Enter Deposits/Payments the utility inside of Medisoft that allows the user to post deposits and apply payments.

EOB comments notes that contain additional information provided by the insurance company on the EOB, such as coverage terminated, no full-time student letter received, or insurance premium not paid/coverage terminated.

ERA electronic remittance advice

Explanation of Benefits (EOB) a statement given to the clinic by the insurance company to explain how the patient's claim was adjudicated.

Fair Debt Collection Practices Act a federal law controlling the collection of debt.

File Maintenance the utility in Medisoft that optimizes the performance of the system, including the processes to purge data, rebuild indexes, pack data, and recalculate balances.

Filter Selections allows the user to specify tasks that will be displayed in the Assignment List.

Final Draft word processing software that interfaces with Medisoft.

follow-up procedures describes the steps of how unpaid accounts will be processed by the office in order to collect the outstanding balance.

footer the bottom section of a report.

Format Grid the section of DCRB where the user adds the fields.

General a tab inside Report Properties that allows the user to make major changes in the appearance of the report or bill; some of the options include changes in margins, paper size, or page orientation.

grid column fields within each Medisoft table that store data.

Groups the function in Work Administrator that allows tasks to be assigned to a pre-defined group of users.

Group Setup an add-on to Security Setup that allows the practice to define groups of users.

guarantor person who is financially responsible for the account and will receive the statement.

guarantor balance the balance due from the person responsible for the patient's account, i.e., the parent of a minor child.

hardship and bad debt write-offs adjustments made to the accounts of patients who cannot pay or those who refuse to pay for which the clinic deems it acceptable to cancel the debt.

Health Care Financing Administration (HCFA) a government agency now called CMS.

header the top section of a report.

Healthcare Common Procedure Coding System (HCPCS) a five-digit coding system beginning with an alpha character created by CMS; a standard code set for reporting professional services, procedures, and supplies.

Health Insurance Portability and Accountability Act (HIPAA) a federal law passed in 1996 to develop standards among providers, health plans, clearinghouses, and employers regarding electronic transactions, security, and privacy.

health plan an organization that provides insurance coverage including employer plans, insurance plans, or government plans.

Hold a claim status used to indicate the claim is not ready to be sent.

hotkeys keys that are set up as shortcuts to accomplish a desired task quickly.

ICD-9-CM abbreviation for International Classification of Diseases, 9th Revision, Clinical Modification. A coding system used to identify signs, symptoms, injuries, diseases, and conditions.

initial balance tape an adding tape that is initially created by adding up the receipts of the day and used to balance the deposits and payments.

Insurance Code the five-digit code assigned to the insurance by Medisoft when it is initially created.

insurance contractual adjustments write-offs made to the patient's account under the agreement of the contract between the healthcare provider and the insurance company.

insured person who owns the insurance policy, also known as subscriber.

internal notes comments entered into Medisoft that help the user to handle the patient and the account more effectively.

KB kilobytes, a storage unit used to define computer hard drive space.

Knowledge Base Medisoft's online collection of articles to provide help to users.

List Rules button to execute the Task Rules List within Work Administrator.

Master File identifies the Medisoft table from which data fields for the Format Grid may be selected.

Medisoft practice management software commonly used by medical offices that allows practices to track patient information, appointments, and accounts receivable.

modifier a two-digit number placed after the five-digit CPT* code to indicate that the description of the service or procedure has been altered.

MSP Medicare Secondary Payer

MultiLink Codes a feature within Medisoft that allows the user to create multiple transactions at the same time.

Multimedia tab the Medisoft Network Professional feature that allows the user to save media in patient cases, such as pictures, X-rays, and medical records.

National Center for Health Statistics (NCHS) the government office that provides U.S. public health statistics, including information on diseases, pregnancies, births, aging, and mortality.

National Provider Identifier (NPI) the lifetime provider number that uniquely identifies a healthcare provider in standard transactions, such as healthcare claims.

New Case the function that adds the insurance information, facility, referring doctor, and other details to the patient.

New Patient the feature that allows users to add patient information such as name, address, and phone number.

New Practice the utility that allows another set of data to be created.

New Task utility in Work Administrator that allows the user to create a new assignment.

non-contract insurance category the section of accounts receivable that has been billed to a non-contract insurance company.

NSF National Standard Format

NUCC National Uniform Claim Committee

OCR optical character reader

Office Hours software within Medisoft used to track patient appointments.

off-site refers to storing the backups at a location other than the office.

Open Practice the utility that allows users to switch from one practice to another.

paper statements statements printed, stuffed, and stamped by the office.

patient the person receiving healthcare services.

patient balance the balance due from the patient/guarantor after all insurance sources have paid.

Patient Day Sheet Medisoft report used to proof daily transactions, showing all transactions posted on patient accounts for the selected time frame.

patient information personal information provided by the patient to the medical office in order for the office to treat the patient and obtain reimbursement for services.

payment money received from insurance, or patients, lowering the patient's balance.

Payment Code a Medisoft code used in deposit/payment entry to apply the payment to a patient's account.

Pending a claim status used to indicate the claim is waiting at the insurance company for additional information.

Permissions the utility inside of Medisoft that assigns tasks to user access levels.

POS place of service

Practice Analysis the most commonly used Medisoft report to analyze information.

practice management system (PMS) software that allows a clinic to manage its daily tasks via a computer.

*CPT is a registered trademark of the American Medical Association.

primary claim a claim sent to the patient's insurance that has first responsibility.

Program Options a comprehensive utility that lets users define settings for Medisoft.

protected health information (PHI) under HIPAA, individually identifiable health information transmitted or maintained in any form or medium, which is held by a covered entity or its business associate.

Ready to Send a claim status used to indicate that the claim needs to be filed either on paper or electronically.

registration the process whereby registration is created when the Medisoft program is initially installed. The sequence of the clinic's name and serial number creates the registration code.

Rejected a claim status used to indicate that the claim was transmitted electronically and an electronic reject was posted to the comment tab inside the claim details.

Rejection Code a Medisoft code that indicates the reason the insurance rejected the charge.

remainder statements statements that print only for balances due from the patient.

remittance advice (RA) term that is used interchangeably with the term explanation of benefits.

Repeat Setup pop-up window under New Task that allows assignments to be set up to repeat automatically.

Report Properties a utility within DCRB that allows definitions and changes to be performed on the report being modified or created.

Report Style the default settings for the Format Grid assigned in the Report Properties of the report created; each report (e.g., labels or lists) has its own characteristics.

Restore Data the process of replacing the existing practice data with a backup copy.

Restore Root Data the process of replacing the existing root data with a backup copy of the root data.

right-click keys shortcuts that can be used inside of Medisoft by clicking the right button on the mouse (see hotkeys).

root data data that is stored in the Medidata folder and shared by all practices in the folder.

Rules items created under the Task Rules List that have circumstances associated to them that will trigger an assignment if met.

scheduling the process of entering breaks and appointments into the schedule.

SCHIP State Children's Health Insurance Program.

secondary claim a claim sent to the patient's insurance that has secondary responsibility.

Security Setup the utility in Medisoft that sets up login rights for users, permission access levels, group assignments, and the ability to reset the user password.

self-pay balance the balance due from the patient/guarantor.

self-pay category the section of accounts receivable that is entirely due from the patient guarantor.

Sent a claim status used to indicate the claim has been sent to the insurance carrier.

Set Program Date function that allows the Medisoft date to be changed.

signature on file (SOF) indicates to the insurance company that the clinic has a copy of the required signature on file for CMS-1500 claim form boxes 12 and 13.

Small Balance Write-off a Medisoft feature allowing the user to mass write off small balances after setting the appropriate parameters.

standard statements statements that print for all patients that have a balance, regardless of who owes the balance, insurance or guarantor.

Statement Management the utility inside of Medisoft used to process and track statements.

statement notes comments entered into Medisoft that will print on the patient statements.

statements invoices sent to patients/guarantors.

superbill a form used by clinics to track the patient's visit, procedures performed, and the diagnoses assigned to the visit.

Take Back Code a Medisoft code used in deposit/payment entry to record the amount the insurance deducts from a payment to compensate for a previous overpayment.

Task Rules List allows the user to view, delete, edit, or create a Rule in Work Administrator.

Task Scheduler utility that allows the user to schedule tasks such as backups, reports, file maintenance, or eligibility verification to be performed after hours.

tertiary claim a claim sent to the patient's insurance that has responsibility after the secondary insurance.

ticklers items within the Collection List.

TOS type of service

TPO Treatment, Payment, and Operations

transaction detail the line in the insurance form that contains the charges on the claim.

Transaction Entry utility inside Medisoft that allows the user to enter charges, payments, adjustments, comments, and track balances.

transaction header a buffer before the transaction detail allowing for increasing and decreasing the margin.

trending the days in AR keeping a running log of the outstanding days in AR.

Users individuals' setup in the Medisoft security utility that allows the program to manage and track activities performed.

View Backup Disks a function that allows the user to view existing backups stored on various types of media; it gives the file name, date, and size of each file contained within a particular backup.

Withhold Code a Medisoft code used in deposit/payment entry to record the amount a contracted insurance company deducts from the provider's payment and may be paid back to the provider at the end of the fiscal period.

Work Administrator utility in Medisoft used to assign, track, and manage clinic work.

Index

D

Daily tasks, 3–17. *See also* Backup
  appointments, scheduling, 4–8
  balance the day, 287–88
  coding/billing procedures, reviewing, 17
  contract payments, 17
  insurance claims, submitting, 10–11, 288
  insurance coverage, verifying eligibility of, 16–17
  mail denials/payments, processing, 8–9
  patient day sheet, 9–10
  reports, 287–88, 290–91
  superbills, developing, 4–8
Data. *See also* Root data
  backing up, 164
  corrupt, 174
  custom, for case information, 32, 51–53
  new set of, creating, 307–8
  pack, 177, 179
  purge, 177
  restoring, 164, 173
  selection questions, 210
Data field, 240
  adding, 256
  moving, 241
Data field properties, 240
  modifying, 241
  previewing, 246
Data filters tab in report properties, 243, 257
Data path, 253
Date
  calendar, 19
  charges creation, 187
  created range, 209
  from range, 209
  setting, 297–98
Days in accounts receivable
  determining, 209–11, 290
  trending, 290, 323
DCRB. *See* Design Custom Reports and Bills (DCRB)
Deductible code, 130
Delay secondary billing, 45–46
Deposit code, 126, 129, 132
Deposit list, 9, 123

Deposit report
  defined, 124
  printing, 134
  sample, 125, 322
Deposits
  applying, 138–39
  capitation, creating, 133
  for capitation payments, creating, 132
  creating new, 125–26, 138
  detail of, 124, 136
  entering new, 137–38
  insurance, creating, 131
  for insurance payments, 129–31
  for patient payments, 126–28
  viewing, 133
Design custom patient data, 52
Design Custom Reports and Bills (DCRB)
  accessing, 234–36
  copying, 252–57
  creating, 247–50
  customizing, 250–52
  defined, 234
  labels, common, 246–47, 294
  opening existing, 237–46
  overview of, 236–37
Destination file name, 165
Destination file path, 165
Detail file, 248
Detail of reports, 236–37
Diagnosis, 4, 35, 61
  codes, 17, 311
  linkage, 72–74
  tab, 35, 38, 43
Dirty claim, 277
Done (claim status), 104, 105
Drop-down menu bars, 16
Drop-down sort button, 106

E

EDI. *See* Electronic Data Interchange (EDI)
Edit report, 277
Edit rule, 269–70
Edit task, 272
Electronic claims, 89–90

Images
    inserting, 251
    loading, 252
Initial balance tape, 124
Insurance. *See also* Claim(s); Primary insur-
        ance; Secondary insurance; Tertiary
        insurance
    codes, 129, 132
    companies, 312
    contract category, 206
    contractual adjustments, 64
    coverage, 16–17
    forms, 245–46
    non-contract category, 206
    payments, 321
    plans, 129–31
    reports, 215–18
Insurance follow-up
    through claim management, 218–19
    through collection list, 219–25
Insured, 35
Internal notes, 65
International Classification of Diseases, 9th Re-
        vision, Clinical Modification (ICD-9-CM), 39

K

Kilobytes (KB), 171
Knowledge Base Online, 53–54, 176, 301–2

L

Labels
    common, 246–47
    patient, 242
    pop-up window for, 249
    printing, 255–57
Ledgers, 249
List only claims that match, 104
List only feature, 107, 108, 116
Lists. *See also* Collections list
    appointment, printing, 7
    assignment, 264, 317–18
    claim management by, 108–9
    creating items, 309–10
    customer report, 234

custom report, 27
    tasks rule, 268–70
    ticklers, list only, 223, 227
Login report, 198
Logos, 250–52
Logout report, 198

M

Mail denials, 8–9
Mail processing, 124–25. *See also* Posting mail
        payments
Manual claims status, 105
Master file, 248
Maximum billing charges, 187
Medicaid, 134
Medicare, 134
Medicare Secondary Payer (MSP)
    defined, 92
    fact sheet, 93–99
    questionnaire, 100–101
Medisoft
    Advanced Patient Accounting, 40, 129
    Basic, 9, 16, 40, 129, 145, 185, 211, 214
    defined, 2
    manual, 53, 176
    Network Professional, 40, 129
    Patient Accounting, 40, 129
    version of, determining, 41
Menu bars. *See* Toolbars
Minimum billing charges, 187
Minimum past due balance, 187
Modifiers, 17, 61, 71–72
Monthly billing charge, 187
MultiLink codes, 61, 74–78
MultiLink transactions, 76
Multimedia tab, 35

N

National Center for Health Statistics (NCHS), 39
National Provider Identifier (NPI), 47
National Standard Format (NSF), 102
National Uniform Claim Committee (NUCC), 84
New case, 286
New patient, 286